Whole Slide Imaging

Anil V. Parwani
Editor

Whole Slide Imaging

Current Applications and Future Directions

Springer

Editor
Anil V. Parwani
Department of Pathology
The Ohio State University Wexner Medical School
Columbus, OH
USA

ISBN 978-3-030-83331-2 ISBN 978-3-030-83332-9 (eBook)
https://doi.org/10.1007/978-3-030-83332-9

This Springer imprint is published by the registered company Springer Nature Switzerland AG
The registered company address is: Gewerbestrasse 11, 6330 Cham, Switzerland

Foreword

The advance of technology is based on making it fit in so that you don't really even notice it, so it's part of everyday life. Bill Gates

When people talk about digital pathology today, they imply whole slide imaging (WSI). That is because WSI has become the dominant imaging modality for digitizing material in the pathology laboratory. WSI has played an integral part in pathology practice for more than two decades now, with some pathology labs already demonstrating success at going *fully digital* for rendering primary diagnoses using WSI instead of glass slides. Current digital pathology systems arose from computer science research projects in the 1990s. Since then, we have witnessed the commercial introduction of sophisticated WSI systems that have productively incorporated advanced optics, digital cameras, robotics, image management, software, cloud computing, and computer vision technology.

This book effectively encapsulates the entire story about WSI from the past, what the status is at present, and delves into the future. Joel Saltz, one of the pioneers in the early development of the first ever WSI scanner, provides a historical account of the field. WSI technology, however, is complex and accordingly can be intimidating for end users to understand. Therefore, readers should welcome the useful chapters by Mohanty and Parwani as well as McClintock that offer a detailed explanation of the hardware, software, and the prerequisite IT infrastructure needed to operate these systems. For WSI to be effective, this technology also needs to be integrated in the pathology lab, which Hartman eloquently lays out in his chapter on workflow.

There are numerous applications for WSI that range from clinical to non-clinical use cases. These are covered in the chapter by Parwani and Mohanty, and also addressed in much more informative detail by global experts in the field such as Singh et al on education, Treanor and Williams on primary diagnosis, McClintock and Cornish on telepathology, Lujan et al on teleconsultation, as well as Raess and Sirintrapun on quality assurance. WSI in cytopathology has been less pervasive due to technical challenges related to focusing and screening workflow. Li and Pantanowitz suitably address these obstacles in their chapter on WSI and cytopathology. The chapters written by Dangott deal with WSI for research and image analysis, two areas where this technology has perhaps had the largest footprint and continues to drive the fields of computational pathology and biomedical informatics forward. We are also on the brink of AI adoption into mainstream pathology clinical practice. This is possible due to advances in computational technology and deep learning. The final chapter in this book by Machiraju and Parwani nicely demonstrates the synergism possible when WSI is coupled with AI.

There is no longer doubt about whether WSI is here to stay or will fade away as another novel fad in the history of pathology. WSI has ushered in a new platform that by allowing us to digitize not just an entire glass slide, but also an entire anatomical pathology lab's routine workload, has transformed the field of pathology. WSI has thereby finally untethered pathologists from their microscopes and delivered pathology care to patients who otherwise would never have benefited from access to expert diagnoses. WSI has also liberated pathology laboratories to leverage WSI in favor of more cost-efficient processes and allowed them to expand their services. Finally, WSI has additionally allowed the field of pathology to remain in the driver's seat for precision medicine and AI. I am certain that you will derive great benefit from this comprehensive book on WSI and likely find yourself returning to it time after time to refer to many of these valuable chapters.

Liron Pantanowitz, MD
University of Michigan, Pathology & Clinical Labs
Ann Arbor, MI, USA

Preface

In recent years, advances in imaging modalities and the ability to analyze these images using digital pathology and artificial intelligence software have created many new opportunities to advance patient care. The conversion of glass slides into a digital format and the electronic communication of digitized images is digital pathology. Digital pathology provides the users with the ability to transfer a microscopic image, between one pathologist and another physician (pathologist or other clinician). Digital pathology has been around for decades and continues to have many applications today in the national as well as global pathology community to be used for primary diagnosis, intraoperative consultation, second opinion consultations, research, quality reviews, tumor boards, and education.

One of the mediums used in digital pathology is whole slide imaging (WSI). WSI technology has several advantages over conventional microscopy; portability (images are often accessible anywhere and at any time), ease of sharing and retrieval of archival images, and the ability to make use of computer-aided diagnostic tools (image analysis algorithms). The automated instrument used for WSI is a scanner equipped with a robotic microscope capable of digitalizing an entire glass slide, using software to merge or stitch individually captured images into a composite digital image. The critical components of an automated WSI system include bar coded slides, hardware (scanner composed of an optical microscope and digital camera connected to a computer), software (responsible for image creation and management, viewing of images, and image analysis where applicable), and network connectivity. The last decade has seen significant technology advances in the evolution of WSI with the ability to rapidly digitize large numbers of slides automatically and at high resolution. Many applications have emerged and, as a result, WSI is increasingly being used in both clinical and research areas. Whole slide imaging technology has evolved to the point where digital slide scanners are currently capable of automatically producing high-quality, high-resolution digital images within a relatively short time – less than one minute per slide.

The focus of this book is to provide up-to-date and practical knowledge in all aspects of whole slide imaging by experts in the field. This includes a historical perspective on the evolution of this technology, technical aspects of making a great whole slide image, the various applications of whole slide imaging, and future applications using WSI for computer-aided diagnosis.

The goal is to provide practical knowledge and address knowledge gaps in this emerging field. This book is unique because it will address an emerging area in pathology for which currently there is only limited information about the practical aspects of deploying this technology. For example, there are no established selection criteria for choosing new scanners and a knowledge base with the key information. The authors of the various chapters have years of real-world experience in selecting and implementing WSI solutions in various aspects of pathology practice. This book will also provide practical tips and pearls to address the selection of a WSI vendor, technology details, implementing this technology and provide an overview of its everyday uses in all areas of pathology.

This book will also provide readers with important information on how to integrate their digital slides with the laboratory information system and streamline their "digital workflow" with the intent of saving time, saving money, reducing errors, improving efficiency and accuracy, and ultimately benefiting patient outcomes.

I am particularly excited about this book and have invited expert contributors to also focus on applications of WSI in the area of artificial intelligence and machine learning techniques such as deep neural networks which may be trained to not only recognize specific patterns on a whole slide image of an H&E slide but in addition AI tools may also help in the interpretation of features in the tissue that are predictive and/or prognostic.

This is an exciting time in pathology, and this book aims to give the readers a look at WSI with a deeper lens and also envision the future of pathology imaging as it pertains to WSI and associated digital innovations. These digital innovations have the potential to change the way clinical diagnosis occurs, with added benefits of shared images and data; increased efficiency and integrated diagnostics; modernized pathology work flows to improve patient care and safety; increased collaboration through multidisciplinary, disease-specific patient care conferences; improved accountability in the work flow; and, finally, cost savings by optimizing staff performance. The possibility of using WSI in computational pathology and artificial intelligence has the promise to open new frontiers in pathology which even I cannot fully imagine but can only dream of. The possibilities are endless, and I want to invite you to share the vision and the possibilities and take a virtual journey into the next generation of amplified and augmented pathology.

Columbus, OH, USA Anil V. Parwani

Contents

Contributors

Jacob T. Abel, MD University of Michigan, Department of Pathology, Ann Arbor, MI, USA

Asmaa Aljuhani, MS in Computer Science Department of Computer Science and Engineering, College of Engineering, The Ohio State University, Columbus, OH, USA

Marilyn M. Bui, MD, PhD Moffitt Cancer Center, Department of Pathology, Tampa, FL, USA

Jany Chan, PhD Department of Computer Science and Engineering, College of Engineering, The Ohio State University, Columbus, OH, USA

Toby C. Cornish, MD, PhD University of Colorado School of Medicine, Department of Pathology, Aurora, CO, USA

James P. Cronin, DVM Department of Veterinary Biosciences, College of Veterinary Medicine The Ohio State University, Columbus, OH, USA

Department of Internal Medicine, College of Medicine, The Ohio State University, Columbus, OH, USA

Bryan Dangott, MD Mayo Clinic – Jacksonville, Department of Laboratory Medicine and Pathology, Jacksonville, FL, USA

Rajarsi Gupta, MD, PhD Department of Biomedical Informatics, Stony Brook University, Health Sciences Center, Stony Brook, NY, USA

Matthew G. Hanna, MD Memorial Sloan Kettering Cancer Center, Department of Pathology, New York, NY, USA

Douglas J. Hartman, MD University of Pittsburgh Medical Center, Department of Pathology, Pittsburgh, PA, USA

Department of Anatomic Pathology, University of Pittsburgh Medical Center, Pittsburgh, PA, USA

Tahsin Kurc, PhD Department of Biomedical Informatics, Stony Brook University, Health Sciences Center, Stony Brook, NY, USA

Zaibo Li, MD PhD Department of Pathology, The Ohio State University Wexner Medical Center, Columbus, OH, USA

Giovanni Lujan, MD College of Medicine, The Ohio State University Wexner Medical Center, Department of Pathology, Columbus, OH, USA

Raghu Machiraju, PhD Department of Computer Science and Engineering, College of Engineering, The Ohio State University, Columbus, OH, USA

Department of Biomedical Informatics, College of Medicine, The Ohio State University, Columbus, OH, USA

Department of Pathology, College of Medicine, The Ohio State University Wexner Medical School, Columbus, OH, USA

David S. McClintock, MD University of Michigan, Department of Pathology, Ann Arbor, MI, USA

Sambit K. Mohanty, MD Department of Pathology and Laboratory Medicine, Advanced Medical Research Institute, Bhubaneswar, Odisha, India

Liron Pantanowitz, MD Department of Pathology, University of Michigan, Ann Arbor, MI, USA

Anil V. Parwani, MD, PhD, MBA Department of Pathology, College of Medicine, The Ohio State University Wexner Medical School, Columbus, OH, USA

Philipp W. Raess, MD, PhD Oregon Health & Science University, Department of Pathology, Portland, OR, USA

Joel H. Saltz, MD, PhD Department of Biomedical Informatics, Stony Brook University, Health Sciences Center, Stony Brook, NY, USA

Rajendra Singh, MD Northwell Health, Department of Pathology, New York, NY, USA

S. Joseph Sirintrapun, MD Memorial Sloan Kettering Cancer Center, Department of Pathology, New York, NY, USA

Arunima Srivastava, PhD Department of Computer Science and Engineering, College of Engineering, The Ohio State University, Columbus, OH, USA

Darren Treanor, MB, BSc(Computing), PhD, FRCPath Leeds Teaching Hospitals NHS Trust, Department of Histopathology,, Leeds, UK

University of Leeds, Leeds, UK

Department of Clinical Pathology, and Department of Clinical and Experimental Medicine, Linköping University, Linköping, Sweden

Center for Medical Image Science and Visualization (CMIV), Linköping University, Linköping, Sweden

Bethany Jill Williams, MBBS BSc Leeds Teaching Hospitals NHS Trust, Department of Histopathology, Leeds, UK

Introduction to Digital Pathology from Historical Perspectives to Emerging Pathomics

Rajarsi Gupta, Tahsin Kurc, and Joel H. Saltz

Introduction

Digital pathology became a vast new frontier in medicine and science ever since glass slide scanners emerged 20 years ago. Nowadays, high-resolution whole slide images (WSIs) of histologic tissue samples are available on demand through virtual microscopy. As the number of glass tissues slides that are converted into WSIs continues to grow, digital pathology is leading to the creation of substantial multidisciplinary research efforts comprised of physicians, scientists, and engineers who are actively collaborating across academia and industry around the world.

Whole slide imaging, virtual microscopy, and digital pathology were driven by the need for telepathology to enable pathologists with the ability to remotely view tissue samples and communicate histopathologic diagnoses. The first applications of telepathology utilized cameras to take pictures and record videos of tissue samples while using robotic light microscopes and satellite communications [1–5]. As we transitioned from the analog to the digital age of data, whole slide imaging and the internet supplanted those technologies in modern telepathology, which were supported by advances in computer hardware, frameworks, networks, and data management to support the capture and storage of high-resolution WSIs. Currently available applications of telepathology include remote microscopic examination for rapid on-site evaluation (ROSE) of cytology samples, primary diagnosis by pathologist with subspecialty expertise, and intradepartmental and outside institutional consultation for urgent, challenging, and difficult cases.

After several decades of development, high-resolution digital WSIs are routinely captured by robust and automated glass slide scanners that are easily stored, shared,

R. Gupta · T. Kurc · J. H. Saltz (✉)
Department of Biomedical Informatics, Stony Brook University, Health Sciences Center, Stony Brook, NY, USA
e-mail: Joel.Saltz@stonybrookmedicine.edu

A. V. Parwani (ed.), *Whole Slide Imaging*,
https://doi.org/10.1007/978-3-030-83332-9_1

and readily viewed with established software systems [3, 6, 7]. The wide availability of WSIs has led to using the terminology, "digital pathology" to refer to scanning slides, archival of tissue images for tumor boards and education, and diagnostic consultation with telepathology [8]. The clinical adoption of digital pathology has been welcomed due to readily apparent opportunities that can meaningfully impact laboratory efficiency and delivering better patient care through rapid remote subspecialty consultation. Other exciting opportunities include improving diagnostic accuracy, increased review for quality assurance and control (QA/QC), and computational image analysis.

Digital pathology also represents a vast frontier for collaborative research among physicians, scientists, and engineers. For example, common steps in a typical surgical pathology research project to evaluate the prognostic and predictive value for biomarker expression may include (1) reviewing diagnostic reports to identify cohorts, (2) identifying formalin-fixed paraffin-embedded (FPPE) tissue samples of interest, (3) requesting glass slides for microscopic review, (4) preparation of non-diagnostic histologic tissue sections for research from FFPE tissue blocks, (5) performing immunohistochemical (IHC) studies, (6) obtaining clinicopathologic data from electronic health records (EHR) or tumor registries, and (7) correlative analyses with clinicopathologic and tumor registry data. In comparison, a straightforward application of digital pathology in the same setting easily saves a lot of time, costs, and resources by supporting cohort discovery via virtual access to tissue samples to ascertain the potential of pursuing a wide variety of research avenues.

Beyond the borders of laboratory medicine, digital pathology has also led to the establishment of pathomics as a result of the emergence of novel computational image analysis methodology driven by scientific and technical expertise in machine learning, artificial intelligence (AI), computer vision, and data science. Currently, sophisticated deep learning computer vision methods are being developed, implemented, and automated to routinely analyze WSIs and harvest quantitative pathomics data in order to develop advanced precision medicine applications for future clinical use. Thus, scalable Pathomics methodology is being increasingly considered for use in clinical trials and research in international academic, industrial, and pharmaceutical partnerships in order to identify patterns and relationships in embedded in massive amounts of clinical, imaging, and laboratory data to help further understand the nuances of complex human diseases.

As the integration of WSIs into clinical and research laboratories increases, it is important to be aware about various technological advances that were needed to establish digital pathology. Before having WSIs at our fingertips with broadband internet was a reality, the development of remote-controlled robotic microscopes that permitted navigation, changing magnification, and adjusting focus were critical to the development of early telepathology applications. Moreover, the fact that we can explore large collections of WSIs so seamlessly have been made possible due to significant improvements in scanning speeds, storage capacity, file compression, software, data transfer, and powerful data management resources and applications [1, 9–11]. Therefore, we provide a brief overview about the first virtual microscope, computational frameworks, and software that paved the way for whole slide imaging and digital pathology en route to the emergence of Pathomics in this chapter [1, 8, 12–18].

Origins of the Virtual Microscope

Our colllective understanding of tissues and cells has been dramatically transformed by light microscopy. The fundamental goal of digital pathology is to further advance our understanding of biology and pathology in the same manner. From a historical perspective, the roots of digital pathology are rooted in optics, robotics, and computers. In this section, we focus on virtual microscopy as a critical component of digital pathology and modern telepathology for viewing WSIs in a feasible and practical manner, which could never be possible without all of the necessary technological innovations that permit us to scan large quantities of glass tissue slides and generate high-resolution WSIs. However, we focus on virtual microscopy and how the current software systems and methods for data management, query, and viewing WSIs in digital pathology arose in the 1990s during the era of spatial dataset research in computer science [19].

The core functionality of a virtual microscope emulates conventional light microscopy. Virtual microscopy enables a person to use a computer to view, pan, and zoom in and out of WSIs in the same way that a glass tissue slide is examined with a microscope. In comparison, early telepathology systems provided support for remote access with either static images or live microscopy [2–5]. Beyond basic functionality, virtual microscopes provide the capability to organize and manage a collection of tissue images for remote access and viewing by concurrent users via a client-server configuration. Implementations of the virtual microscope have made it possible to efficiently catalog WSIs, share information, and perform collaborative consultation to remotely examine tissue samples for telepathology applications, where concurrent users can access the same image or the same set of images.

The main challenge of implementing a virtual microscope in the 1990s was the difficulty of achieving interactive viewing of images that did not fit in the memory of a computer that had relatively limited memory, disk storage space, and I/O bandwidths. There were also low network bandwidths, so it was not feasible to read an entire image and transfer it to a remote client. To work around these limitations, captured images were stitched together to create multi-gigabyte WSIs to work with the first glass tissue slide scanners, which were also slow at that time [20]. Thus, it was necessary to use distributed memory computational clusters with one or more disks that were attached to each cluster node to provide a request-response capability to (1) retrieve and reduce data on the server depending on the client request and (2) send the reduced data to the client side to achieve acceptable response times. This approach required methods and tooling for the careful placement of image data across the system, as well as orchestration of I/O, data filtering, and reduction operations to minimize data retrieval overheads and latency.

The first virtual microscope system that was capable of achieving interactive viewing functionality utilized high-performance computing, which was publicly demonstrated at the American Medical Informatics Association (AMIA) conferences in 1997 and 1998 [9, 20]. The development of this virtual microscope system arose from a computer science research project that targeted the management, visualization, and analysis of large datasets from sensors [21, 22]. The novel

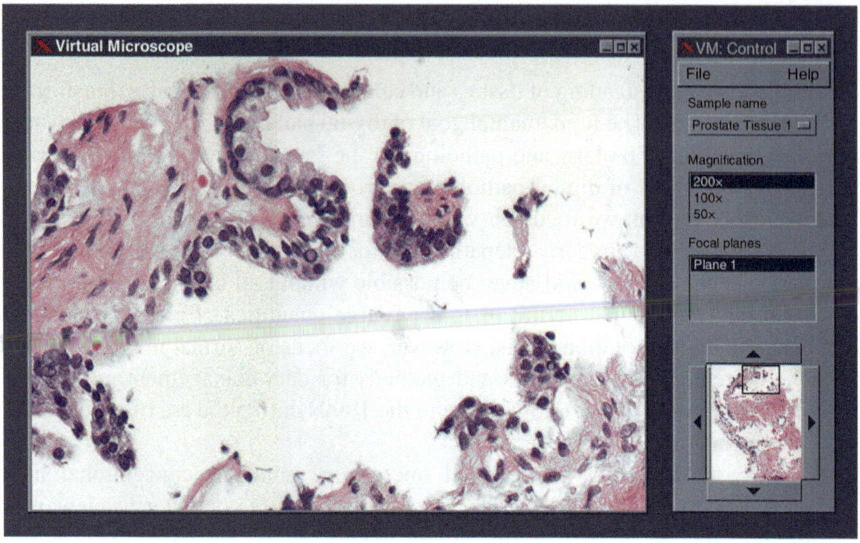

Fig. 1 1997–1998 era virtual microscope client

focus of this project was processing extremely large datasets with intensive computing to develop techniques and tools to analyze images in an extensible software platform. Until that time, the supercomputing community primarily focused on optimization to increase computational speed for data that would fit into distributed computer memory.

The first virtual microscope is shown in Fig. 1 and received the best application paper award from AMIA in 1997. By the late 1990s, it was increasingly recognized that the amount of data that was beginning to be captured by sensors on instrumentation like satellites was rapidly exceeding several orders of magnitude beyond the capacity of computer memory. The amount of data was even larger than aggregate memory on a high-performance computer with distributed memory.

Development of Computational Frameworks and Software

As the computational requirements associated with large-scale data became increasingly appreciated, the systems software group in the computer science department at the University of Maryland at College Park developed several prototype software systems to traverse datasets of images captured at multiple resolutions in the late 1990s and early 2000s. These software systems performed customized computations with sub-setting operations that rendered data for visualization and sent the output to clients to be displayed [21–23]. The scientific applications that motivated the development of these prototypes included the management and analysis of digital images from space telescopes to study changing global vegetation, seismic surveys, and subsurface oil reservoirs for Earth science. Figure 2 shows a representative screenshot from a project supported by the National Science Foundation (NSF) to

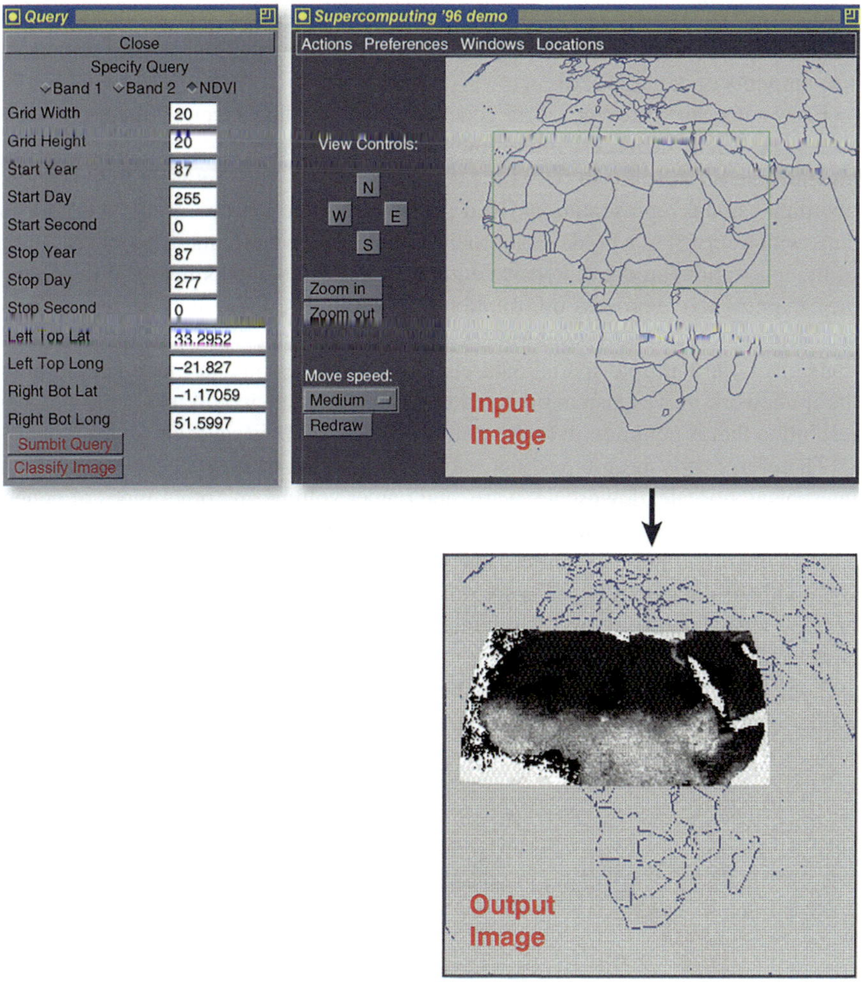

Fig. 2 NSF grand challenge in land cover dynamics

analyze the changes in global vegetation by using high-resolution satellite images by creating input data to develop models to study hydrology, carbon, and the global biogeochemical cycle.

These efforts were also driving the development of software systems and applications for digital pathology. Datasets in virtual microscopy were recognized as being very rich and complex at multiple scales of magnification for both normal and cancer-associated histology, which vary substantially across organ sites. Digital pathology was as computationally demanding as analyzing high-resolution satellite data, if not much more, due to the high degree of variability of the morphologic appearance of normal and diseased tissues and cells. Therefore, software systems for virtual microscopy were implemented to run on distributed memory computer clusters and supercomputers with many disks and processors, where the nature of the computational framework resembled Hadoop or Apache Spark to deal with massive amounts of data [24–26].

Early software prototypes were generalized models that executed mapping operations between different multidimensional coordinate systems (e.g., three-dimensional mesh space to two-dimensional image space or between two different two-dimensional representations) and performed reduction operations on mapped data, which served as a predecessor to the popularized MapReduce model [24]. One of the innovations in data-intensive computational frameworks involved designing the capability to (1) process information from multiple coordinate systems, (2) process data captured at different levels of spatial resolution, and (3) perform computations involving multiple spatial datasets. During the design and implementation of the framework, it was also anticipated that some datasets would have non-uniform resolution that is common in both satellite imagery and virtual microscopy.

Therefore, early prototypes were able to support a broad range of methods to interpolate, upscale, downscale, warp, and render volume and other types of generalized reduction or aggregation functions. The computational frameworks were also capable of combining data sources and performing in situ data visualization, which was used for data analysis in many other types of scientific research applications besides virtual microscopy. A schematic depicting one of these early systems is shown in Fig. 3.

Even though pathology images were typically limited to manually captured photomicrographs at the time, digital pathology was an early target application domain

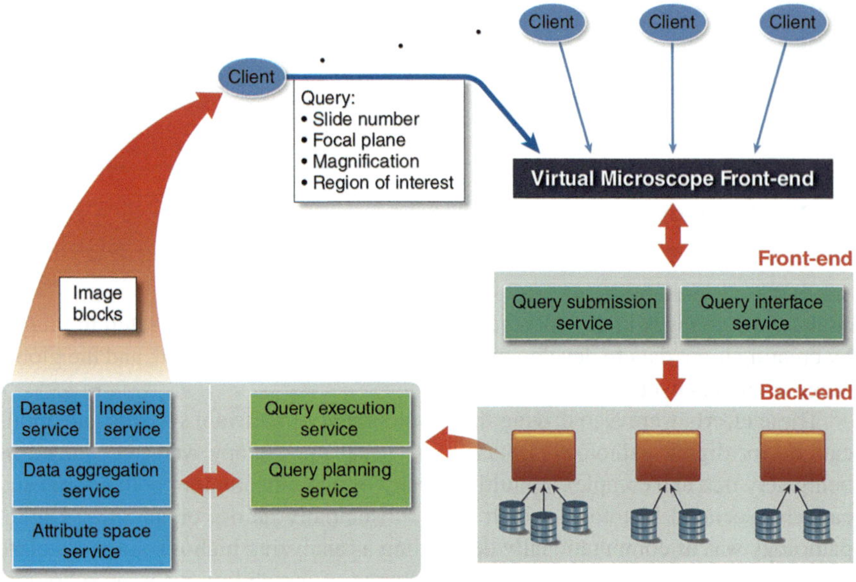

Fig. 3 Active data repository used to support whole slide digital microscopy

for this computational framework since it was clear that the widespread digitization of glass tissue slides would ultimately prove to be of great importance in medicine and science. Digital pathology was a natural application for this computational framework since processing and visualizing WSIs is very resource intensive. Basic operations such as panning and zooming were implemented with mapping and reduction operations. For example, zooming operations were viewed as reductions on image data by subsampling image pixels to fit in the viewer window at a given magnification and resolution.

Even though the first virtual microscope application was developed and described from 1997 to 2003, the fundamental concepts for computational demands and core functionality are still the same in modern whole slide imaging systems [9, 20, 27]. Users must be able to traverse WSIs by panning and zooming, overlay manual and computer-generated annotations, and collaboratively interact with the same set of WSIs. This data-intensive computational framework provided the building blocks to implement the virtual microscope system [21, 22]. However, additional optimizations were still needed to achieve high performance for this core set of tasks due to the relatively primitive nature of the hardware at that time, during when virtual microscopy was considered a relatively heroic computational effort and accomplishing these fundamental tasks to support navigating histologic images of tissues was considered monumental.

A popular high-performance computer system architecture was one in which each processor managed its own hard drives. This simplified the implementation and operating system requirements of the computer system. However, it required careful placement and management of the data and precise orchestration of I/O and computations. In order to reduce disk storage requirements and I/O retrieval costs, WSIs were partitioned into patches that were stored in compressed files in the virtual microscope system. These image patches were de-clustered across processor clusters or supercomputers to achieve computational and I/O load balance in order to achieve interactive level performance. This approach made it possible to utilize relatively inexpensive disks and aggregate I/O bandwidth from multiple storage units.

The virtual microscope software would partition a data request to view regions of WSIs at a desired zoom level into patches, overlap disk retrieval, and then assemble the image to be sent to the client in order to reduce I/O overheads. An R-tree index was implemented to quickly find the image patches that satisfied a given request [28]. In order to minimize network transfer overheads, the virtual microscope system implemented client-side caching to request regions of an image that were not in the client cache. Two versions of the virtual microscope were tested and implemented [27], where the first version was developed with the assumption that the system would be deployed on a homogeneous distributed memory system with tightly coupled nodes over a switch, whereas the second version was built on a software component architecture called DataCutter [10, 29].

In the DataCutter implementation, operations such as index lookup, data retrieval, data compression, data decompression, data subsampling, and data assembly would be implemented as individual components and loosely coupled to each other via a streaming component framework. This implementation was based on the recognition of the emerging grid computing paradigm, where even a moderate size computing environment could consist of a heterogeneous collection of storage and computation devices. Moreover, a component-based implementation would allow new computational capabilities by either adding components and/or modifications to individual components without having to maintain a single code base. In some ways, this implementation resembled microservice architectures that have become very popular in cloud computing and distributed computing environments.

In terms of software, both open-source and commercial virtual microscopy systems have proliferated in recent years. These software systems are typically built with advanced web and cloud computing technologies that include JavaScript modules for enhanced client-side functionality and microservice-based implementation through containerization technologies. For example, the Quantitative Imaging in Pathology (QuIP) platform [30] is a fully containerized open-source system software that was developed by an academic collaboration between Emory University and Stony Brook University. Individual containers implement core functionalities, such as data management, visualization, security, and data manipulation. The containers interact with each other in a loosely coupled manner via well-defined services and interfaces to enable user interaction through internet applications. The design and implementation of QuIP has leveraged and adapted the techniques developed since the early 2000s for data management, interactive exploration of images, and viewing the results of various types of image analyses in the context of modern web and cloud computing technologies.

QuIP is one of many examples of open-source systems for virtual microscopy [31–37], as shown in Fig. 4. Other notable open-source software systems include the Digital Slide Archive[34] and Cytomine [35], which are web-based, containerized technologies and service architectures. Popular alternatives that provide desktop functionality include the Pathology Image Informatics Platform for Visualization, Analysis, and Management (PIIP) [36] and QuPath (University of Edinburgh, Edinburgh, UK) [32]. In addition, vendors of commercial slide scanners also offer their own proprietary virtual microscopy software. Alongside these options, there are also an increasing number of specialized commercial software products for viewing digital images and performing image analysis, such as HALO (Indica Labs, Corrales, New Mexico, USA), Aperio GENIE (Vista, California, USA), HistoRx AQUA Analysis (Branford, Connecticut, USA), and Visiopharm (Hoersholm, Denmark).

These open-source and commercial systems generally support a wide array of functions that surpass core image retrieval and visualization capabilities. All of the viewers are designed to give users the ability to freely explore any part of WSIs by panning and zooming to recapitulate the experience of using traditional light microscopes to examine glass tissue slides. These software applications also provide interfaces that permit viewing, organizing, and annotating large collections of WSIs. Since image analysis is beginning to play a much larger role in digital pathology, most modern software packages also support viewing computational analyses as well. Software packages that incorporate data analysis typically allow users to display the results of image analysis in an additional companion viewer or overlaid as

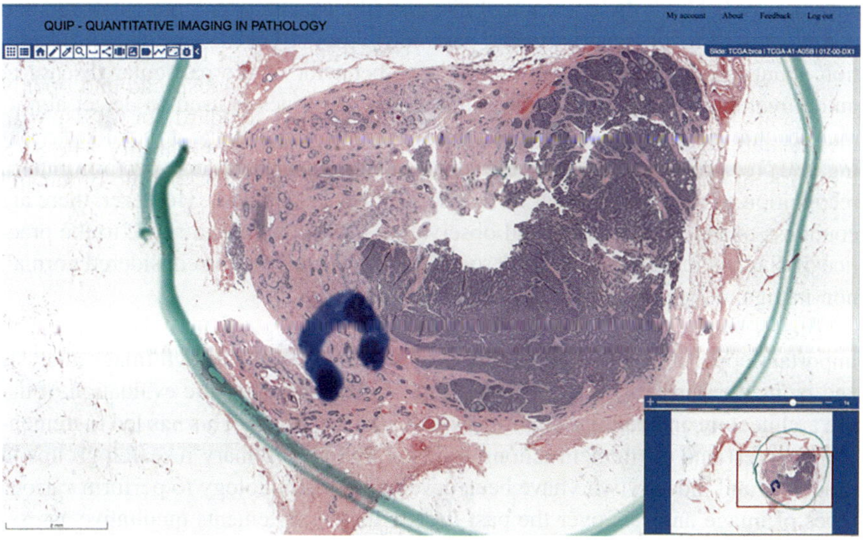

Fig. 4 QuIP digital pathology software. The WSI is from a glass tissue slide of breast cancer from the publicly available the Cancer Genome Atlas (TCGA). Breast cancer, TCGA-A0SB-01Z-00-DX1

additional layers on WSIs. Typical examples of image analysis that can be displayed include segmentation and classification of various microarchitectural components of tissues that are described in the next section.

Frontiers of Computational Pathology and Pathology Informatics

Tissue samples are routinely obtained and sent to clinical laboratories like cytology and surgical pathology for diagnostic testing Tissue samples that are obtained during clinical trials and biomarker discovery studies are typically processed in research histology laboratories. Typically, FFPE tissue sections are stained with hematoxylin and eosin (H&E) and/or various biomarkers for specialized IHC and immunofluorescence (IF) testing as part of diagnostic workups to classify and subclassify a wide spectrum of benign and malignant diseases. Histopathologic features of disease and associated biomarker expression are used to predict disease progression and guide treatment by identifying drug targets. Even though there have been many important discoveries and considerable advances, a comprehensive understanding about diseases like cancer still remains elusive. In this section, we succinctly describe the emerging field of Pathomics that combines virtual microscopy, image analysis, and biomedical informatics to characterize various aspects of tissue and cells with computational image analyses.

One of the main objectives of pathologists is to systematically examine tissue samples with the goal of identifying various histopathologic features of tissues and cells associated with the presence of diseases like cancer, which are cataloged and communicated in diagnostic surgical pathology reports. This data provides information about tumor classification and biologic behavior of the particular disease to guide treatment. The microscopic examination of tissues is used to detect abnormalities that is based on acquiring extensive medical knowledge, specialized training, and precious experience over the course of many years in order to perform pattern recognition to delineate normal from diseased tissues and cells. However, there are countless nuances, semantics, and observation biases that are intrinsic to the practice of diagnostic histopathology across the spectrum of what is considered normal, non-malignant, and overtly malignant disease.

This is where WSIs, computational pathology, and pathomics data represents important opportunites to gain further insight into diseases through image analysis and biomedical informatics by augmenting traditional diagnostic evaluation of tissue architecture and cellular features with quantitative datat. This has led to tremendous interest and excitement among growing multidisciplinary research groups in academia and industry who have been developing methodology to perform various types of image analysis over the past decade that complements qualitative assessment by pathologists in order to provide pathologists with clinical decision support (CDS) tools. Image analysis in digital pathology primarily focuses on segmentation and classification tasks to identify and characterize various aspects of tissue microanatomy, populations of cells, and phenotypic features of nuclei. Pathomics analyses have been performed in various types of tissues to calculate the color, size, shape, and texture of cells and larger microanatomic regions and structures in order to quantitatively measure a wide pectrum of phenotypic features of disease (see [8, 13, 15, 38–49] for algorithmic development related to semi-automated and automated image analysis and [12, 18] for recent white papers that provide practical guides to whole slide imaging and image analysis).

Briefly, classical image analysis of WSIs extracts pixel-level, object-level, or semantic-level-based features. Segmentation algorithms identify and delineate the boundaries of objects based on statistical variations in color intensity and texture, data clustering, binary classifiers, and with probabilistic/non-probabilistic machine learning methods, which is then used to classify various aspects of pathology images [38, 41, 43, 44, 46, 47, 49–55]. Pixel-level analyses typically analyze features like color, boundaries, contrast, texture, size, and shape. In comparison, object-level analyses focus on characteristics like nuclei, nucleoli, mitoses, and microanatomic structures, such as glands, ducts, blood vessels, and nerves. Semantic-level features classify different types of tissue based on the microanatomic configuration of different kinds of cells, which can be used to differentiate tumor versus non-tumor tissues, determine the presence or degree of dysplasia, and identify infiltrates of immune cells [50–54, 56–61].

One of the main areas where computational pathology has been utilized is the measurement and scoring the IHC biomarker expression. IHC biomarkers are a cost-effective approach that is used to label cells that express a particular protein. This is of particular interest in surgical pathology and clinical research when looking for molecular genetic anomalies in diseases like cancer. Since IHC biomarkers can cells based on the expression of proteins that may be impacted by gene amplification, mutation, deletion, translocation, and virally mediated alterations, IHC testing is routinely performed for diagnostic classification, identifying potential drug targets, and predicting disease progression and clinical outcomes. However, there are several challenges in using digital pathology algorithms to measure IHC biomarker expression due to nuances in calculating percentage of "positive" cells that are labeled by a particular IHC marker. Typical obstacles include the heterogeneous expression of biomarkers by a particular cell of interest, non-specific staining, and variations in the color intensity of the label due to differences in biomarker specificity, pattern of expression, and staining intensity [62–64]. Even though it appears relatively simple to perform a targeted analysis of cells that typically appear brown in color due to the use of the chromogen, 3,3′-diaminobenzidine (DAB), algorithmic analyses must intrinsically account for these sources of variability within the appropriate histologic context.

Pathologists spend many years learning about the strengths, nuances, and limitations of the IHC biomarkers that they regularly utilize and interpret to provide diagnostic and prognostic information to clinicians. Despite the challenges, there is great interest in algorithmic approaches to help complement human interpretation since IHC is used in constantly in daily practice. If reliable and robust computational methodology can be implemented to help further automate laboratories, digital pathology will become a very important factor that improves efficiency, decreases observer variability, and reduces costs [8]. Measuring IHC with digital pathology is an active area of computational pathology where methods are being continuously developed and refined so that biomarker scoring algorithms can be reliably implemented in the near future. En route to developing algorithms to quantify IHC expression, conventional machine learning algorithms have been used to perform cell segmentation by using combinations of median filtering, thresholds, watershed segmentation, contour models, and shape dictionaries, among a wide variety of other Pathomics variables [41, 42, 46, 47, 49, 50, 55–57, 65–69]. However, these methods often require detailed adjustments of various parameters and settings to avoid under- and oversegmentation in order to account for differences in nuclear, cytoplasmic, and membranous staining across a constantly growing library of IHC biomarkers.

The transition from light microscopes to virtual microscopy has led to the incorporation of deep learning and computer vision in image analysis to develop automated AI algorithms to analyze and harvest Pathomics data from WSIs. Deep learning and AI have grown substantially in popularity due to remarkable advances in machine learning, computer vision, increased computing capacity, and the near omnipresence of technologies like smartphones, cameras, digital images, and video. Recent developments in deep learning applications for computational pathology have demonstrated the capability to quantitatively analyze WSIs to perform tumor detection, as well as diagnostic classification, grading, and staging [8, 18, 40, 57, 70–98], along with the classification of a wide spectrum of other salient histologic features that can help predict the presence of gene mutations from WSIs (see recent papers [19, 46, 56, 57, 66–75, 99–120]).

A very important advantage of deep learning applications in pathomics tissue analytics is that relatively robust performance can be achieved with decreased requirements for fine-tuning traditional image analysis parameters (i.e., variations in tissue processing and colors with H&E and IHC staining). Thus, there are many research groups that are actively working to develop, test, and refine deep leaning computer vision applications in Pathomics to systematically and uniformly harvest quantitative measurements of various histopathologic features of diseases from WSIs. Since WSIs typically contain hundreds of thousands to millions of cells within the context of heterogeneous and diverse histologic landscapes, it was natural for investigators to investigate the potential of deep learning algorithms in Pathomics. Beyond harvesting massive amounts of pathomics data from WSIs, deep learning is also being implemented in identifying overt and subtle non-linear relationships and patterns within billions upon billions points of pathomics data that cannot be analyzed with conventional statistical approaches.

Even though we are gaining the ability to perform sophisticated image analysis with deep learning, we must also state the importance of due diligence and systematic studies to measure the performance of these algorithms in terms of accuracy, precision, and robustness. The typical workflow in developing these kinds of algorithms includes design, annotating WSIs, development of deep learning models, testing, validation in an independent dataset, and iterative refinement before deployment with appropriate QA/QC mechanisms, which is no different than what would be expected in the development and implementation in any kind of laboratory testing. As fascinating as it is to see the kinds of analyses that can be performed with deep learning pathomics applications, we must remember that these computational methods have limitations and biases based on the quality of the training dataset and spectrum of variability of the data points that the models use during training. In other words, we need to understand that deep learning models are not infallible and will occasionally fail, especially within the context of interpreting the complexity of the histologic microenvironment in healthy and diseased tissues.

The opportunities that are presented by deep learning in digital pathology to perform automated image analysis on a large scale have led to the creation of large collections of institutional, private, and publicly available WSIs. The most famous repository is the Cancer Genome Atlas (TCGA), which serves as an extraordinary source of WSIs to the international research community while providing corresponding molecular, radiologic, survival, and other anonymized clinical metadata [43, 44, 70, 76, 77, 121–123]. The public availability of TCGA WSIs has been critical to the recent explosion of interest in computational pathology and numerous correlative studies that link Pathomics analyses with genomics, imaging, treatment, and survival data in more than 30 different types of cancer.

Computational pathology is also being used to help understand the role of a wide range of hierarchical regulatory pathways in cancer, such as cell signaling by studying the spatial relationships of different populations of cells within the context of gene expression in the histologic landscape of cancer pathology. As a result of these studies, significant efforts are being dedicated to computational pathology to discover novel digital pathology biomarkers to predict clinical outcomes and potentially help select treatment strategies based on favorable response. Thus, the importance of computational pathology cannot be understated in precision medicine initiatives that will inevitably require quantitative measurements in order to define and compare phenotypic differences in cancer tissue samples. In this manner, Pathomics analytics is very useful for performing standardized and uniform analyses that catalog different regions of tissue, cell populations, and nuclear characteristics along with a characterization of spatial properties and relationships in the tumor microenvironment, which can then be used to systematically explore the biological behavior of cancer in individual patients.

Pathomics methods are potentially meeting and possibly exceeding current limitations in performance due to increased involvement of pathologists in generating high-quality annotated data and testing in multiple independent datasets that are being validated with reference data [108]. For example, many groups are investigating the role of using deep learning to identify tumor-infiltrating lymphocytes (TILs) in cancer to support the role of precision medicine in immunotherapy to treat cancer [65, 81, 99, 124–128]. Figures 5 and 6 show examples of using deep learning

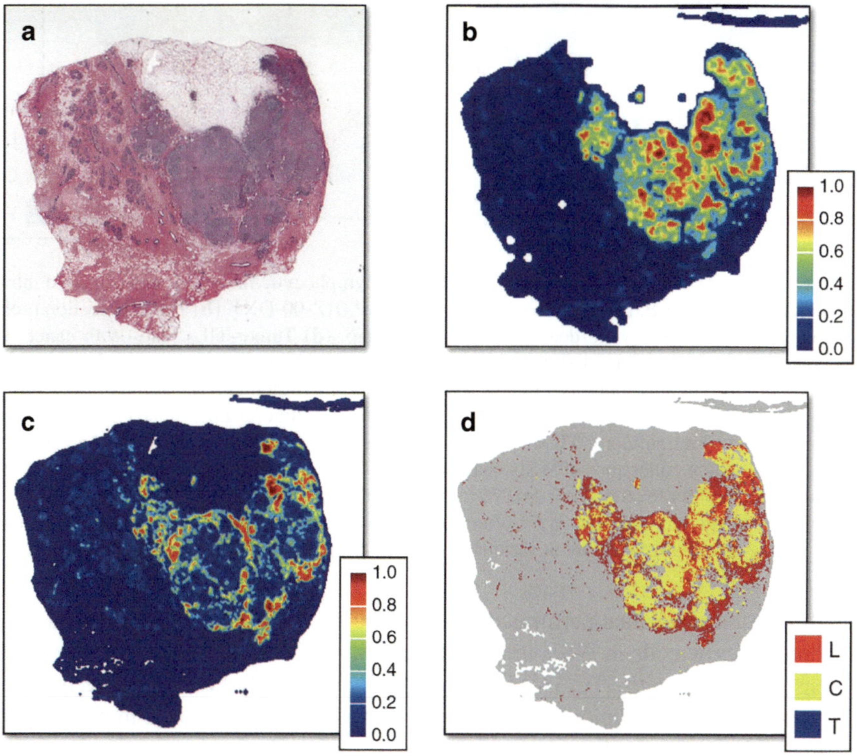

Fig. 5 Spatial tumor-TILs analyses showing the abundance and distribution of TILs in breast cancer. (**a**) H&E, breast cancer, TCGA-A2-A0CL-01Z-00-DX1. (**b**) Tumor detection probability map. (**c**) Lymphocyte detection probability map. (**d**) Tumor-TILs maps with cancer in yellow and lymphocytes in red. (L lymphocytes, C cancer; and T non-tumor non-lymphocyte background tissue). This figure demonstrates the ability to implement automated tumor and lymphocyte detection with the goal of analyzing the spatial distribution of tumor immune responses. In this case, we observe abundant intratumoral and peritumoral TILs that are diffusely distributed throughout the tumor. Relative probabilities are used to ascertain prediction certainty in order to quickly evaluate the overall performance of the algorithms within the context of the corresponding H&E WSI

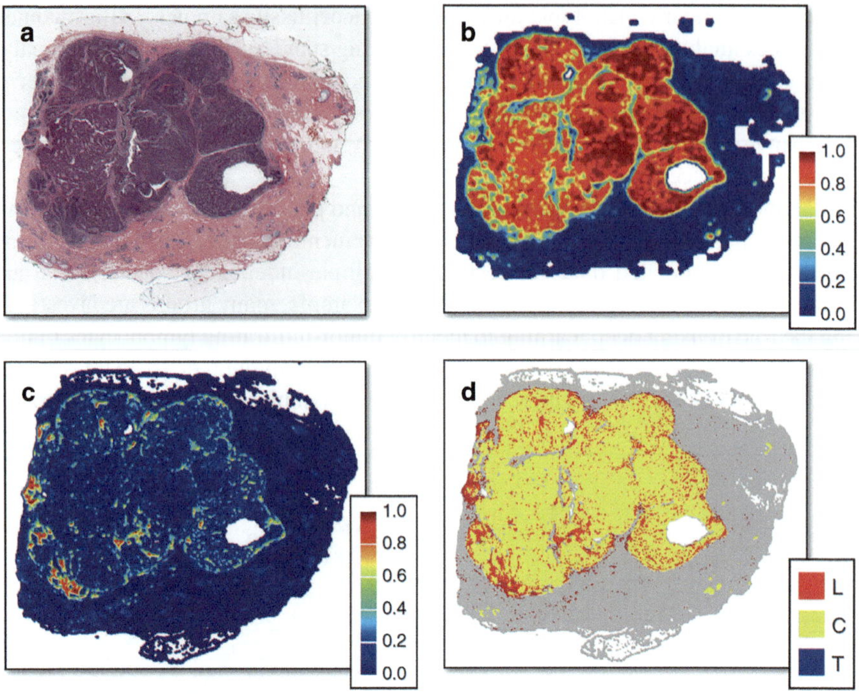

Fig. 6 Tumor-TILs map showing mostly peritumoral lymphocytic infiltrates with scattered intratumoral TILs. (**a**) H&E, breast cancer, TCGA-A2-A0SP-01Z-00-DX1. (**b**) Tumor detection probability map. (**c**) Lymphocyte detection probability map. (**d**) Tumor-TILs maps with cancer in yellow and lymphocytes in red. (L lymphocytes, C cancer; and T non-tumor non-lymphocyte background tissue). The distribution of tumor immune responses is qualitatively different from Fig. 5 with a more muted immune response. We observe mostly peritumoral TILs in localized areas containing scattered intratumoral TILs. Pathomics analyses like Tumor-TILs mapping can easily be performed in large collections of WSIs in a scalable fashion to virtually analyze tissue samples for each patient in order to stratify candidates for immunotherapy. These kinds of Pathomics analyses can also be integrated with other types of image analysis methods in order to systematically extract and catalog quantitative data about various phenotypic properties of tissues, cells, and nuclei

Pathomics analyses that performed automated detection of tumor regions and lymphoplasmacytic cells in WSIs in order to identify TILs in more than 1000 WSIs of breast cancer from the TCGA [78, 99, 124]. Even though these are basic types of Pathomics analyses, tumor-TILs Pathomics clearly show how tumor immune interactions are quite variable and heterogeneous within the boundaries of the tissue that are identified as positive for breast cancer (tumor depicted in yellow and lymphocytes depicted in red in the bottom right panels in Figs. 5 and 6). Analyses like this have never been performed on such a large scale but clearly show the potential of Pathomics to help characterize the functional immune status of the tumor microenvironment on a per patient sample basis and how much it can vary, which may potentially affect treatment response and survival.

Digital pathology currently encompasses whole slide imaging, telepathology, and computational pathology/Pathomics. While computational pathology is an extremely active research area, the penetration of these methods into the clinical practice has been limited. However, FDA approval for primary diagnosis has created a lot of excitement about Pathomics applications that can be clinically useful for precision medicine applications [129]. Therefore, one can reasonably expect that current Pathomics research initiatives are laying the foundation for the future when automated AI-driven Pathomics algorithms with rapidly increasing computational power are analyzing large collections of readily available WSIs to harvest all kinds of quantitative data about cancer and other diseases. The true impact of digital pathology will be felt when pathology informatics aggregates and integrates pathomics data for downstream correlative analyses with laboratory, imaging, genomic, treatment, survival, and other clinical data in order to identify patterns and relationships that can provide clinical insight to improve patient care and treatment.

As seen in Figs. 5 and 6, tumor-TILs analyses generate a readily interpretable figure that can help pathologists evaluate the functional immunologic status of the tumor microenvironment. Furthermore, pathologists can look at these kinds of Pathomics analyses to identify regions of interest for further microscopic examination and provide novel types of information to clinicians to help guide treatment (e.g., tumor immune interactions in tissue samples may help select and stratify candidates for immunotherapy). One can also envision further enhancing tumor-TILs analyses by combining the tumor detection algorithm with capabilities to perform tumor subclassification as well in an effort to study how the histologic subtype influences tumor immune interactions within the context of tumor heterogeneity. Similarly, one can combine tumor-TILs analyses with nuclear segmentation and cell classification to study the distributions of different populations of tumor cells and identify specific phenotypic features in subpopulations of tumor cells that are present in metastases and recurrence. Other readily available opportunities also include the combination of using advanced computational methods to quantify IHC biomarker expression with automated tumor detection in emerging multiplex IHC platforms that use multiple biomarkers in panels to label different types of cells with designated colors in a single tissue section.

The advancements in digital pathology have been remarkable in the last 20 years. With the increasing availability of WSIs, digital pathology has given birth to computational pathology, Pathomics, and pathology informatics, which will undoubtedly play important roles to quantify various aspects of traditional microscopic examination of tissues while helping perform complex types of correlative analyses with diverse types of healthcare data to improve treatment and clinical outcomes. Similar to how IHC also emerged in diagnostic pathology in the last 20 years and revolutionized the histologic subclassification of tumors by providing the ability to study the expression of a large number of biomarkers that were used to correlate genomics and molecular data with in situ protein expression, Pathomics appears to be heading the same directions as we collectively aim to refine our understanding about different molecular subtypes of common and uncommon cancers and other diseases. We also see how IHC biomarkers that were once used for diagnostic evaluation are now being revisited to further explore their prognostic value and ability to serve as potential therapeutic drug targets, so Pathomics will likely return to incorporate lessons learned from fundamental research with traditional image analysis methodology to couple with the incredible capabilities of machine learning and AI Pathomics applications. Therefore, we end this section with full awareness about how computational pathology and pathology informatics will likely follow the trajectory of IHC with the intention of providing a concrete example of how digital pathology and Pathomics will become indispensable tools for the practice of pathology to help improve various aspects of healthcare in the age of precision medicine. Although these technologies are still early in their development cycles, it is incredibly exciting to consider how pathomics data will transform medicine through advanced data analytics by providing calculated projections about patient survival, likelihood of disease recurrence, and progression in the very near future.

Conclusions

The world of digital pathology has flourished in the last 20 years to give humankind an unprecedented look into the microscopic world of tissue biology through virtual microscopy of high-resolution WSIs. Therefore, we must appreciate our privilege of having stable web-based virtual microscopy software that allows us to instantly view WSIs with modern broadband internet, which supports the immediate transfer of massive amounts of data. After significant contributions by the research community in academia, industry, and the government, digital pathology is on the cusp of delivering significant returns on investment with image analysis tools and Pathomics tissue analytics workflows that complement the modern practice of surgical pathology and precision medicine initiatives. As high-throughput commercial slide scanners become more common in clinical laboratories, WSIs will fundamentally transform the practice of pathology in many ways. Therefore, we hope that our description about the first virtual microscope and the related developments in infrastructure that support the needs of digital pathology and modern telepathology helps preserve a deep appreciation for the pioneering efforts in this field. Furthermore, we need to be grateful for having the ability to be able to access digital high-resolution WSIs of tissue samples at our fingertips since access to virtual tissue samples is leading the way to providing patients with rapid primary diagnoses and consultations for difficult, rare, and emergent cases along side the incredible opportunities to further the boundaries of our knowledge through Pathomics.

Thus, we hope to have provided a bird's eye view of the past, present, and future of digital pathology. Machine learning and AI applications in digital pathology likely represent the pioneering work towards having actively learning algorithms that function as clinical decision support tools for pathologists that will constantly harvest, aggregate, integrate, and analyze diverse types of Pathomics data with data from the electronic heathcare records in order to refine patient stratification and improve treatment selection, clinical outcomes, and survival. Due to ubiquitous advanced forms of technology in today's world, it is not hard to conceive a nearby future where Pathomics data from the infinite, multidimensional, and complex microscopic universe of tissue pathology will lead to transformative discoveries that can revolutionize our understanding about how cancer forms, progresses, and metastasizes so that we can better treat patients. In parallel, we look forward to the increasing role of pathology informatics in precision medicine as this kind of data starts being utilized to identify subtle and complex patterns to discover biomarkers, spatial relationships of various types of cells in the tumor microenvironment, and correlations between quantified histopathologic features, clinical outcomes, and treatment response that cannot be performed by human beings.

Visual images will always play an important role in communication and learning in every facet of human life. Even though it is easy to get lost in all of the excitement of computational pathology, deep learning, computer vision, and pathomics data informatics, we must always pay our respects to all of the pioneers who developed whole slide imaging and virtual microscope systems that evolved from nascent efforts in the 1990s and early 2000s to provide us with remote access to high-resolution images by paving the roads to the thriving and dynamic ecosystem of digital pathology and its role in the future of healthcare and individualized precision medicine.

References

1. Hedvat CV. Digital microscopy: past, present, and future. Arch Pathol Lab Med. 2010;134(11):1666–70.
2. Weinstein R, Holcomb M, Krupinski E. Invention and early history of telepathology (1985–2000). J Pathol Inform. 2019;10(1):1–1.
3. Weinstein RS. Prospects for telepathology. Hum Pathol. 1986;17(5):433–4.
4. Weinstein RS, et al. Telepathology: a ten-year progress report. Hum Pathol. 1997;28(1):1–7.
5. Weinstein RS, Bloom KJ, Rozek LS. Telepathology. Long-distance diagnosis. Am J Clin Pathol. 1989;91(4 Suppl 1):S39–42.
6. Bashshur RL, et al. The empirical foundations of telepathology: evidence of feasibility and intermediate effects. Telemed e-Health. 2017;23(3):155–91.
7. Williams S, et al. Telepathology for patient care: what am I getting myself into? Adv Anat Pathol. 2010;17(2):130–49.
8. Nam S, et al. Introduction to digital pathology and computer-aided pathology. J Pathol Transl Med. 2020;54(2):125–34.
9. Afework A, et al. Digital dynamic telepathology–the virtual microscope. In Proceedings of the AMIA symposium. 1998. American Medical Informatics Association.
10. Beynon M, et al. DataCeutter: middleware for filtering very large scientific datasets on archival storage systems. In IEEE symposium on mass storage systems. 2000.
11. Beynon MD, et al. Distributed processing of very large datasets with DataCutter. Parallel Comput. 2001;27(11):1457–78.
12. Aeffner F, et al. Introduction to digital image analysis in whole-slide imaging: a white paper from the digital pathology association. J Pathol Inform. 2019;10:9–9.
13. Bui MM, et al. Digital and computational pathology: bring the future into focus. J Pathol Inform. 2019;10:10.
14. Farahani N, et al. International telepathology: promises and pitfalls. Pathobiology. 2016;83(2–3):121–6.
15. Ghaznavi F, et al. Digital imaging in pathology: whole-slide imaging and beyond. Ann Rev Pathol Mech Dis. 2013;8(1):331–59.
16. Jr., D.W. Digital pathology gives rise to computational pathology. Medqor healthcare informatics – technology outlook 2017 [cited 2020 May 29]; Available from: http://www.clpmag.com/2017/10/digital-pathology-gives-rise-computational-pathology/.

17. Park S, et al. The history of pathology informatics: a global perspective. J Pathol Inform. 2013;4(1):7.
18. Zarella MD, et al. A practical guide to whole slide imaging: a white paper from the digital pathology association. Arch Pathol Lab Med. 2019;143(2):222–34.
19. Pantanowitz L, et al. Twenty years of digital pathology: an overview of the road travelled, what is on the horizon, and the emergence of vendor-neutral archives. J Pathol Inform. 2018;9:40.
20. Ferreira R, et al. The virtual microscope. Proc AMIA Annu Fall Symp. 1997:449–53.
21. Chang C, et al. T2: a customizable parallel database for multi-dimensional data. ACM SIGMOD Rec. 1998;27(1):58–66.
22. Chang C, et al. Titan: a high-performance remote-sensing database. In Proceedings 13th international conference on data engineering. 1997.
23. Ferreira R, et al. Object-relational queries into multidimensional databases with the active data repository. Parallel Proc Lett. 1999;9(02):173–95.
24. Dean J, Ghemawat S. MapReduce: simplified data processing on large clusters. Communications of the ACM. 2008;51(1):107–13. https://doi.org/10.1145/1327452.1327492.
25. White T. Hadoop: the definitive guide. 2012: " O'Reilly Media, Inc.".
26. Zaharia M, et al. Spark: cluster computing with working sets. HotCloud. 2010;10(10–10):95.
27. Çatalyürek Ü, et al. The virtual microscope. IEEE Trans Inf Technol Biomed. 2003;7(4):230–48.
28. Beckmann N, et al. The R*-tree: an efficient and robust access method for points and rectangles. In Proceedings of the 1990 ACM SIGMOD international conference on Management of data. 1990.
29. Beynon M, et al. Distributed processing of very large datasets with DataCutter. Parallel Comput. 2001;27(11):1457–2478.
30. Baig F, et al. SparkGIS: resource aware efficient in-memory spatial query processing. In proceedings of the 25th ACM SIGSPATIAL international conference on advances in geographic information systems. 2017. ACM.
31. Allan C, et al. OMERO: flexible, model-driven data management for experimental biology. Nat Methods. 2012;9(3):245–53.
32. Bankhead P, et al. QuPath: open source software for digital pathology image analysis. Sci Rep. 2017;7(1):16878.
33. Foran DJ, et al. ImageMiner: a software system for comparative analysis of tissue microarrays using content-based image retrieval, high-performance computing, and grid technology. J Am Med Inform Assoc. 2011;18(4):403–15.
34. Gutman DA, et al. The digital slide archive: a software platform for management, integration, and analysis of histology for cancer research. Cancer Res. 2017;77(21):e75–8.
35. Marée R, et al. Cytomine: an open-source software for collaborative analysis of whole-slide images. Diagn Pathol. 2016;1(8):1395.
36. Martel AL, et al. An image analysis resource for cancer research: PIIP—pathology image informatics platform for visualization, analysis, and management. Cancer Res. 2017;77(21):e83–6.
37. Williams E, et al. Image data resource: a bioimage data integration and publication platform. Nat Methods. 2017;14:775.
38. Cooper L, et al. Feature-based registration of histopathology images with different stains: an application for computerized follicular lymphoma prognosis. Comput Methods Prog Biomed. 2009;96(3):182–92.
39. Hamilton PW, et al. Digital pathology and image analysis in tissue biomarker research. Methods. 2014;70(1):59–73.
40. Hamilton PW, et al. Automated tumor analysis for molecular profiling in lung cancer. Oncotarget. 2015;6(29):27938–52.
41. Irshad H, et al. Methods for nuclei detection, segmentation, and classification in digital histopathology: a review—current status and future potential. IEEE Rev Biomed Eng. 2014;7:97.

42. Janowczyk A, Madabhushi A. Deep learning for digital pathology image analysis: a comprehensive tutorial with selected use cases. J Pathol Inform. 2016;7(1):29.
43. Kothari S, et al. Biological interpretation of morphological patterns in histopathological whole-slide images. ACM-BCB ... : the ... ACM conference on bioinformatics, computational biology and biomedicine acm conference on bioinformatics, computational biology and biomedicine, 2012. 2012: p. 218–225.
44. Kothari S, et al. Pathology imaging informatics for quantitative analysis of whole-slide images. J Am Med Inform Assoc. 2013;20(6):1099–108.
45. Madabhushi A, et al. Computer-aided prognosis: predicting patient and disease outcome via quantitative fusion of multi-scale, multi-modal data. Comput Med Imaging Graph. 2011;35(7–8):506–14.
46. Madabhushi A, Lee G. Image analysis and machine learning in digital pathology: challenges and opportunities. Med Image Anal. 2016;33:170–5.
47. Xing F, et al. Transfer shape modeling towards high-throughput microscopy image segmentation. Med Image Comput Comput Assist Interv. 2016;9902:183–90.
48. Xing F, et al. deep learning in microscopy image analysis: a survey. IEEE transactions on neural networks and learning systems, 2017. p. 1–19.
49. Xing F, Yang L. Robust nucleus/cell detection and segmentation in digital pathology and microscopy images: a comprehensive review. IEEE Rev Biomed Eng. 2016;9:234–63.
50. Hou L, et al. Unsupervised histopathology image synthesis. arXiv [cs.CV], 2017.
51. Hou L, et al. Robust histopathology image analysis: to label or to synthesize? Proceedings of the IEEE conference on computer vision and pattern recognition, 2019. p. 8533–42.
52. Hou L, et al. Sparse autoencoder for unsupervised nucleus detection and representation in histopathology images. Pattern Recogn. 2019;86:188–200.
53. Hou L, et al. Patch-based convolutional neural network for whole slide tissue image classification. Proceedings of the IEEE Conference on Computer Vision and Pattern Recognition (CVPR), 2016. p. 2424–2433.
54. Hou, L., et al. Automatic histopathology image analysis with CNNs. In 2016 New York scientific data summit (NYSDS). 2016. IEEE.
55. Wang F, et al. A data model and database for high-resolution pathology analytical image informatics. J Pathol Inform. 2011;2(1):32.
56. Al-Milaji Z, et al. Integrating segmentation with deep learning for enhanced classification of epithelial and stromal tissues in H&E images. Pattern Recogn Lett. 2017;
57. Al-Milaji Z, et al. Integrating segmentation with deep learning for enhanced classification of epithelial and stromal tissues in H&E images. Pattern Recogn Lett. 2019;119:214–21.
58. Cheng CL, et al. Enabling digital pathology in the diagnostic setting: navigating through the implementation journey in an academic medical centre. J Clin Pathol. 2016;69(9):784–92.
59. Corredor G, et al. A watershed and feature-based approach for automated detection of lymphocytes on lung cancer images. Medical Imaging 2018: Digital Pathology, 2018. 10581: 105810R.
60. Corredor G, et al. Spatial architecture and arrangement of tumor-infiltrating lymphocytes for predicting likelihood of recurrence in early-stage non–small cell lung cancer. Clin Cancer Res. 2019;25(5):1526–34.
61. Murthy V, et al. Center-focusing multi-task CNN with injected features for classification of glioma nuclear images. IEEE Winter Conference on Applications of Computer Vision (WACV), 2017: p. 834–841.
62. Troncone G, Gridelli C. The reproducibility of PD-L1 scoring in lung cancer: can the pathologists do better? Transl Lung Cancer Res. 2017;6(Suppl 1):S74–s77.
63. Valous NA, et al. Spatial intratumoral heterogeneity of proliferation in immunohistochemical images of solid tumors. Med Phys. 2016;43(6):2936–47.
64. Veillard A, Kulikova MS, Racoceanu D. Cell nuclei extraction from breast cancer histopathologyimages using colour, texturee, scale and shape information. In diagnostic pathology. 2013. BioMed Central.

65. Amgad M, et al. Joint region and nucleus segmentation for characterization of tumor infiltrating lymphocytes in breast cancer. In medical imaging 2019: digital patehology. 2019. International Society for Optics and Photonics.
66. Janowczyk A, et al. A resolution adaptive deep hierarchical (RADHicaL) learning scheme applied to nuclear segmentation of digital pathology images. Comput Methods Biomech Biomed Eng Imag Vis. 2018;6(3):270–6.
67. Mahmood F, et al. Deep adversarial training for multi-organ nuclei segmentation in histopathology images. arXiv [cs.CV]. 2018.
68. Sirinukunwattana K, et al. Locality sensitive deep learning for detection and classification of nuclei in routine Colon cancer histology images. IEEE Trans Med Imaging. 2016;35(5):1196–206.
69. Vu QD, et al. Methods for segmentation and classification of digital microscopy tissue images. Front Bioeng Biotechnol. 2019;7:53.
70. Cruz-Roa A, Gilmore H, Basavanhally A, et al. Accurate and reproducible invasive breast cancer detection in whole-slide images: A Deep Learning approach for quantifying tumor extent. Sci Rep. 2017;7:46450:1–14. https://doi.org/10.1038/srep46450.
71. Djuric U, et al. Precision histology: how deep learning is poised to revitalize histomorphology for personalized cancer care. NPJ Precis Oncol. 2017;1(1):22.
72. Golatkar A, Anand D, Sethi A. Classification of breast cancer histology using deep learning. In International conference image analysis and recognition. 2018. Springer.
73. Kather JN, et al. Deep learning can predict microsatellite instability directly from histology in gastrointestinal cancer. Nat Med. 2019;25(7):1054–6.
74. Vandenberghe ME, et al. Relevance of deep learning to facilitate the diagnosis of HER2 status in breast cancer. Sci Rep. 2017;7:45938.
75. Wang D, et al. Deep learning for identifying metastatic breast cancer. arXiv preprint arXiv:1606.05718, 2016.
76. Cooper LA, et al. PanCancer insights from the cancer genome atlas: the pathologist's perspective. J Pathol. 2018;244(5):512–24.
77. Cruz-Roa A, et al. High-throughput adaptive sampling for whole-slide histopathology image analysis (HASHI) via convolutional neural networks: application to invasive breast cancer detection. PLoS One. 2018;13(5):e0196828.
78. Le H, et al. Utilizing automated breast cancer detection to identify spatial distributions of tumor infiltrating lymphocytes in invasive breast cancer. arXiv e-prints, 2019.
79. Aresta G, et al. BACH: grand challenge on breast cancer histology images. arXiv preprint arXiv:1808.04277, 2018.
80. Dong N, et al. Reinforced auto-zoom net: towards accurate and fast breast cancer segmentation in whole-slide images. In: Deep learning in medical image analysis and multimodal learning for clinical decision support. Cham: Springer; 2018. p. 317–25.
81. Donnem T, et al. Strategies for clinical implementation of TNM-immunoscore in resected nonsmall-cell lung cancer. Ann Oncol. 2016;27(2):225–32.
82. Galon J, et al. Cancer classification using the immunoscore: a worldwide task force. J Transl Med. 2012;10:205.
83. Hagos YB, Mérida AG, Teuwen J. Improving breast cancer detection using symmetry information with deep learning. Image analysis for moving organ, breast, and thoracic images. 2018. p. 90–7.
84. Huang H, et al. Cancer diagnosis by nuclear morphometry using spatial information. Pattern Recognit Lett. 2014;42:115–21. https://doi.org/10.1016/j.patrec.2014.02.008.
85. Kather JN, et al. Predicting survival from colorectal cancer histology slides using deep learning: a retrospective multicenter study. PLoS Med. 2019;16(1):e1002730.
86. Kather JN, et al. Topography of cancer-associated immune cells in human solid tumors. elife. 2018;7:e36967.
87. Kibbe W, Klemm J, Quackenbush J. Cancer informatics: new tools for a data-driven age in cancer research. Cancer Res. 2017;77(21):e1–2.
88. Kwak JT, et al. Multimodal microscopy for automated histologic analysis of prostate cancer. BMC Cancer. 2011;11:62.

89. Le H, et al. Pancreatic cancer detection in whole slide images using noisy label annotations. In: Medical Image Computing and Computer Assisted Intervention – MICCAI 2019. Cham: Springer Publishing. 2019, pp. 541–49. https://doi.org/10.1007/978-3-030-32239-7_60.
90. Lin H, et al. ScanNet: a fast and dense scanning framework for metastastic breast cancer detection from whole-slide image, in 2018 IEEE Winter Conference on Applications of Computer Vision (WACV). 2018. p. 539–546.
91. Litjens G, et al. 1399 H&E-stained sentinel lymph node sections of breast cancer patients: the CAMELYON dataset. GigaScience. 2018;7(6):giy065.
92. Liu Y, et al. Artificial intelligence-based breast cancer nodal metastasis detection. Arch Pathol Lab Med. 2019;143(7):859–68. https://doi.org/10.5858/arpa.2018-0147-OA. Epub 2018 Oct 8.
93. Luo X, et al. Comprehensive computational pathological image analysis predicts lung cancer prognosis. J Thorac Oncol. 2017;12(3):501–9.
94. Mobadersany P, et al. Predicting cancer outcomes from histology and genomics using convolutional networks. Proc Natl Acad Sci U S A. 2018;115(13):E2970–9.
95. Nawaz S, Yuan Y. Computational pathology: exploring the spatial dimension of tumor ecology. Cancer Lett. 2016;380(1):296–303.
96. Nazeri K, Aminpour A, Ebrahimi M. Two-stage convolutional neural network for breast cancer histology image classification. In international conference image analysis and recognition. 2018. Springer.
97. Ren J, et al. Recurrence analysis on prostate cancer patients with Gleason score 7 using integrated histopathology whole-slide images and genomic data through deep neural networks. J Med Imaging (Bellingham). 2018;5(4):047501.
98. Wang X, et al. Prediction of recurrence in early stage non-small cell lung cancer using computer extracted nuclear features from digital H&E images. Sci Rep. 2017;7(1):13543.
99. Abousamra S, et al. Learning from thresholds: fully automated classification of tumor infiltrating lymphocytes for multiple cancer types. arXiv e-prints, 2019.
100. Achi HE, et al. Automated diagnosis of lymphoma with digital pathology images using deep learning. Ann Clin Lab Sci. 2019;49(2):153–60.
101. Albarqouni S, et al. AggNet: deep learning from crowds for mitosis detection in breast cancer histology images. IEEE Trans Med Imaging. 2016;35(5):1313–21.
102. Bejnordi BE, et al. Diagnostic assessment of deep learning algorithms for detection of lymph node metastases in women with breast cancer. JAMA. 2017;318(22):2199–210.
103. Buitrago PA, Nystrom NA, Gupta R, Saltz J. Delivering scalable deep learning to research with bridges-AI. In: Crespo-Mariño J, Meneses-Rojas E. (eds) High Performance Computing. CARLA 2019. Communications in Computer and Information Science. Springer, Cham. 2020;1087. https://doi.org/10.1007/978-3-030-41005-6_14.
104. He K, Zhang X, Ren S and Sun J, Deep Residual Learning for Image Recognition. 2016 IEEE Conference on Computer Vision and Pattern Recognition (CVPR). 2016;770–78, https://doi.org/10.1109/CVPR.2016.90.
105. Khosravi P, et al. Deep convolutional neural networks enable discrimination of heterogeneous digital pathology images. EBioMedicine. 2018;27:317–28.
106. Korbar B, et al. Deep learning for classification of colorectal polyps on whole-slide images. J Pathol Inform. 2017;8:30.
107. Linder N, et al. Deep learning for detecting tumour-infiltrating lymphocytes in testicular germ cell tumours. J Clin Pathol. 2019;72(2):157–64.
108. Hagos YB, Merida AG, Teuwen J. Image Analysis for Moving Organ, Breast, and Thoracic Images. Springer; Cham, Switzerland: Improving breast cancer detection using symmetry information with deep learning. 2018:90–7.
109. Moeskops P, Wolterink JM, van der Velden BHM, Gilhuijs KGA, Leiner T, Viergever MA, and Išgum I. Deep learning for multi-task medical image segmentation in multiple modalities. In Unal G, Ourselin S, Joskowicz L, Sabuncu MR, Wells W (Eds.), Medical Image Computing and Computer-Assisted Intervention - MICCAI 2016 - 19th International Conference, Proceedings. (Lecture Notes in Computer Science (including subseries Lecture Notes in Artificial Intelligence and Lecture Notes in Bioinformatics)). Istanbul, Turkey. Springer Verlag. 2016;9901 LNCS:478–86). https://doi.org/10.1007/978-3-319-46723-8_55.

110. Nirschl JJ, et al. A deep-learning classifier identifies patients with clinical heart failure using whole-slide images of H&E tissue. PLoS One. 2018;13:e0192726.
111. Radford A, Metz L, Chintala S. Unsupervised representation learning with deep convolutional generative adversarial networks. 2016.
112. Senaras C, et al. DeepFocus: detection of out-of-focus regions in whole slide digital images using deep learning. PLoS One. 2018;13(10):e0205387.
113. Webb S. Deep learning for biology. Nature. 2018;554(7693):555–7.
114. Koelzer VH, et al. Precision immunoprofiling by image analysis and artificial intelligence. Virchows Arch. 2019;474(4):511–22.
115. Qaiser T, Tsang Y-W, Taniyama D, Sakamoto N, Nakane K, Epstein D, Rajpoot N. Fast and accurate tumor segmentation of histology images using persistent homology and deep convolutional features. Med Image Anal. 2019;55:1–14. https://doi.org/10.1016/j.media.2019.03.014.
116. Sirinukunwattana K, et al. Gland segmentation in colon histology images: the glas challenge contest. Med Image Anal. 2017;35:489–502.
117. Sirinukunwattana K, et al. Locality sensitive deep learning for detection and classification of nuclei in routine colon cancer histology images. Med Imag. 2016;35:1196–206.
118. Sirinukunwattana K, Snead DR, Rajpoot NM. A stochastic polygons model for glandular structures in Colon histology images. IEEE Trans Med Imaging. 2015;34(11):2366–78.
119. Snead DRJ, et al. Validation of digital pathology imaging for primary histopathological diagnosis. Histopathology. 2016;68(7):1063–72.
120. Veta M, et al. Assessment of algorithms for mitosis detection in breast cancer histopathology images. Med Image Anal. 2015;20(1):237–48.
121. Cancer Genome Atlas Network. Comprehensive molecular characterization of human colon and rectal cancer. Nature. 2012;487(7407):330.
122. Cancer Genome Atlas Research Network. Comprehensive molecular characterization of gastric adenocarcinoma. Nature. 2014;513(7517):202.
123. Thorsson V, et al. The immune landscape of cancer. Immunity. 2018;48(4):812.
124. Saltz J, et al. Spatial organization and molecular correlation of tumor-infiltrating lymphocytes using deep learning on pathology images. Cell Rep. 2018;23(1):181.
125. Althobiti M, et al. Heterogeneity of tumour-infiltrating lymphocytes in breast cancer and its prognostic significance. Histopathology. 2018;73(6):887–96.
126. Hendry S, et al. Assessing tumor-infiltrating lymphocytes in solid tumors: a practical review for pathologists and proposal for a standardized method from the international immuno-oncology biomarkers working group: part 2: TILS in melanoma, gastrointestinal tract carcinomas, non-small cell lung carcinoma and mesothelioma, endometrial and ovarian carcinomas, squamous cell carcinoma of the head and neck, genitourinary carcinomas, and primary brain tumors. Adv Anat Pathol. 2017;24(6):311–35.
127. Salgado R, et al. The evaluation of tumor-infiltrating lymphocytes (TILs) in breast cancer: recommendations by an international TILs working group 2014. Ann Oncol. 2015;26(2):259–71.
128. Savas P, et al. Clinical relevance of host immunity in breast cancer: from TILs to the clinic. Nat Rev Clin Oncol. 2016;13(4):228.
129. FDA allows marketing of first whole slide imaging system for digital pathology. https://www.fda.gov/news-events/press-announcements/fda-allows-marketing-first-whole-slide-imaging-system-digital-pathology, 2017.

Whole Slide Imaging Hardware, Software, and Infrastructure

David S. McClintock, Jacob T. Abel, and Toby C. Cornish

Introduction

Imagine the following scenario:

> You are a pathologist. You arrive at your desk in the morning, hot cup of coffee in hand, ready to start the day's sign out. You login to your computer; dual 32-inch, 6K displays light up the room. You fire up your digital pathology image management system and review your worklist, cases automatically triaged by priority. You open the first case, a new biopsy, and review the preselected regions of interest on the digital H&E stained slides. You are prompted to review the associated digital IHC stains and confirm your diagnosis. You review the prefilled synoptic report, make a couple of edits, run a final quality check, and then sign out the case. Five minutes have passed – you take a sip of your (still) hot coffee and move on to the next case.

This scenario demonstrates a fully digital sign-out workflow, augmented by expert-driven software and optimized for pathologist efficiency. Unfortunately, it does not reflect current workflows available for pathologists (circa 2020–2021) but instead denotes the future potential for improving both the quality and performance of one's typical anatomical pathology (AP) practice.

So how do we get here? What is needed in order to achieve this vision, one that not only makes life easier for pathologists but also, most importantly, improves diagnostic accuracy, quality, and turnaround time for patients? To start, none of this is possible without having a completely digital workflow, one where practically every glass slide is digitized and made available for machine learning (ML)

D. S. McClintock (✉) · J. T. Abel
University of Michigan, Department of Pathology, Ann Arbor, MI, USA
e-mail: dsmcclin@umich.edu; jtabel@umich.edu

T. C. Cornish
University of Colorado School of Medicine, Department of Pathology, Aurora, CO, USA
e-mail: toby.cornish@cuanschutz.edu

A. V. Parwani (ed.), *Whole Slide Imaging*,
https://doi.org/10.1007/978-3-030-83332-9_2

and artificial intelligence (AI) algorithms. These tools, created by pathology experts, will be integrated within and drive the clinical workflow, including case triage, ordering additional stains, recommending additional testing (e.g., molecular/genomics), highlighting and annotating diagnostically important regions of interest, quantifying histopathologic features (e.g., mitoses, necrosis, tumor volume), integrating pertinent clinical information (prior cancer history, other lab values, radiology features, etc.), and finally, creating a standardized, enhanced report for both clinicians and patients.

Digital pathology (DP) is defined by the Digital Pathology Association as "a blanket term that encompasses tools and systems to digitize pathology slides and associated meta-data, their storage, review, analysis, and enabling infrastructure" [1]. At the heart of digital pathology is whole slide imaging (WSI), an innovative technology that scans a standard histologic glass slide and generates a high magnification "whole slide" image. While WSI devices have been around for over 20 years [2–4], only in the past 5 years have conditions been met to more seamlessly integrate them within the AP laboratory's clinical workflow [5–10]. Much like how a pathologist cannot simply purchase a microscope and start signing out cases, the same is true of the transition to digital pathology – acquiring a WSI device does not immediately enable a digital workflow. Instead, one must understand the underlying technology, hardware, and software options, in addition to the information technology (IT) infrastructure required, to successfully implement whole slide imaging systems.

Whole Slide Imaging Technology

Whole Slide Imaging Fundamentals

Whole slide imaging is the process of creating a single high-resolution digital image from a glass slide. The devices that digitize glass slides into WSIs have been generally referred to as "slide scanners," "virtual microscopes," and/or "whole slide imaging devices" over the past 20 years [11–13]. Slide scanners evolved from home-brewed motorized microscopes that began to appear in research laboratories in the 1990s. The first commercially available whole slide imaging device, the Bacus Labs' BLISS, was essentially a fully motorized Olympus BX-51 upright microscope equipped with a CCD camera and custom software designed for acquiring a series of high power fields and stitching them together [14]. The BLISS was developed in the mid-1990s and was available commercially later in that decade. While today's slide scanners still have much in common with the BLISS, they have evolved over the past 20-plus years into purpose-built instruments to address a range of clinical, research, education, quality, and industry use cases [3, 4, 15–18].

While the actual scanning of slides was the initial focus of whole slide imaging, this has transitioned over the years to its software, image management system, and the whole slide image itself. In fact, similar to how the telecommunications and the internet can be represented by the abstraction layers of the Open Systems Interconnection (OSI) model [19, 20], from the physical layer to the application layer, whole slide imaging can be represented by its own layered model. In the WSI layer model (Fig. 1), the hardware, represented by the slide scanner and its constitutive elements, is at the base, with software elements, including the whole slide image itself and the image management system, comprising the upper half of the model. Over time, the emphasis in digital pathology will shift primarily from foundational WSI hardware to application and system integration, interoperability, and usability.

A whole slide image, once created, serves as a virtual image object that can be interpreted and viewed using specialized software (commonly called a "viewer," more on this below). Overall the goal is to allow the pathologist to view a whole slide image in a similar manner as one would view a physical microscope slide. WSIs are typically stored as sets of smaller images, commonly referred to as tiles [12, 21]. Each tile is composed of a two-dimensional series of pixels, or "picture elements," which are the most granular component of any digital image. A high-definition computer monitor or television can display images that are 1920 × 1080 pixels, or two million pixels in total. By comparison, a single WSI scanned at an equivalent magnification of 40× contains pixels numbering in the billions, making

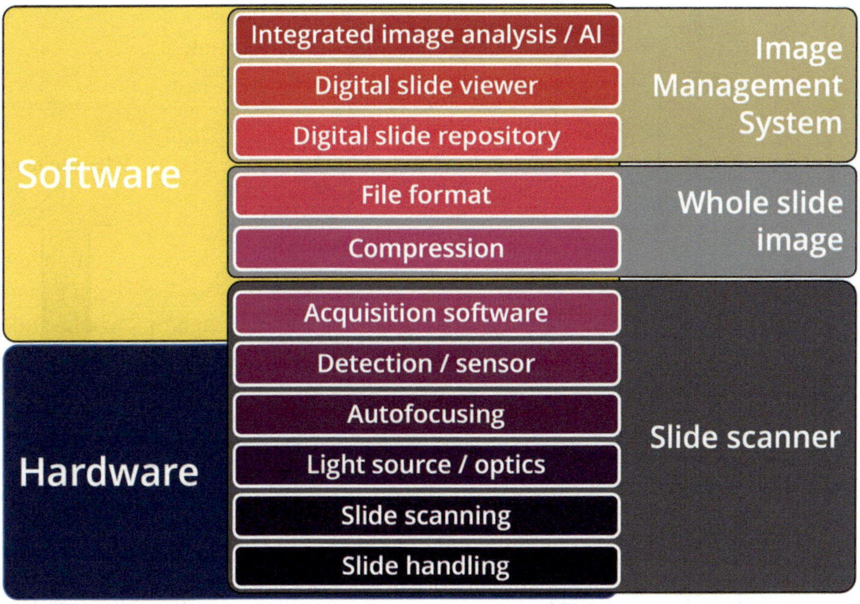

Fig. 1 WSI layer model. This model of WSI technology was inspired by the Open Systems Interconnection (OSI) model of computing. The WSI layer model organizes the components of a WSI system from the lowest (physical) layers through intermediate software and finally the highest (application) layers with which users will interact. The model also classifies the layers as hardware and software (on the left) and organizes the layers into system components (on the right)

it impractical to load and view a WSI as a single, static image due to human, hardware, and network limitations [22]. To overcome these limitations, WSI file formats were developed in order to simulate the viewing of whole slide images like that of a physical slide.

WSI File Format

WSI files are written to permanent storage (such as hard disks) in specific file formats. Unfortunately, due to a lack of standardization by vendors, a wide variety of different WSI file formats exist, and these are frequently proprietary formats. Most, but not all, of the vendor formats are based around the "tiled pyramid" paradigm. In the "tiled pyramid" approach, the WSI file contains the base image layer (the full resolution scan) as well as a number of pre-calculated zoom levels which are typically scaled by a factor of 1/4 or 1/2 at each level (Fig. 2) [22–24]. The number of zoom levels present in this type of WSI file varies as it depends on the size of the base level image and the scaling between levels. While at first glance this arrangement may appear wasteful, the additional levels typically increase the file size by less than 25% while significantly improving retrieval speed. In part, this is because each of the levels is further partitioned into tiles of equal size (commonly around

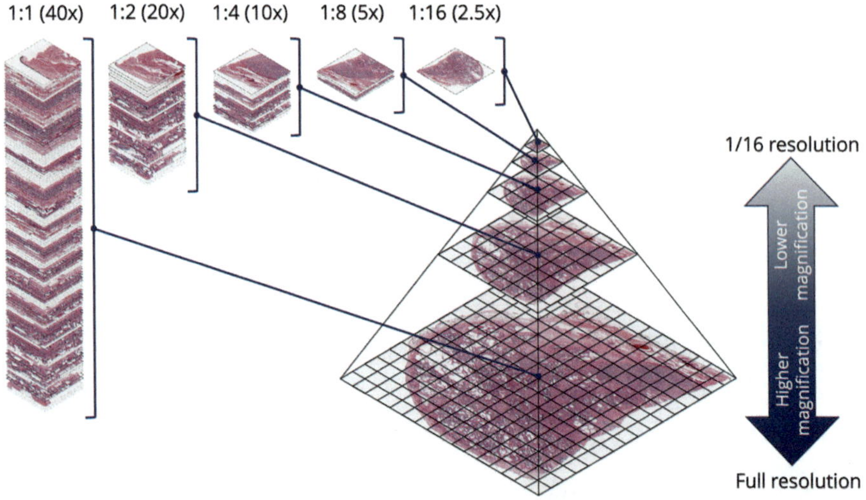

Fig. 2 WSI pyramid. Whole slide images are typically represented in a pyramid structure with each level in the pyramid representing a different pre-calculated zoom level. The base level represents the full resolution image. Moving up the pyramid, each subsequent layer is digitally subsampled to create a lower magnification view, ending at the lowest magnification image at the apex of the pyramid. Note that each layer is a ratio of the original resolution (shown here as a factor of 2) and approximately equivalent to a specific magnification (not shown to scale). Each level is further divided into small tiles of a fixed size (not shown to scale). Since the tiles are of a fixed size, the base level is composed of the largest number of tiles, with each subsequent level being composed of fewer and fewer tiles as illustrated

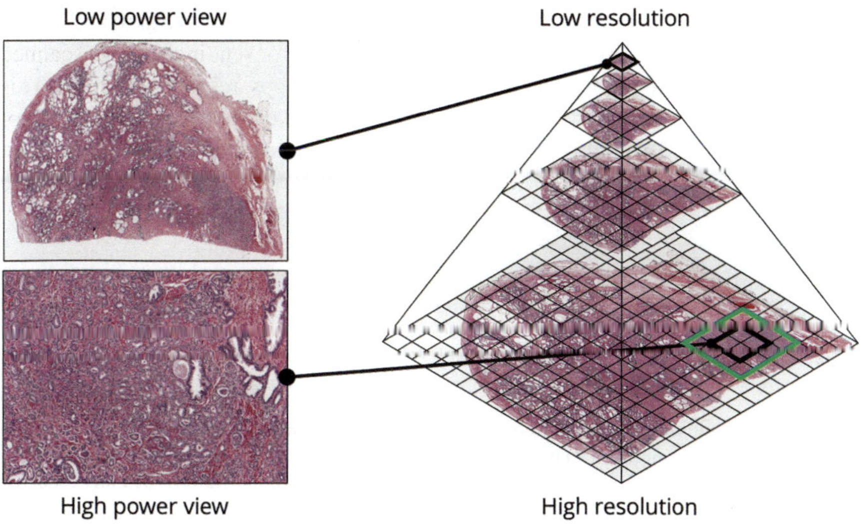

Fig. 3 WSI fields of view represent specific areas in the WSI pyramid. At the apex of the WSI pyramid, the lowest resolution tile(s) are sent to the WSI viewer and represent the microscopic equivalent of low power views (top). Similarly, to get a high power view, only the specific high-resolution tiles of the requested field of view are sent to the WSI viewer (black diamond). Note that some WSI viewers, in anticipation of where a pathologist will look next, may pre-fetch tiles adjacent to the desired field of view (green diamond) in order to provide a more seamless viewing experience

256 × 256 pixels). This allows a WSI viewer to retrieve only those tiles that are actively being displayed to the user from the most appropriate level in the pyramid (Fig. 3). These two factors permit fast and dynamic interaction with WSIs while minimizing the amount of image data transferred across the network. Delivery of image tiles inadvertently led to the "pixelation" phenomenon that plagued early WSI systems. This occurs when navigating a WSI on an underpowered computer or slow network connection, where "blocky" low power WSI tiles persist while higher power data slowly fills in the image (Fig. 4) [25, 26]. Fortunately, with modern networks, servers, computers, and WSI viewers, this issue has largely been mitigated, with state-of-the-art viewers providing extremely fluid and seamless performance.

In order to optimize storage needs, almost all WSI files are compressed to some degree, reducing the amount of data being stored or transmitted. In general, there are two forms of compression, lossless and lossy. Lossy compression involves an irreversible removal of data (in the case of whole slide imaging, this is usually pixels or color data) from the WSI file [27]. In contrast, lossless compression retains all the original data elements in some form, and the file is able to be reverted into its original state. While one would think that lossless compression would always be preferred, the degree of compression possible with lossless methods is limited. Some examples of compression methods used for WSI files include lossy methods such as JPEG and JPEG2000, as well as lossless methods such as Lempel-Ziv-Welch (LZW) [28]. The former methods make use of subsampling, while the latter

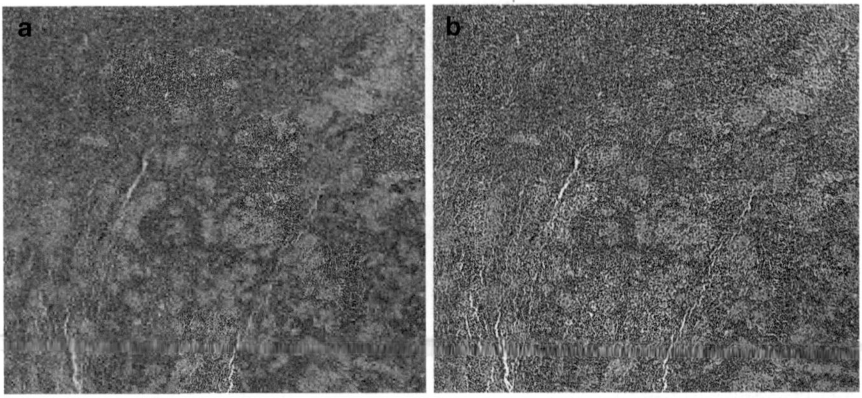

Fig. 4 Whole slide imaging loading artifact. (**a**) Zooming from low to high power using an underpowered computer or network may result in individual image tiles to appear pixelated or blurry while the data for that field of view is transmitted from the WSI to the viewer. (**b**) Fully rendered field of view with all high power tiles loaded

encodes the same data in a more efficient manner [27]. The performance of a compression process is usually reported as a ratio, where a typical result using JPEG compression is 1:15–1:20 and JPEG2000 compression would be 1:30–1:50 (i.e., the compressed WSI is 1/30th to 1/50th the size of the original raw file) [22].

The majority of WSI file formats are based on the TIFF or Tagged Image File Format. TIFF is an open file format that was originally developed to store scanned multipage documents by the Aldus Corporation (later bought by Adobe Systems) [29]. TIFF as a format for WSIs was popularized by Aperio, who used it for their SVS file (see below). Several characteristics of the TIFF format made it attractive for WSIs. The first is that it is one of the few image file formats that supports the storage of multiple images (called pages) within a single container. For a WSI, these pages store levels in the image pyramid, as well as metadata such as the label image, thumbnail, and macro images. Pages can also be used to represent z-level images and fluorescence channels. TIFF is also very attractive because of its flexibility. It supports custom metadata ("tags") as well as a variety of color spaces, bit depths/data types, and compression schemes. TIFF also permits images to be stored in a tiled format, which is key to both storing and retrieving WSIs. Notably, the original TIFF format was designed around 32-bit integers, which created a size limit of 4 GB. To overcome this limitation, WSI files larger than 4 GB use the BigTIFF file format which uses 64-bit integer offsets. BigTIFF arose to accommodate WSIs and a number of people contributed to the format, foremost of whom was Ole Eichhorn while he was at Aperio [30].

The Leica Aperio SVS file was the first TIFF-based WSI format and remains the best exemplar of this type. Because it was an early, widespread and openly documented file format, SVS has become a de facto standard for WSIs, with many smaller vendors targeting this format to achieve interoperability. The SVS format contains a number of custom TIFF tags as well as a specific order and relationship between the pages that represent the WSI pyramid and the optional label image, macro image, and thumbnail. SVS supports standard TIFF compression schemes (none, LZV, and JPEG) as well as JPEG2000, which is nonstandard. In contrast, two of the file formats used by Hamamatsu scanners (.vms and. vmu) are actually directories of multiple image files along with an index file that outlines their mapping to the overall WSI. The .vms format stores the image data as JPEGs, while the.vmu file uses a nonstandard file format [31]. Another directory-based file format, Deep Zoom Images (DZI), was created as a general purpose large image format by Seadragon Software, which was later purchased by Microsoft and is no longer supported as of October 2021 [32]. In the DZI format, tiles exist as separate images (typically JPEGS) and are organized in one directory per level. DZI is popular for use with the open-source, web-based OpenSeadragon viewer [33], but managing tens of thousands of files per WSI can be challenging.

For most users, extensive knowledge of the finer points of WSI file formats is not necessary. However, it is important to recognize the larger differences between the various formats. This becomes critical when discussing storage of the WSI files, as well as when selecting any viewing, image management, interfacing, or image analysis software. While first and third-party software is available to convert between some formats, this is not always the case. These factors have impeded cross-compatibility and system interoperability over time and are only recently beginning to be overcome (see "DICOM" section). This introduces an additional layer of complexity when constructing or utilizing large databases of WSI files from multiple scanners, multiple institutions, or over long time periods.

DICOM in Whole Slide Imaging

DICOM (Digital Imaging and Communications in Medicine) is the fundamental and universal standard for digital medical imaging [34]. At its base DICOM is a communication standard, facilitating image interchange through extensive use of image metadata while at the same time not mandating internal image formats. DICOM also addresses imaging workflow by uniquely identifying information as objects, with information objects defined for images, patients, studies, reports, fiducials, etc. Once an image object is defined within the standard, it can be acted upon by DICOM-compliant devices and information systems, allowing a wide range of programmed workflows.

In the mid-2000s, the DICOM Working Group 26 (WG-26) was charged with supporting and developing the use of DICOM in the pathology domain, and considerable progress has been made in supporting pathology images, including WSIs [34, 35]. To this end, WG-26 has authored two supplements to the DICOM standard that relate to WSI, Supplement 122 in 2008 and Supplement 145 in 2010. Supplement 122 added new information objects, concepts, and relationships within DICOM to support pathology workflows, e.g., the concept of a specimen, the concept of a container, and the relationship that an image can be acquired from a specimen that itself came from a container, which can give rise to additional specimens. Supplement 145 described the information object model for WSIs, including its pyramidal representation where high-resolution images at the base are digitally subsampled to create lower resolution images moving up towards the apex.

More recently, WG-26 has coordinated with hardware and software vendors to demonstrate interoperability in a series of Digital Pathology Connectathons within the United States and Japan [36]. While DICOM promises a standards-driven future in pathology imaging, its clinical use in pathology is still limited. At the time of this writing, no FDA-cleared digital pathology systems actually employ it natively [37]; however, at least one high-throughput WSI device (Leica Aperio GT 450 DX) outputs DICOM natively [38] and has been cleared for diagnostic use (CE IVD) in both Asia and Europe [39, 40].

Whole Slide Imaging Systems: Hardware

Whole Slide Imaging Devices

Over the years, multiple types of WSI devices have been developed, with devices distinguished by the following major features: 1) slide capacity, 2) slide loading and handling, 3) slide format, 4) magnification and spatial resolution, 5) scanning and focus strategy, 6) scanning speed, and 7) imaging modalities supported [28, 41]. Currently, most scanners support or have optimized some of these features within a single device; however, no one device has been made that can "do it all." For example, a high-throughput scanner may have fast scanning speeds and excellent autofocusing, but may only support bright-field microscopy on traditional 1″ × 3″ slides at a single magnification. In this section, the pertinent technical parameters surrounding WSI device use will be discussed.

Slide Capacity

Early slide scanners, like the aforementioned Bacus Labs' BLISS, had a capacity of only one slide. While this sufficed for low-throughput use cases (e.g., image analysis of tissue microarray slides), companies quickly realized that increased slide capacity, in the order of hundreds of slides per batch, was needed to support a variety of digital pathology use cases. Currently, WSI devices can be purchased that support anywhere from 1 to 1000 slides per batch, although these typically follow a bimodal distribution, favoring low- and high-capacity devices.

On the low end of capacity, current major WSI devices support between 1 and 20 slides. These scanners are made primarily for small pathology practices, specific low volume use cases (e.g., frozen sections, telepathology, research, education), or for those looking to ease into digital pathology with a lower cost solution. In general, these devices do not produce the fastest scans; however, they offer a wider range of options, such as magnification scanned, manual focus adjustments, multiple image modalities supported, etc., as compared to higher capacity devices. These scanners also typically support both automatic and manual scans, the latter allowing users to fine-tune and adjust scanning options (e.g., tissue detection, field of view, focal points, etc.) in order to achieve the best scan possible.

On the high end of capacity, current major WSI devices support between 100 and 1000 slides, with most having maximum capacities ranging between 100 and 400 slides. These scanners are primarily aimed towards large pathology practices, industry, large-scale research/slide scanning services, and other use cases that require large-scale scanning. Of all of the WSI devices available, these have the fastest speeds, although most typically allow only a single image modality (bright-field microscopy) and magnification option per batch (40× equivalent). Unlike their low-capacity cousins, high-capacity WSI devices operate best in automatic scanning mode, with some devices only supporting automated scanning (no manual mode available).

Of note, high-capacity WSI devices, on average, have large footprints and, at the time of this writing, do not support parallel scanning, where multiple slides can be scanned concurrently in a single device. This leads to many practices purchasing much more scanning capacity than is needed to support their daily workload. For example, if one's anatomic pathology lab workflow requires 6 scanners to complete a daily workload of 1000 slides and each scanner can hold 450 slides, an excess capacity of 1700 slides has been created. Not counting the unnecessary upfront capital costs, the excess capacity created by a lack of parallel scanning results in increased physical lab space, electricity/utilities, and full-time equivalent (FTE) workers needed to support loading and unloading the extra scanners. Therefore, before purchasing WSI devices, the effects of redesigning anatomic pathology laboratory workflows to better support and optimize digital pathology should be considered [42].

Slide Loading and Handling

A key feature that differentiates slide scanners is the method of loading slides. Slide loading can be broadly divided into two methods: slide trays and slide cassettes (or magazines). The choice of slide loading method dictates the slide formats that can be scanned, the work required to load and unload a batch of slides, and aspects of downstream slide handling in the device. It follows therefore that the slide loading mechanism significantly impacts its appropriateness for a given use case.

Slide Trays

The concept of slide trays originated with motorized microscope stages, some of which featured removable multislide "trays." Slide trays are typically flat pieces of machined aluminum possessing recessed areas slightly larger than the glass slides they contain (Fig. 5a). The slides may be held in place using a clip, spring tension, or just gravity. Slide trays, unlike some slide cassettes, are not interchangeable between vendors or with histology equipment.

Slide trays have a number or advantages when compared to slide cassettes. The most notable advantage is that they are inherently a more flexible format than cassettes. Because the internal arrangement of slides in a tray can be altered while maintaining the outside dimensions of the tray, different slide trays can be designed to accommodate varying numbers and sizes of slides. Thus slide trays permit large format glass slides such as traditional whole mount slides (2″ × 3″) or larger in addition to standard 1″ × 3″ slides (Fig. 5c).

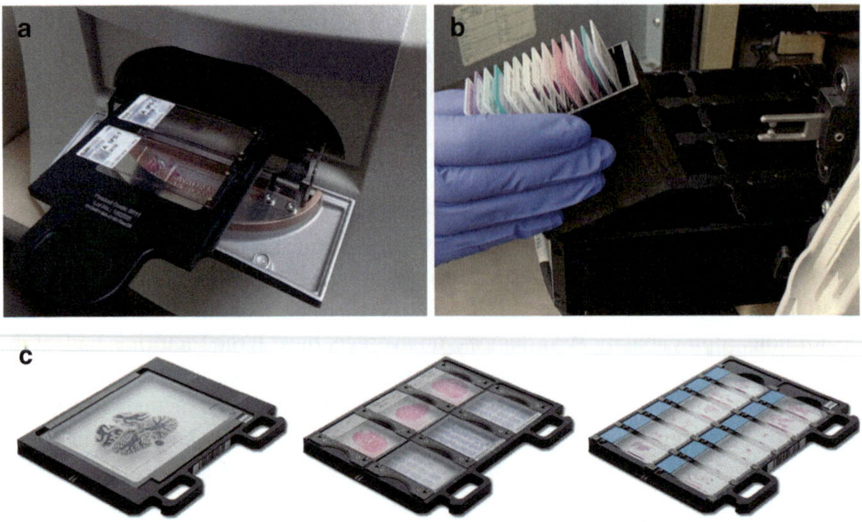

Fig. 5 Slide trays and cassettes used for whole slide imaging. Broadly speaking, WSI scanners are loaded using either slide trays or cassettes. (**a**) Example of a four-position slide tray being loaded into a desktop slide scanner. One advantage of slide trays is that the slides never leave the tray, which serves essentially as a microscope stage during the imaging process. (**b**) Example of a slide cassette being loaded into a high-capacity scanner. An advantage for using slide cassettes is the ability to load many hundreds of slides into a single WSI device. (**c**) Slide trays offer a range of slide formats. Here, interchangeable slide trays allow the same slide scanner to scan either twelve 1″ × 3″ slides (left), six 2″ × 3″ slides (middle), or one 6″ × 8″ slide (right) depending on the tray used (images in (**c**) courtesy of Huron Digital Pathology, used with permission)

Slide trays also benefit from their simplicity. The tray itself acts in a manner analogous to a microscope stage with the slides remaining in the tray at all times and the entire tray being translated under the objective. This significantly reduces the complexity of the scanner and the likelihood of dropped slides, broken slides, and mechanical failure. Slide trays are also more tolerant of imperfections, such as slides with overhanging labels, crooked coverslips, and even wet cytoseal (i.e., "goopy" frozen section slides). Some scanners with slide trays may even tolerate double thick slides, including those that were broken and subsequently glued back together.

Slide trays have a number of potential disadvantages as well. Trays have a lower slide density than cassettes, which usually translates to lower capacity scanners. Although there have been exceptions, most scanners that use slide trays accept only one tray at a time. The capacity of these trays ranges from 1 to 20 slides, and a capacity of 2 to 6 slides is most commonly seen. Loading and unloading of slide trays is also a slower process compared to loading and unloading most slide cassettes, which can translate to more FTEs needed in the lab.

Slide Cassettes

Slide cassettes evolved from early stand-alone slide autoloaders ("slide hotels") that held large numbers of slides and were capable of feeding these slides to motorized stages mounted on traditional microscopes. While slide hotels are still in use (primarily in research labs), modern slide scanners have integrated their slide storage and most have adopted slide cassettes for this purpose. Slide cassettes, also called magazines, racks, or baskets, are designed to hold between 10 and 40 slides each, and multiple cassettes are loaded into a scanner to achieve capacities of 100 to 1000 slides (Fig. 5b).

Slide handling within a slide scanner is more complex with cassettes than with slide trays because the slides must be removed from the cassette and placed on a separate stage before the slide can be imaged. At a minimum, the slide must be moved at least 3 inches to clear the magazine, but the actual distance and path traveled during imaging vary considerably among the various designs on the market. Depending on the design of the slide path, the time it takes to move the slide from the cassette to the stage may actually be quite significant in relation to the scan time, reducing the effective throughput of a slide scanner. To eliminate the impact of the slide path on scanner throughput, some vendors have gone to great lengths to minimize the distance a slide travels, while others have implemented mechanisms that eliminate the contribution of this distance. One approach is to physically queue a slide in a location adjacent to the stage. Keeping a slide "on deck" allows slides to be moved in and out of slide cassettes while the slide on the stage is being scanned. It also allows the scanner to perform macro imaging and apply tissue detection and other pre-processing to the "on deck" slide.

The design of the slide cassette itself has changed considerably over time. Early slide cassettes were engineered specifically for use in slide scanners, but these proprietary designs have been gradually replaced by cassette formats already in wide use for hand staining, autostaining, and autocoverslipping of slides. This move has significantly reduced the cost of the cassettes, but more importantly, it has created the opportunity for directly transferring slides from automatic coverslippers to the slide scanner without needing to handle slides individually.

Slide Format

As mentioned previously, the way in which a scanner loads and handles slides is one of the major determinants of its slide format compatibility. Slide format, as used here, denotes the physical dimensions of the slide being scanned. The most widely used slide format available (and the vast majority of the slides produced in most labs) is the traditional 1″ × 3″ (25 mm × 77 mm) slide. As expected, every WSI device available supports this slide format. Other than the traditional slide format, a double slide, "whole mount," or 2″ × 3″ (51 mm × 77 mm) format, is the second most common format and is supported by select WSI devices. This double slide format can be found in both cassette and tray-based loading configurations;

however, in the case of the former, the cassettes are specially modified to support the larger slide size. Lately, double slide formats have gained popularity within prostate and genitourinary pathology given the additional information provided by the larger slides [43, 44].

Large format slides, here defined as any slide larger than the 2″ × 3″ double slide format, severely limit the number of potential scanners available for use. Due to the large slide size, these scanners require either a tray-based slide loading and handling system or a mounted camera on a microscope with a robotic stage in order to be able to capture slides up to 6″ × 8″ (152 mm × 203 mm). While these scanners were primarily marketed for research applications early on, histology technology has improved [45] and the clinical utility of using large format slides for cancer diagnosis is now pushing clinical laboratories to better support them [46, 47].

Magnification and Spatial Resolution

The light path in WSI devices mirrors that found in traditional light microscopes. Light originates in a lamp (now typically an LED source) and passes through the condenser lens, through the sample (glass slide), and into the objective. The objective is composed of a variable number of high-quality lenses and has a defined numerical aperture that, in combination, contributes a known amount of magnification (e.g., 2×, 4×, 10×, 20×, 40×, etc.) and resolving power (ability to discern fine details), respectively. In a traditional microscope, the light then travels to the eyepiece which contributes additional magnification, in most cases 10×. Thus when one views a slide using a 20× objective, the image is in fact being observed at 200× total magnification.

In WSI devices, however, the 10× microscope eyepieces are replaced by a digital image sensor with micrometer-scale pixels. Here, the post-objective light path may vary considerably, and the additional lenses used in the scanner must be carefully matched to the pixel size of the charge-coupled device (CCD) or complementary metal oxide semiconductor (CMOS) camera chip/sensor. The relationship between the size of the image projected onto the sensor and the size of the sensor's wells that collect light at each pixel determines the spatial resolution of the WSI device [48]. For example, if a WSI device with a 5 μm CCD sensor scans a slide with histopathologic features 1 μm apart, the image projected onto the sensor does not have enough optical resolution for the features to be digitally distinguishable. However, if that image is magnified by a 20× objective prior to hitting the sensor, the features are now 20 μm apart and can thus be accurately captured and resolved by the 5 μm sensor. While the reality of this situation is more complex, in principle one can improve the spatial resolution of the images produced by the slide scanner by either increasing the magnification of the objective or decreasing the pixel size of the camera sensor [48].

With WSIs, spatial resolution is customarily expressed in micrometers per pixel (μm/pixel or mpp), which for the current generation of WSI devices is approximately 0.5 mpp for 20× equivalent magnification scans and 0.25 mpp for 40× equivalent magnification scans. Given that each WSI device typically uses a different combination of light sources, lenses, objectives, and camera sensors, WSI spatial resolution may differ from instrument to instrument even if they use the exact same objective. For this reason, when describing the magnification of WSIs, it is best to use the term "equivalent" and include the number of micrometers per pixel as there is no universal standard for 20× or 40× magnification [48].

Scanning and Focus Strategy

While traditional microscopes have a full set of objectives, most whole slide imaging devices only have a single objective, typically either of 20× or 40× magnification. As mentioned above, certain WSI devices use a doubling lens that allows the use of a lower magnification objective to achieve greater spatial resolution images and higher equivalent magnifications (e.g., up to 80×) without sacrificing scanning speed. Of note, the typical scanning objective has gone through some interesting modifications in the past. For example, the first WSI vendor to create a sub-one-minute WSI device in the mid-2000s developed a custom 80-objective lens that could scan an entire slide in a single pass [49, 50].

When scanning glass slides, there are two main approaches for creating WSIs: tile scanning and line, or linear array, scanning (Fig. 6). In tile scanning, the WSI device scans the slide as a series of rectangular overlapping tiles in a raster pattern until the slide has completed scanning (Fig. 6a). Depending on the scanning device, the tiles are assembled into a WSI either concurrently or after scanning is finished. In line scanning, the WSI devices scan the slide as a series of long, narrow overlapping strips, advancing laterally across the slide in this fashion until the slide has completed scanning (Fig. 6b). As with tile scanning, the strips can be assembled into a WSI either concurrently or after the scanning is finished. In both tile and line scanning, the resulting images (tiles or strips) are stitched together into a single large image, i.e., the whole slide image, by the WSI device acquisition software.

So why are there two primary approaches to scanning slides? Why not just one? To start, it is important to remember that whole slide imaging is a new technology as compared to the microscope. The first patents for WSI devices were awarded for tile-based scanning (Bacus Laboratories, 2000 & 2001), followed soon after by

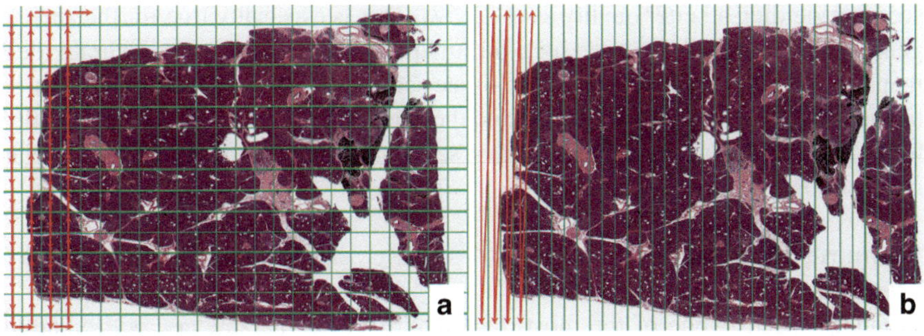

Fig. 6 Approaches to slide scanning. There are two primary slide scanning approaches, tiling and linear array (line scanning). (**a**) The red arrows demonstrate a typical tiling approach, where each green square represents a single tile captured. (**b**) The red arrows demonstrate a typical line scanning approach, where each long green rectangle represents a line captured

linear array scanning (Aperio Technologies, 2004) [51]. Between 2001 and 2013, there were 293 patents granted for digital pathology, with different companies investing significantly in DP and pursuing different technological approaches [51]. Innovation continues to this day for WSI, including new scanners, acquisition methods, focusing strategies, etc., as evidenced by the continuous annual release of new WSI hardware and/or software.

One of the primary reasons whole slide imaging as a technology has been successful is because the scanning process produces an image from three-dimensional tissue sections that, in general, is mostly in focus. The way in which a WSI device adjusts focal planes during image acquisition is directly related to the scanning approach. Both tiling and line scanning utilize image-based autofocusing techniques, either by moving the objective lens the proper distance to and from the tissue section to achieve focus or by moving the stage position in the z-direction (perpendicular to the slide) [52]. In an ideal state, the WSI device would adjust focus continuously for every tile present on the slide. However, while that would definitely produce a high quality in focus slide, it would also take significantly longer than the current standard of <1 minute per slide.

Instead, WSI devices employ autofocus strategies that sample the slide in order to maximize scanning speed without sacrificing overall focus quality [52]. For tile-based scanning, focal points are selected with the assumption that the immediate tiles surrounding the focal point are within the same focal plane, whereas for line scanning, only a few focal points are chosen with the assumption that focus will not vary much along the strip itself. Unfortunately, these assumptions are not always true, leading to some slides having major areas out of focus due to significant topographical changes in the tissue section. While one typically can rescan the slide, manually choosing more focal points to account for these three-dimensional changes with low-volume scanners, this is not practical, or even possible, for some high-volume scanners. For this reason, autofocus strategies are a prime area of research and development for decreasing scan speed and increasing scan quality [53–56]. Further, efforts to improve tissue preparation and to minimize tissue thickness for glass slides can also help with focusing issues, with thinner, more consistent tissue sections yielding a better quality scan [2, 57]. This is especially true for the current generation of clinically focused high-throughput scanners. Only with accurate focal maps reflecting the topography of the tissue section, along with better coordination between software, robotics, lighting, and the camera sensors, can diagnostic quality, high-resolution scans be achieved at fast scanning speeds with minimal technician intervention.

Scanning Speed

Scan Times

Scanning speed is one of the most quoted WSI device parameters, with vendors touting this figure as a premier benchmark and competing for the chance to say that their slide scanner is the fastest. For many years, scanning speed was considered to be one of the limiting factors, if not the primary one, for why clinical workflows could not be supported by whole slide imaging, thus relegating use cases to mainly research and education. However, with recent advances in high-throughput scanning, scanning speeds are no longer the bottleneck to pathology workflows they once were.

Fundamentally, the speed at which a whole slide image is created is given as the scan time, measured in seconds or minutes. In general, scan times are captured by measuring the time it takes to scan a 15 mm × 15 mm area on a glass slide. This 15 mm × 15 mm area has become the de facto standard WSI reference tissue size by which all vendors state their scan times for each scanner, typically differentiating between whether the scan was captured at a 20× or 40× equivalent magnification. Importantly, what has not become standardized among vendors is the actual time points used for measuring the scan time – some vendors state the actual time it takes to scan the reference tissue size, while others state the time it takes from the start of the scan process to when one can view the slide, aka the "time to view." Unfortunately, either of these techniques is currently valid, and users basing purchasing decisions on this parameter should query vendors specifically on how their WSI device scan times are calculated.

As laboratories have begun to integrate whole slide imaging into their workflows, scanning hundreds to thousands of slides per day, scan times have been replaced or augmented with the parameter "throughput." With throughput, the emphasis has shifted from the time it takes to scan a single slide to the number of slides able to be scanned per hour or per day. For example, two recently released WSI devices, the Pannoramic 1000 by 3DHistech and the Aperio GT450 by Leica, boast throughputs of 100 and 81 slides per hour, respectively [38, 58]. Similar to slide capacity, throughput can be divided into high and low categories for WSI devices, with at least five scanners currently marketed as high-throughput devices (Fig. 7). Besides fast scan times, high-throughput devices have added on-device one button operation, continuous scanning capabilities (ability to load/unload slides without disrupting the scanning process), enhanced automatic tissue detection and autofocusing algorithms, and deeper integration with health information systems to provide positive patient identification. Overall, one should expect throughput to replace scan time as one of the primary ways to categorize WSI devices as digital pathology is more widely adopted and integrated into anatomical pathology laboratories.

Z-Stacking and Extended Depth of Focus

An oft-cited limitation of whole slide imaging is the single plane of focus that traditional WSI devices produce. Ideally a slide scanner would deliver a WSI with all tissue on the slide perfectly in focus. In reality, due to the three-dimensional nature of tissue sections, scanners may approach this ideal, but they do not fully achieve it. Issues with out-of-focus areas are exacerbated in cytology preparations which tend to be even thicker and more heterogeneous. Despite this fact, published validation studies have not found significant issues with the current state of focus in WSI, and these out-of-focus areas do not appear to affect the ability of pathologists to arrive at the correct diagnosis in histopathology preparations [59, 60]. However, it should be noted that digital pathology systems have not yet received FDA clearance for

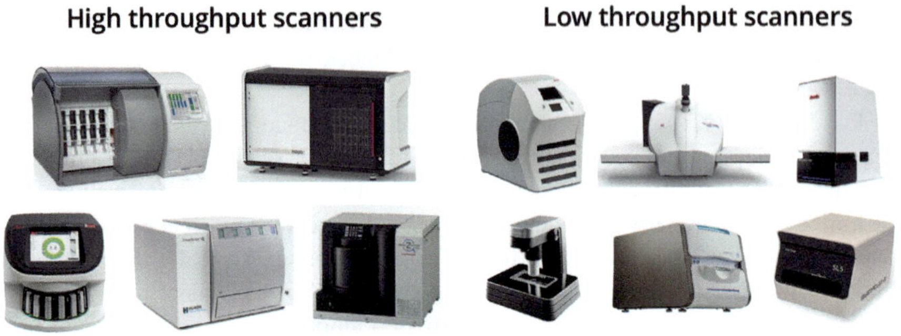

Fig. 7 Example whole slide imaging devices, categorized by throughput, circa 2021. High-throughput scanners are noted for their higher slide capacities, fast scan times (<1 min/slide), one-button operation, and continuous loading capabilities. Scanners pictured: (top) Philips Ultra Fast Scanner, 3DHistech Pannoramic 1000; (bottom) Leica GT450, Huron TissueScope iQ, and Hamamatsu NanoZoomer S360. Low-throughput scanners are noted for their lower slide capacities, versatility in operation and magnification, smaller physical footprint, and lower cost. Scanners pictured: (top) Leica CS2, 3DHistech Pannoramic MIDI II, MoticEasyScan One; (bottom) Grundium Ocus, Roche DP200, Mikroscan SL5. Each WSI device image courtesy of the device vendor, images used with permission

cytology and certain hematopathology preparations, and the impact of a single plane of focus on clinical diagnosis is not as well studied in these areas.

To overcome the limitations of a single plane of focus, some WSI devices have implemented "Z-stacking" (aka z-axis scanning). Z-stacking is a method in which multiple additional image planes above and below the "optimal" focus plane are captured, retained, and made available for viewing by the user (Fig. 8). Typically, multiple focal planes are captured at fixed intervals along the vertical (z) axis and then stacked one atop the other to produce a single, multiplanar composite image. The viewer software can then simulate the ability to focus by scrolling (moving up and down) through the different planes stored in the WSI file. This allows the pathologist to bring different cellular features into focus.

Currently, z-stacks can be captured in two different ways. The first method captures multiple WSI planes of the entire slide. In this method, the size of the WSI increases linearly by the total number of planes captured (e.g., five planes captured would result in a file size five times greater). Scan times will also increase substantially; however, since loading and unloading times are still only performed once, the actual scan time will only increase by the time needed to capture each additional plane. Alternatively, z-stacks can be limited to specific regions of interest. While this method has the advantage of smaller file sizes and quicker scan times, current methods require manual selection of these regions of interest. Automatic selection of these areas is not yet available in commercial platforms, and it is unclear when this will be developed and implemented.

Extended depth of focus (or extended depth of field; EDOF) is an alternative to Z-stacking that presents a compromise between discarding all out-of-plane information and retaining multiple planes of focus. There are a number of EDOF

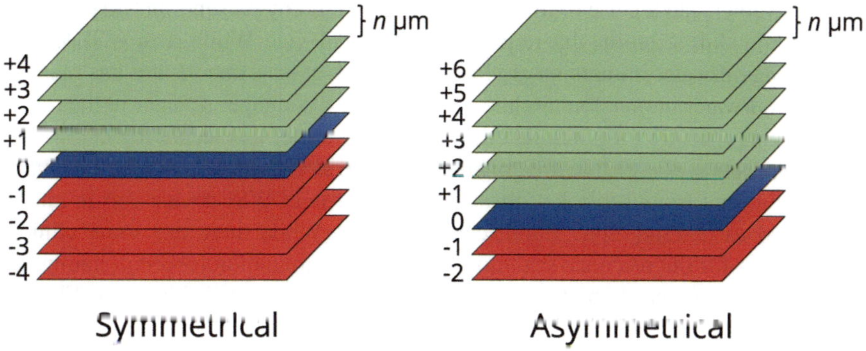

Fig. 8 Approaches to Z-stacking. During the process of slide scanning, additional planes are captured at fixed distances (n micrometers) above (green) and below (red) the optimal focal plane (blue). In both of these examples, a total of nine planes are captured and stored in the resultant whole slide image. The symmetrical example captures an equal number of planes above and below the optimal plane of focus, while the asymmetrical example does not require these quantities to be equal. Asymmetrical Z-stacking may better reflect the distribution of useful focal planes on a glass slide. Not all scanners are capable of Z-stacking, and those that do may not support an asymmetrical distribution of focal planes

implementations, but all share the common goal of incorporating in-focus information from multiple focal planes into a single image. As with Z-stacking, EDOF requires that multiple planes are imaged, but EDOF computationally combines in-focus information from planes into a single flat image. Thus, while the imaging time for EDOF and Z-stacking are similar, the WSI produced by EDOF is the same size as a non-z-stacked WSI.

Image Modalities

Unlike radiology, which has a variety of different imaging modalities, most mainstream WSI devices can only capture images in two primary imaging modalities: bright-field (traditional light) and fluorescence microscopy. Image modality, as used here, is defined as the method used to capture images in WSI, specifically as it relates to the combination of the energy source, optics, camera sensors, and image output (note that our definition of modality differs from DICOM, which would classify all of these as "slide microscopy"). Bright-field microscopy is by far the most common image modality used in both the practice of pathology and by extension, WSI devices. To date, all Food and Drug Administration (FDA) De Novo granted and 510(k) cleared WSI devices use bright-field microscopy.

Oil/water immersion-capable WSI devices are specialty devices that can support either bright-field or fluorescence imaging and are sold as research use only within the United States. Oil or water immersion WSI devices are equipped with, as the name implies, either oil or water immersion lenses capable of capturing images at up to 100× maximum equivalent magnification, which is especially useful for hematopathology blood smears and tissue sections. Automatic dispensing and management of immersion fluids present a non-trivial challenge in an enclosed device like a slide scanner, and the use of immersion fluids essentially presents an "all-or-none" scenario for slide scanning that requires a dedicated device. While most WSI devices supporting oil/water immersion are low throughput, at least one vendor has plans to offer an oil/water immersion module for their high-throughput scanner in the future [58], paving the way for potential clinical applications of this technology.

Fluorescence whole slide imaging can be added as an option to at least one high-throughput and to multiple low-throughput bright-field WSI devices, or it can be purchased as a stand-alone fluorescence scanner. While there are some clinical applications for fluorescence scanning (e.g., direct immunofluorescence staining in renal, transplant, and dermatopathology, fluorescent in situ hybridization (FISH)), the majority of use cases reside in research. Additional specialized modalities can be found with some of these imaging systems, such as dark-field, polarized, and phase contrast imaging. Ultimately, until WSI and digital pathology gain widespread adoption, fluorescence and oil/water immersion scanning are unlikely to become common high-throughput clinical options.

Finally, additional image modalities are gaining attention within the digital pathology space, including multispectral imaging, hyperspectral imaging, stimulated Raman histology (SRH), infrared spectroscopy, and microscopy with ultraviolet surface excitation (MUSE) [61–63]. While these technologies are not technically whole slide imaging (they are not "scanning" traditional glass slides), the end products are similar to whole slide images. Notably, technologies like SRH and MUSE scan tissue directly and are slide-free, eliminating the need for tissue processing and glass slides. Overall, if able to be mass produced and integrated into clinical workflows, these potentially disruptive technologies could revolutionize the practice of anatomical pathology.

Workstations

Within the WSI pixel pathway (discussed elsewhere in this book), the WSI workstation is not given much consideration [64]. To date, only one of the two WSI systems authorized by the FDA has specified a workstation as a required part of their clearance, primarily due to the vendor not including an image management system in their device submission [65]. The other high-throughput WSI system is a standalone device with an on-board computer and thus does not require, per its FDA De Novo granted designation, a separate connected workstation for its operation [66]. However, even for this system, a workstation is typically bundled with the scanner in order to access the image management system upon WSI device installation.

For most other (non-FDA) WSI systems, a workstation is included with the device, either due to the need for device-specific hardware controllers or to run scanner-specific operations software. Workstations are invariably Microsoft Windows-based PCs, typically with high-powered CPUs, discrete graphics, and larger amounts of random-access memory (RAM). These workstations often are rigorously managed by the vendor to ensure that operating system and other software updates (e.g., antivirus, drivers, etc.) do not negatively impact device performance. Generally, while features will vary per WSI device, most software required to operate the device allows for choosing which cassette/tray/slides to scan, prefilling slide metadata, selecting magnification, adjusting scannable regions, selecting focal points, choosing the file destination, etc. Some vendors may also include workstations to facilitate telepathology and live-view functionality with their scanners, especially seen with hybrid scanners (see Chapter "Whole Slide Imaging and Telepathology" for a more in-depth discussion). Of note, given the rise of cybersecurity concerns within large hospital systems, one should check with their Information Assurance team to ensure outside vendor workstations conform with proper security controls.

Displays

Displays are an extremely important component of a WSI system as they provide the visual gateway to the digital slide. There are three main types of displays from a digital pathology perspective: 1) consumer-off-the-shelf (COTS), 2) professional-grade (PG), and 3) medical-grade (MG) displays [67]. Most people are well aware of COTS displays as these comprise the vast majority of displays produced, typically bundled with PCs or available separately from a variety of technology-focused to general purpose retail outlets. COTS displays are usually lower cost (e.g., $100 to $2000); however, over the past 5–10 years, they have markedly increased in quality, narrowing the gap between them and their higher cost PG and MG cousins. In contrast, PG displays are marketed not to the general public, but instead to specific professions in need of very high-quality displays with specific performance metrics, such as graphics design, photography, video production, animation, etc. Finally, MG displays are similar to PG displays in that they are generally composed of higher quality components than COTS displays and include medically relevant features, such as being easily washable/disinfected, conformant to medical imaging standards, long lasting (> 5 years maintained performance), more easily calibrated, etc.

When deciding on which display to use for digital pathology, there are a number of potential features to consider, including display panel type, size, aspect ratio, resolution, luminance, contrast ratio, color depth, color gamut, refresh rate, viewing distance, etc. While a thorough discussion of each of these parameters is present elsewhere [67, 68], there unfortunately is a lack of research regarding which features, and by extension which display types, are the most important to the practice of digital pathology [67]. As a case in point, early display use for whole slide imaging was primarily dictated by the vendor, with high-end COTS or PG displays used in order to better market the system. However, recent trends in digital pathology have been to use MG displays as systems move through the FDA submission process [65, 66, 69, 70].

Of note, unlike the workstation, displays play an important role within the WSI pixel pathway. Specific displays are required to be validated in conjunction with the

WSI device and image management system for primary diagnosis. In fact, in both WSI systems authorized by the FDA, a specific model MG display must be sold with the WSI device in order for that system to maintain its FDA status; using any other display, regardless of its grade (COTS, PG, or MG), automatically means a clinical laboratory must validate the entire system as a laboratory-developed test (LDT) [64, 67]. Given that most new displays, COTS or otherwise, are of superior quality and specifications than those of the two MG displays included for with FDA authorized WSI systems, it will be interesting to see over the next 5 years if laboratories choose to pursue the LDT versus the FDA route.

Whole Slide Imaging: Software

Once a WSI is captured from the glass slide, the file is compressed, saved, and then sent either to the local workstation or to a networked server. Depending on one's use case, the software required to organize, manage, and view WSI can vary significantly, ranging from simple folder-based local file storage to complex image management systems interfaced with the laboratory information system (LIS) or electronic health record (EHR). Further, in order to view a WSI, one must have a compatible image viewer, typically provided by the WSI vendor due to the proprietary nature of the WSI image file format. Additionally, optional software components are available, such as image analysis and AI platforms, research WSI solutions, WSI-based education systems, and enhanced reporting solutions. The following section will review the major WSI software topics including viewers, image management systems, and adding value to whole slide imaging through AI.

The Viewer

Of all the software associated with whole slide imaging systems, the viewer is arguably the most important component. For many pathologists, the viewer represents the proverbial "first impression" they have with a WSI system and can make or break their opinion on its quality, ease of use, and functionality. Historically, WSI vendors have provided dedicated viewers for their WSIs, either bundling them with the system or providing them as free downloads for all to use. Typically, these viewers have existed as stand-alone Microsoft Windows-based applications, although more recently vendors have started to provide web-based viewers in order to support cross-platform compatibility. Of note, two software vendors have recently gained FDA clearance for their viewers to be used with the FDA-granted (Paige.AI FullFocus viewer with the Philips Intellisite Pathology Solution) and FDA-cleared (Sectra Digital Pathology Module with the Leica Aperio AT2 DX) WSI systems [71, 72].

The look and feel of different viewers can vary remarkably from vendor to vendor. They may have different sets of tools and options for panning, zooming, rotating, measuring, annotating, taking/exporting snapshots, color control, image analysis, and more. Even when two different viewers have the same functionality, the user interface and, thus, the user experience may differ between them. As file formats vary between different vendors, a given viewer may be limited in its ability to open WSI files from a competitor. This becomes a significant issue if the WSI devices in a department come from different vendors, many times resulting in multiple viewers being used; however, as DICOM becomes more widespread, this issue will eventually be minimized. Notably, it is vital when evaluating a WSI system that the viewing software be appraised as critically as the scanner itself.

Although beyond the scope of this discussion, some institutions may choose to purchase a third-party viewing solution or even to develop their own viewing software using open-source tools, such as OpenSlide and OpenSeadragon [33, 73, 74]. This allows for increased customization with respect to the needs of a particular department and can be helpful when dealing with multiple vendor file formats. However, using different viewing software than what was bundled with the scanner will require further validation and may limit the ability of the WSI vendor to support an institution's digital pathology needs.

Image Management Systems

For early whole slide imaging, image management was a manual process, relying on human intervention to either prepopulate slide information and file destinations within the slide scanning software or relabel and reorganize them afterwards. In the mid to late 2000s, as both WSI devices and AP LISs started to support barcoding and positive patient identification, early digital pathology image management software was born. In the early 2010s, WSI vendors began working with LIS vendors to interface their systems, opening the door for image management systems (IMS) to use patient-, case-, and image-specific metadata to organize and manage WSI into meaningful groups [28]. Of note, image management systems may or may not include its own image repository, i.e., location where the slides are stored, and interestingly enough, the image repository is not deemed an essential part of the pixel pathway (64). Today there are multiple companies offering image management systems for a variety of intended uses, in particular for clinical, research, and educational purposes.

Clinical Image Management Systems

Clinical image management systems are a fairly recent, but important, addition to the IMS landscape. While initial WSI vendor-based IMSs were able to organize and manage WSIs based on case accession numbers and slide identifiers, it was only after high-throughput WSI devices were released that additional features, such as clinical worklists and workflow management, were added. Even as the WSI device manufacturer space contracted in the late 2000s/early 2010s, clinical image management began to grow as a separate business outside of WSI device manufacturers. To date, there are more than 15 IMS vendors offering some form of clinical image management for whole slide imaging [75].

While all clinical image management systems include an WSI image viewer, they vary regarding most other features. In general, the following features can be found in some combination in most clinical IMSs: (1) case management, (2) pathologist worklists, (3) workflow management, (4) DICOM conformance, (5) tumor board/multidisciplinary conference management, (6) image analysis/AI algorithm integration, (7) LIS/ EHR integration, (8) vendor-neutral archive (VNA) and/or enterprise picture archiving and communications system (PACS) integration, (9) image sharing and collaboration tools, (10) teleconsultation tools, and (11) other image management (e.g., electron microscopy, immunofluorescence, and gross images).

The presence of proprietary WSI file formats and their associated viewers has been a major contributing factor in stifling adoption of whole slide imaging and WSI data exchange [76]. A significant benefit resulting from the growth of clinical IMS platforms has been increased discussions and progress surrounding WSI/IMS vendor interoperability. Further, as clinical image analysis and AI platforms have emerged, new partnerships between these vendors have formed, allowing for the seamless integration of diagnostically relevant algorithms within clinical workflows [77, 78]. While there is still much to be done in regard to both IMS and AI algorithm development, there are early adopter pathology practices today paving the way forward and sharing their experiences of "going digital" [5, 6, 79].

Research and Education Image Management Systems

Unlike clinical IMSs, research and education IMSs have gone through multiple phases of development and iterations over the years due to being the initial primary use cases for whole slide imaging. For research IMSs, there are a number of advanced features that exist beyond the typical slide organizational tools common to all, such as (1) integrated image analysis (e.g., for tissue microarrays, IHC marker development, etc.); (2) image analysis development tools; (3) clinical trial support, including case management and clinical trial fulfillment software; (4) industry support for biopharma and other related companies; and (5) supervised and unsupervised machine learning algorithm creation platforms, including deep learning.

In the education space, image management systems have only recently begun to expand out from simple folder-based slide management integrated into institutional learning management systems. Unfortunately for most, investing in a separate education IMS above and beyond the simple image management tools the WSI vendor provides is a luxury since, in the authors' experiences, educational programs are not nearly as well funded as research or clinical initiatives. That said, there are a number of education IMS features worth mentioning: (1) multiformat WSI viewers and/or WSI file converters (from proprietary to open formats); (2) on-premises or cloud-based platforms with included storage that allows for many simultaneous connections (slide seminars, histology lab units, etc.); (3) pathology case creation tools with integrated gross, microscopic, and whole slide images; (4) simulated pathology case environments; and (5) virtual slide boxes/digital slide repositories [80, 81].

Adding Value Through Software

As the adoption of whole slide imaging, and by extension, digital pathology, has increased, discussion at many healthcare institutions has begun regarding how pathology images should be managed at the enterprise level. While radiology has been the prototypical image-based medical specialty setting the standard for image management, healthcare enterprises have seen a flood of additional imaging over the past decade from practically every medical specialty. However, while these specialties generally are dealing with smaller, static images (e.g., dermatology, family medicine, gastroenterology), known video formats (surgery, neurology), and other departmental radiologic-based imaging (echocardiograms, prenatal ultrasounds), whole slide imaging has the potential to disrupt current enterprise image management with its new file types incompatible with clinical enterprise universal viewers and massive storage needs (see below).

After going digital in the late 1990s/early 2000s, radiology found success with clinicians wanting to review their patients' radiologic imaging. In that regard, besides eliminating film (and its associated equipment, chemicals, etc.), radiology built out a robust imaging infrastructure with a significant return on investment through the development of DICOM-conformant imaging devices, feature-rich PACS, and most recently, interoperable vendor neutral archives in order to promote image sharing [82–85]. In that regard, radiology demonstrated itself to be a write-once, read-often specialty with readily justifiable (and funded) clinical imaging use cases.

Conversely, at its heart, anatomic pathology as a field has traditionally been a write-once, read-once specialty, with the vast majority of AP cases signed out never viewed or accessed again by pathologists or by clinicians. Whether this is due to a lack of central access, a lack of histopathology training, or simply a lack of interest by clinicians is not known. However, combined with the significant startup, implementation, and storage costs associated with full adoption of whole slide imaging [86, 87], it means the business case for implementing whole slide imaging will most likely not come from the enterprise or the non-pathology medical community.

Returning to the initial scenario presented at the beginning of this chapter, one can see that a major driving force for adding value through the adoption of whole slide imaging is its place on the road towards adopting artificial intelligence. Machine learning and artificial intelligence platforms represent a large subset of digital pathology software applications gaining prominence, with at least one pathology AI vendor to date receiving FDA Breakthrough Device designation status [88]. While the utility of AI within pathology has been described in detail [89–92], only through its integration with digital pathology platforms will digital pathology gain the mechanism to consistently add value through improved diagnostics, optimized efficiency, and improved patient safety. Further, only after WSI data has been collected in sufficient quantity will the pathology community be better able to determine how best to use it, how best to store it, and, ultimately, how long to keep it.

Whole Slide Imaging: Infrastructure

IT infrastructure is an often overlooked component when making the transition to a digital workflow. In this section, the related, but distinct, infrastructure components of networking and storage will be described. An easy way to conceptualize storage is to ask the question "how much data will you produce," while networking is a question of "how fast do you need your data" (also known as bandwidth). Data is measured in bits and bytes (where 8 bits = 1 byte, bits abbreviated "b" and bytes "B"), but due to the size of WSI files, these are typically given in prefixed SI format (International System of Units), with the most frequently used prefixes being kilo-, mega-, giga-, tera-, and peta-, corresponding to 10^3, 10^6, 10^9, 10^{12}, and 10^{15}, respectively [93]. As an example, an average single, compressed WSI file scanned at 40x equivalent resolution contains about 1.25 gigabytes (GB) of data. This number can trend upwards if higher quality settings are enabled on the scanner, if Z-stacking is used, or if the slide contains a large square area of tissue (e.g., resection specimens, cytology, and blood smears). By comparison, a typical radiology breast MRI study uses about 300 MB of space, and only CT studies with extremely large numbers of "slices" reach the data requirements of a single WSI [94]. Since even small biopsies can have multiple sections on a single slide and additional data is used for color encoding, the data requirements for digital pathology typically exceed those of radiology on a case-by-case basis by at least an order of magnitude. Unlike data storage, which is measured in bytes, networking bandwidth is defined by the bit-rate of networking medium and is thus measured in bits, e.g. 100 Mbps (megabits per second). Of note, in addition to the raw storage and bandwidth requirements for digital pathology IT infrastructure, pathology practices must also consider the upfront and maintenance costs associated with supporting this infrastructure (outlined below).

Networking

There are multiple connections for which specific networking bandwidths are recommended when setting up WSI devices. Given that WSIs are measured in MB and GB, WSI vendors typically recommend network speeds of 1–10 Gbps for the physical connection between a single WSI device and the data center/server housing the image repository. Because WSI devices currently do not support parallel scanning, this means that each device will require its own networked connection at the recommended bandwidth. Vendors also recommend the same 1–10 Gbps (ideally closer to 10 Gbps) for physical connections between the image management system and the image repository.

Fortunately, the network bandwidth required for serving up WSIs to individual pathologist workstations is much less than that required for sending a newly scanned WSI file to the image repository (1–40 Mbps vs. 1–10 Gbps, respectively) [95]. This is in large part due to the pyramidal structure of WSI files (only a small portion of the slide is served up at any given time) in addition to the fact that each pathologist will only view a subset of the total number of slides scanned. Nevertheless, the ability to rapidly view digital slides in a seamless manner is crucial for pathologist efficiency and satisfaction [10].

Depending on specific use cases, additional factors affecting networking may come into play. If an institution or practice is distributed throughout multiple physical sites, a connection over a wide area network (WAN) is required. Further, if practicing telepathology among these sites (either via WSI or via live-view microscopy), a fast networking connection able to support 1080p (~5 Mbps) or 4K (~25 Mbps) video with near 100% uptime is required at each potential site/workstation. Tumor boards present their own unique problems in that the presentation room, typically not under a pathologist's control, requires not only a fast network connection to its workstation but also the proper videoconferencing software/hardware to support WSI screen sharing. Most recently with the SARS-CoV-2 (COVID-19) global pandemic, performing remote sign out and working from home have become increasingly common, straining network bandwidth from local ISPs and forcing people to upgrade their connections [96].

Finally, as image analysis and artificial intelligence platforms use increases, one must consider the network connections between these systems, the IMS, and the image repository. For most healthcare systems, this shouldn't be an issue since these servers/systems will be housed and supported in large, well-connected data centers. However, for smaller pathology practices relying on local servers, small business internet service providers, and/or potentially cloud-based services, their network bandwidth could easily become a rate-limiting step in their workflow. Using a cloud-based or other off-site storage method will necessarily demand fast upload speeds (>50 Mbps minimally, ideally >100 Mbps or even >500 Mbps) not always available in all areas. Overall, it is vital during the validation of one's digital pathology system that all use cases, physical sites, and respective network topologies be considered and tested. For additional information regarding additional networking parameters for WSI, please refer to the Networking section of Chap. 7, "Whole Slide Imaging and Telepathology."

Storage

The cost and scale of storage for digital pathology can be quite dramatic and are frequently underappreciated. As an example, a large academic institution producing 800,000 slides per year at an approximate 1.25 GB/slide (40x equivalent magnification, current accepted estimate for average slide size) would generate 1 PB of data per year. Doubling this storage calculation to account for best IT practices and system redundancy yields, for that institution, 2 PB of required storage per year in order to fully adopt WSI. Although theoretically one could purchase a large quantity of storage in the form of external or internal hard drives in a retail setting, this is both unfeasible and technically irresponsible for clinical use cases in digital pathology.

When discussing storage options in the many TB to PB scale, one size definitely does not fit all. Instead, one must distinguish between the different performance levels of storage as they relate to one's use cases. In the IT space, storage performance levels are thought of conceptually as temperatures, namely, as "hot," "warm," and "cold" storage that refers to the relative accessibility of the data [97]. Hot storage refers to data frequently accessed and rapidly retrieved, whereas cold storage refers to data that is rarely accessed and, by default, slow to retrieve. As expected, warm storage falls in between these two extremes, being accessed less frequently than hot storage but still accessed frequently enough to require faster retrieval than cold storage.

Given that WSI, as seen in the example above, has the potential of requiring massive amounts of storage (PB) per year, WSI data should be optimally stored within a specialized data center to ensure near 100% network access and continuous support in the face of any technical difficulties. Besides the cost of raw storage itself, data center overhead typically includes the following: cooling, power (uninterruptible power supply and generators), fire suppression, security, equipment maintenance/replacement, networking (tiered pricing by speed), and staff to run the data center 7 days a week, 24 hours a day, 365 days a year (7×24×365). Within data centers, the temperature of the storage tier is directly proportional to both the cost of the storage and its support, with hot storage the most expensive and cold the most economical. Thus, when deciding on how to set up one's storage options for WSI, determining how one's storage is to be used and its associated performance level is just as important as the amount of storage required.

In addition to the type of data storage performance needed, additional factors to take into consideration are system uptime/downtime, system redundancy and the potential for data loss, and the need for disaster recovery plans. System uptime refers to the amount of time a system is fully operational, or "up" per unit of time, whereas downtime is the opposite, referring to the amount of time a system has lost service, or "down" [98]. Uptime is generally given as a percentage (e.g., 99.7% uptime per year) or as hours/days of downtime (e.g., <26 hours of downtime per year). Concurrent with the concept of uptime is system redundancy, where a system is operationally duplicated (typically at an alternate facility) and continuously synced in order to avoid data loss in the event of unplanned downtime. In the event of a major hardware/software failure, or worse, destruction of one's data center facility, a disaster recovery (DR) plan lists and prioritizes the order in which systems are to be restored [99]. Those systems with the highest priority and greatest redundancy will be restored first, minimizing potential data loss and maintaining uptime goals. For any given system, its uptime, system redundancy, potential for data loss, and disaster recovery are ultimately managed by assigning it to a defined data center service tier (Table 1) [98].

To put this all together, one must consider how the storage will be used, not just how often it will be accessed, when determining the type of storage required (Table 2). For example, the pathology practice mentioned above may potentially require 2 PB of total (redundant) storage per year, but it doesn't need to store all of these slides at the same performance/service tier. Instead, this site could decide to store only the most recent 2 months of WSIs, actively used for sign out, at the hot/gold tier, and then transfer those into warm/silver tier for 4 months, followed

Table 1 Example data center service tiers

Service tiers	Gold	Silver	Bronze
Service/ support availability	24 × 7 × 365	6 days/week	5 days/week
Uptime target	99.7%	99%	98%
System redundancy	Required	Strongly recommended	Optional
Disaster recovery	Within 24-48 hours	Within 7-30 days	> 1 month

Most data centers will offer multiple service tiers (here designated by the value of rare metals, but otherwise may vary per data center), with different support criteria defined per tier. This list has been simplified for presentation purposes, with most data centers providing a wide array of different support criteria. Note that data centers may offer even higher tiers, e.g., platinum in this example, with even higher uptime targets and faster disaster recovery

Table 2 Example pricing values for different performance levels and data center service tiers for storage

Performance level	Service tiers (cost/TB)			
	Annual price with disaster recovery (DR)			w/o DR
	Gold	Silver	Bronze	Bronze
Hot	$3,500	$2,000	$1,800	$1,500
Warm	$1500	$900	$750	$500
Cold	$700	$450	$350	$100

Performing whole slide imaging for primary diagnosis will require hot and/or warm storage at gold or silver tier service levels, whereas archived cases or those being stored for educational or research purposes may be designated as cold storage with a silver or bronze tier service level. While disaster recovery is optional for the bronze service tier, it is strongly recommended for best IT practices. Note, pricing is supplied as a generic estimate from circa 2020; actual costs will differ

by a final transfer to the cold/bronze with DR tier. By the numbers, this equates to approximately 330 TB of hot/gold storage, 670 TB of warm/silver storage, and 1 PB of cold/bronze storage per year, at a total annual cost of $2,108,000. If over time the site decided that warm/gold storage was sufficient for their practice instead of hot/gold, with offloading to cold/bronze storage immediately afterwards (skipping warm/silver storage), this cost could decrease by almost 50% to

Table 3 Performance level and data center service tier recommendations

Performance level	Service tier		
	Gold	Silver	Bronze
Hot	High accessibility High speed High support (Best performance)	High accessibility High speed Moderate support	High accessibility High speed Limited support
Warm	Moderate accessibility Moderate speed High support	Moderate accessibility Moderate speed Moderate support	Moderate accessibility Moderate speed Limited support
Cold	Low accessibility Low speed High support	Low accessibility Low speed Moderate support	Low accessibility Low speed Limited support (Lowest cost)

Depending on one's use cases, there are advantages and disadvantages to choosing one performance level or service tier for digital pathology storage over another. Understanding these options will help when creating retention policies for different classes of WSI data

$1,079,500. Of note, data storage and service tier pricing vary significantly between storage providers, institutions, by storage volume used, and even by year purchased, so it's best to fully explore one's options prior to making a final decision on storage.

Finally, all of one's specific use cases for digital pathology must be considered in combination with the different IT aspects of storage/data centers in order to properly create retention policies for digital pathology (Table 3). For example, decision-making regarding when it is "safe" to archive clinical cases can be fraught with difficulty. While a blanket recommendation for archival solely based on the age of a case may sound good initially, the need to access an old case will vary depending on one's practice and specific specimen types (e.g., lookbacks in gynecological cytology, re-examination of biopsy material after a surgical resection is performed, re-examination of the primary tumor at the time of a suspected metastasis, etc.). Further, from a regulatory perspective, to date a pathology practice in the United States does not need to keep WSI files after sign out as long as the physical glass slides are retained [100]. This means a practice could decide to opt out of storing its WSI data after a very short retention period, markedly reducing costs. In the end, one must take into account all potential use cases (clinical, research, and education) in addition to understanding the IT infrastructure in order to optimize one's WSI data storage experience [101].

Conclusions

For the past 20 years, WSI technological advances have fueled early adopters to embrace digital pathology. Only recently, however, has the WSI industry developed enough from a hardware, software, and infrastructure standpoint to adequately support pathology organizations going fully digital. With the current slate of high-throughput scanners, robust viewers, image management systems, wider use of DICOM, high-speed networks, fast abundant storage, regulatory approval, and promising value-added use cases made possible through artificial intelligence, it is no longer a question of "if" but instead "when" one will implement whole slide imaging.

References

1. Abels E, Pantanowitz L, Aeffner F, Zarella MD, Laak J, Bui MM, et al. Computational pathology definitions, best practices, and recommendations for regulatory guidance: a white paper from the digital pathology association. J Pathol. 2019;249(3):286–94.
2. Yagi Y, Gilbertson JR. Digital imaging in pathology: the case for standardization. J Telemed Telecare. 2005;11(3):109–16.
3. Ho J, Parwani AV, Jukic DM, Yagi Y, Anthony L, Gilbertson JR. Use of whole slide imaging in surgical pathology quality assurance: design and pilot validation studies. Hum Pathol. 2006;37(3):322–31.
4. Pantanowitz L, Sharma A, Carter A, Kurc T, Sussman A, Saltz J. Twenty years of digital pathology: an overview of the road travelled, what is on the horizon, and the emergence of vendor-neutral archives. J Pathol Inform. 2018;9(1):40.
5. Stathonikos N, Nguyen TQ, Spoto CP, Verdaasdonk MAM, van Diest PJ. Being fully digital: perspective of a Dutch academic pathology laboratory. Histopathology. 2019;75(5):621–35.
6. Retamero JA, Aneiros-Fernandez J, del Moral RG. Complete digital pathology for routine histopathology diagnosis in a multicenter hospital network. Arch Pathol Lab Med. 2020;144(2):221–8.
7. Vodovnik A, Aghdam MF. Complete routine remote digital pathology services. J Pathol Inform. 2018;9(1):36.
8. Food and Drug Administration. FDA allows marketing of first whole slide imaging system for digital pathology [Internet]. FDA. FDA; 2020 [cited 2020 Aug 18]. Available from: https://www.fda.gov/news-events/press-announcements/fda-allows-marketing-first-whole-slide-imaging-system-digital-pathology.
9. Food and Drug Administration. 510(k) Premarket Notification-Aperio AT2 DX System [Internet]. [cited 2020 Aug 18]. Available from: https://www.accessdata.fda.gov/scripts/cdrh/cfdocs/cfpmn/pmn.cfm?ID=K190332.
10. Hanna MG, Reuter VE, Hameed MR, Tan LK, Chiang S, Sigel C, et al. Whole slide imaging equivalency and efficiency study: experience at a large academic center. Mod Pathol. 2019;32(7):916–28.
11. Zheng P-P, van der Weiden M, Kros JM. Fast tracking of co-localization of multiple markers by using the nanozoomer slide scanner and NDPViewer. J Cell Physiol. 2014;229(8):967–73.
12. Catalyurek U, Beynon MD, Chang C, Kurc T, Sussman A, Saltz J. The virtual microscope. IEEE Trans Inf Technol Biomed. 2003;7(4):230–48.
13. Gilbertson JR, Ho J, Anthony L, Jukic DM, Yagi Y, Parwani AV. Primary histologic diagnosis using automated whole slide imaging: a validation study. BMC Clin Pathol. 2006;6(1):4.
14. Bacus J. BLISS System [Internet]. [cited 2020 Aug 18]. Available from: http://jamesbacus.com/page10.html

15. Montalto MC. An industry perspective: an update on the adoption of whole slide imaging. J Pathol Inform. 2016;7(1):18.
16. Boyce B. Whole slide imaging: uses and limitations for surgical pathology and teaching. Biotech Histochem. 2015;90(5):321–30.
17. Griffin J, Treanor D. Digital pathology in clinical use: where are we now and what is holding us back? Histopathology. 2017;70(1):134–45.
18. Pantanowitz L, Sinard JH, Henricks WH, Fatheree LA, Carter AB, Contis L, et al. Validating whole slide imaging for diagnostic purposes in pathology: guideline from the College of American Pathologists Pathology and Laboratory Quality Center. Arch Pathol Lab Med. 2013;137(12):1710–22.
19. International Organization for Standardization. ISO/IEC 7498-4:1989 – Information technology – Open Systems Interconnection – Basic Reference Model: Naming and addressing [Internet]. ISO Standards Maintenance Portal. ISO Central Secretariat; 1989 [cited 2020 Aug 18]. Available from: http://standards.iso.org/ittf/PubliclyAvailableStandards/s014258_ISO_IEC_7498-4_1989(E).zip.
20. OSI model. In: Wikipedia [Internet]. 2020 [cited 2020 Aug 18]. Available from: https://en.wikipedia.org/w/index.php?title=OSI_model&oldid=973511610.
21. Ferreira R, Moon B, Humphries J, Sussman A, Saltz J, Miller R, et al. The virtual microscope. Proc AMIA Annu Fall Symp. 1997:449–53.
22. NEMA. DICOM Whole Slide Imaging (WSI) [Internet]. [cited 2020 Aug 18]. Available from: http://dicom.nema.org/Dicom/DICOMWSI/.
23. Daniel C, Macary F, García Rojo M, Klossa J, Laurinavičius A, Beckwith BA, et al. Recent advances in standards for collaborative digital anatomic pathology. Diagn Pathol. 2011;6(Suppl 1):S17.
24. Marques Godinho T, Lebre R, Silva LB, Costa C. An efficient architecture to support digital pathology in standard medical imaging repositories. J Biomed Inform. 2017;71:190–7.
25. Singh R, Chubb L, Pantanowitz L, Parwani A. Standardization in digital pathology: supplement 145 of the DICOM standards. J Pathol Inform. 2011;2(1):23.
26. Herrmann MD, Clunie DA, Fedorov A, Doyle SW, Pieper S, Klepeis V, et al. Implementing the DICOM standard for digital pathology. J Pathol Inform [Internet]. 2018 Nov 2 [cited 2020 May 27];9. Available from: https://www.ncbi.nlm.nih.gov/pmc/articles/PMC6236926/.
27. Taubman DS, Marcellin MW. Introduction to JPEG2000. In: Taubman DS, Marcellin MW, editors. JPEG2000 image compression fundamentals, standards and practice [internet]. Boston, MA: springer US; 2002. p. 399–415. Available from: doi:https://doi.org/10.1007/978-1-4615-0799-4_9.
28. Zarella MD, Bowman D, Aeffner F, Farahani N, Xthona A, Absar SF, et al. A practical guide to whole slide Imaging: a white paper from the digital pathology association. Arch Pathol Lab Med. 2018;143(2):222–34.
29. TIFF, Revision 6.0 [Internet]. 2009 [cited 2020 Aug 18]. Available from: https://www.loc.gov/preservation/digital/formats/fdd/fdd000022.shtml.
30. BigTIFF version of libtiff library [Internet]. [cited 2020 Aug 18]. Available from: http://bigtiff.org/.
31. Hamamatsu format [Internet]. [cited 2020 Aug 16]. Available from: https://openslide.org/formats/hamamatsu/.
32. Deep Zoom [Internet]. [cited 2020 Aug 18]. Available from: https://docs.microsoft.com/en-us/previous-versions/windows/silverlight/dotnet-windows-silverlight/cc645050(v=vs.95).
33. OpenSeadragon [Internet]. [cited 2020 Aug 18]. Available from: https://openseadragon.github.io/.
34. DICOM Standards Committee, Working Groups 26, Pathology. Digital Imaging and Communications in Medicine (DICOM) Supplement 122: Specimen Module and Revised Pathology SOP Classes [Internet]. 2008 [cited 2020 Aug 18]. Available from: https://www.dicomstandard.org/News/ftsup/docs/sups/sup122.pdf.
35. DICOM Standards Committee, Working Groups 26, Pathology. Digital Imaging and Communications in Medicine (DICOM) Supplement 145: Whole Slide Microscopic Image

IOD and SOP Classes [Internet]. 2010 [cited 2020 Aug 18]. Available from: https://www.dicomstandard.org/News/ftsup/docs/sups/sup145.pdf.
36. Clunie D, Hosseinzadeh D, Wintell M, De Mena D, Lajara N, Garcia-Rojo M, et al. Digital imaging and communications in medicine whole slide imaging connectathon at digital pathology association pathology visions 2017. J Pathol Inform [Internet]. 2018 Mar 5 [cited 2020 Aug 9];9. Available from: https://www.ncbi.nlm.nih.gov/pmc/articles/PMC5869966/.
37. Herrmann MD, Clunie DA, Fedorov A, Doyle SW, Pieper S, Klepeis V, et al. Implementing the DICOM standard for digital pathology. J Pathol Inform. 2018;9:37.
38. Leica Biosystems Division of Leica Microsystems Inc. Aperio GT 450 - Automated, High Capacity Digital Pathology Scanner [Internet]. Leica Biosystems. [cited 2020 Aug 9]. Available from: https://www.leicabiosystems.com/digital-pathology/scan/aperio-gt-450/.
39. Press Trust of India. Leica Biosystems launches Aperio GT 450 DX in Asia enabling high volume clinical labs to scale up digital pathology operations. Business Standard India [Internet]. 2020 May 12 [cited 2020 Aug 12]; Available from: https://www.business-standard.com/article/pti-stories/leica-biosystems-launches-aperio-gt-450-dx-in-asia-enabling-high-volume-clinical-labs-to-scale-up-digital-pathology-operations-120051200223_1.html.
40. Leica Biosystems. Leica Biosystems Unveils its Aperio GT 450 DX Digital Pathology Scanner and Delivers Excellence to Leeds Teaching Hospitals NHS Trust, UK [Internet]. 2020 [cited 2020 Aug 12]. Available from: https://tissuepathology.com/2020/08/11/leica-biosystems-unveils-its-aperio-gt-450-dx-digital-pathology-scanner-and-delivers-excellence-to-leeds-teaching-hospitals-nhs-trust-uk/.
41. Hanna MG, Parwani A, Sirintrapun SJ. Whole slide imaging: technology and applications. Adv Anat Pathol. 2020;27(4):251–9.
42. McClintock DS, Lee RE, Gilbertson JR. Using computerized workflow simulations to assess the feasibility of whole slide Imaging full adoption in a high-volume histology laboratory. Anal Cell Pathol Amst. 2012;35(1):57–64.
43. Montironi R, Cimadamore A, Massari F, Montironi MA, Lopez-Beltran A, Cheng L, et al. Whole slide imaging of large format histology in prostate pathology: potential for information fusion. Arch Pathol Lab Med. 2017;141(11):1460–1.
44. Montironi R, Cheng L, Lopez-Beltran A, Scarpelli M. Quantitative image analysis on histologic virtual slides for prostate pathology diagnosis, response to chemopreventive agents, and prognosis. Eur Urol Focus. 2017;3(4):467–9.
45. Bryant P, Haine N, Johnston J, Ntiamoah P. Application of large format tissue processing in the histology laboratory. J Histotechnol. 2019;42(3):150–62.
46. Tot T. Cost-benefit analysis of using large-format histology sections in routine diagnostic breast care. Breast. 2010;19(4):284–8.
47. Foschini MP, Baldovini C, Ishikawa Y, Eusebi V. The value of large sections in surgical pathology. Int J Breast Cancer [Internet]. 2012 [cited 2020 Aug 18];2012. Available from: https://www.ncbi.nlm.nih.gov/pmc/articles/PMC3512286/.
48. Sellaro TL, Filkins R, Hoffman C, Fine JL, Ho J, Parwani AV, et al. Relationship between magnification and resolution in digital pathology systems. J Pathol Inform. 2013;4(1):21.
49. DMetrix Ultra-rapid, Dependable Digital Slide Scanning [Internet]. 2012 [cited 2020 Aug 12]. Available from: https://www.youtube.com/watch?v=pDKMnIgdtCo.
50. Weinstein RS, Descour MR, Liang C, Barker G, Scott KM, Richter L, et al. An array microscope for ultrarapid virtual slide processing and telepathology. Design, fabrication, and validation study. Hum Pathol. 2004;35(11):1303–14.
51. Cucoranu IC, Parwani AV, Vepa S, Weinstein RS, Pantanowitz L. Digital pathology: a systematic evaluation of the patent landscape. J Pathol Inform. 2014;5(1):16.
52. Montalto MC, McKay RR, Filkins RJ. Autofocus methods of whole slide imaging systems and the introduction of a second-generation independent dual sensor scanning method. J Pathol Inform. 2011;2(1):44.
53. McKay RR, Baxi VA, Montalto MC. The accuracy of dynamic predictive autofocusing for whole slide imaging. J Pathol Inform. 2011;2(1):38.

54. van der Graaff L, van der Graaff L, van Leenders GJLH, Boyaval F, Stallinga S, Stallinga S. Computational imaging modalities for multi-focal whole-slide imaging systems. Appl Opt. 2020;59(20):5967–82.
55. Liao J, Jiang Y, Bian Z, Mahrou B, Nambiar A, Magsam AW, et al. Rapid focus map surveying for whole slide imaging with continuous sample motion. Opt Lett. 2017;42(17):3379–82.
56. Jiang S, Bian Z, Huang X, Song P, Zhang H, Zhang Y, et al. Rapid and robust whole slide imaging based on LED-array illumination and color-multiplexed single shot autofocusing. Quant Imaging Med Surg. 2019;9(5):823–31.
57. Yagi Y, Gilbertson JR. A relationship between slide quality and image quality in whole slide imaging (WSI). Diagn Pathol. 2008;3 Suppl 1:S12.
58. 3DHistech Ltd. Pannoramic 1000 [Internet]. 3DHISTECH Ltd. [cited 2020 Aug 17]. Available from: https://www.3dhistech.com/products-and-software/hardware/pannoramic-digital-slide-scanners/pannoramic 1000/.
59. Mukhopadhyay S, Feldman MD, Abels E, Ashfaq R, Beltaifa S, Cacciabeve NG, et al. Whole slide imaging versus microscopy for primary diagnosis in surgical pathology: a multicenter blinded randomized noninferiority study of 1992 cases (pivotal study). Am J Surg Pathol. 42, no. 1. 2018:39–52. https://doi.org/10.1097/PAS.0000000000000948.
60. Borowsky AD, Glassy EF, Wallace WD, Kallichanda NS, Behling CA, Miller DV, et al. Digital whole slide imaging compared with light microscopy for primary diagnosis in surgical pathology: a multicenter, double-blinded, randomized study of 2045 cases. Arch Pathol Lab Med [Internet]. 2020 Feb 14 [cited 2020 Aug 8]; Available from: https://www.archivesofpathology.org/doi/10.5858/arpa.2019-0569-OA.
61. Ortega S, Halicek M, Fabelo H, Callico GM, Fei B. Hyperspectral and multispectral imaging in digital and computational pathology: a systematic review [invited]. Biomed Opt Express. 2020;11(6):3195–233.
62. Hollon TC, Lewis S, Pandian B, Niknafs YS, Garrard MR, Garton H, et al. Rapid intraoperative diagnosis of pediatric brain tumors using stimulated Raman histology. Cancer Res. 2018;78(1):278–89.
63. Qorbani A, Fereidouni F, Levenson R, Lahoubi SY, Harmany ZT, Todd A, et al. Microscopy with ultraviolet surface excitation (MUSE): a novel approach to real-time inexpensive slide-free dermatopathology. J Cutan Pathol. 2018;45(7):498–503.
64. Abels E, Pantanowitz L. Current state of the regulatory trajectory for whole slide imaging devices in the USA. J Pathol Inform. 2017;8(1):23.
65. Food and Drug Administration. 510(k) Substantial Equivalence Determination Decision Summary: K190332 [Internet]. Food and Drug Administration; 2019 [cited 2020 Aug 18]. Available from: https://www.accessdata.fda.gov/cdrh_docs/reviews/K190332.pdf.
66. Food and Drug Administration. De Novo Decision Summary: DEN160056 [Internet]. Food and Drug Administration; 2017 [cited 2020 Apr 27]. Available from: https://www.accessdata.fda.gov/cdrh_docs/reviews/DEN160056.pdf.
67. Abel JT, Ouillette P, Williams CL, Blau J, Cheng J, Yao K, et al. Display characteristics and their impact on digital pathology: a current review of pathologists' future "microscope". J Pathol Inform. 2020;11(1):23.
68. Samei E, Krupinski EA, editors. The handbook of medical image perception and techniques. 2nd ed. Cambridge; New York: Cambridge University Press; 2019. p. 522.
69. Food and Drug Administration. 510(k) Substantial Equivalence Determination Decision Summary: K193054 [Internet]. Food and Drug Administration; 2020 [cited 2020 Aug 18]. Available from: https://www.accessdata.fda.gov/cdrh_docs/reviews/K193054.pdf.
70. Food and Drug Administration. 510(k) Substantial Equivalence Determination Decision Summary: K172922 [Internet]. Food and Drug Administration; 2017 [cited 2020 Aug 18]. Available from: https://www.accessdata.fda.gov/cdrh_docs/reviews/K172922.pdf.
71. Business Wire. Paige Receives FDA Clearance for the FullFocus™ Viewer for Digital Pathology [Internet]. 2020 [cited 2020 Aug 18]. Available from: https://www.businesswire.com/news/home/20200721005369/en/Paige-Receives-FDA-Clearance-FullFocus%E2%84%A2-Viewer-Digital.

72. Food and Drug Administration. 510(k) Premarket Notification-Sectra Digital Pathology Module [Internet]. [cited 2020 Aug 18]. Available from: https://www.accessdata.fda.gov/scripts/cdrh/cfdocs/cfpmn/pmn.cfm?ID=K193054.
73. Norgan AP, Shah KK, Juskewitch JE, Maleszewski JJ. Open-source whole slide image preparation and viewing pipeline. Arch Pathol Lab Med. 2018;142(12):1454–5.
74. OpenSlide [Internet]. [cited 2020 Aug 18]. Available from: https://openslide.org/.
75. DPA: Digital Pathology Association [Internet]. [cited 2020 Aug 9]. Available from: https://digitalpathologyassociation.org/software-vendors.
76. Besson S, Leigh R, Linkert M, Allan C, Burel J-M, Carroll M, et al. Bringing open data to whole slide imaging. Digit Pathol 15th Eur Congr ECDP 2019 Warwick UK April 10–13 2019 Proc Eur Congr Digit Pathol 15th 2019 Warwick U K. 2019 Apr;2019:3–10.
77. Philips Teams up with Visiopharm to Boost Breast Cancer Diagnosis Objectivity Through Computational Pathology [Internet]. 2016 [cited 2020 Aug 18]. Available from: https://www.businesswire.com/news/home/20160621005195/en/Philips-Teams-Visiopharm-Boost-Breast-Cancer-Diagnosis.
78. Inspirata and IBEX Medical Analytics Announce New Technical Partnership at the European Congress of Pathology, Nice [Internet]. GlobeNewswire News Room. 2019 [cited 2020 Aug 18]. Available from: http://www.globenewswire.com/news-release/2019/09/09/1912498/0/en/Inspirata-and-IBEX-Medical-Analytics-Announce-New-Technical-Partnership-at-the-European-Congress-of-Pathology-Nice.html.
79. Evans AJ, Salama ME, Henricks WH, Pantanowitz L. Implementation of whole slide imaging for clinical purposes: issues to consider from the perspective of early adopters. Arch Pathol Lab Med. 2017;141(7):944–59.
80. University of Michigan Department of Pathology. Virtual Slide Box [Internet]. 2020 [cited 2020 Aug 18]. Available from: https://www.pathology.med.umich.edu/slides/.
81. Digital Pathology Association. Whole Slide Imaging Repository [Internet]. 2020 [cited 2020 Aug 18]. Available from: https://digitalpathologyassociation.org/whole-slide-imaging-repository.
82. Dumery B. Digital image archiving: challenges and choices. Radiol Manage. 2002;24(3):30–8; quiz 39–41
83. De Backer AI, Mortelé KJ, De Keulenaer BL. Picture archiving and communication systemspart one: filmless radiology and distance radiology. JBR-BTR. 2004;87(5):234–41.
84. Ortiz AO, Luyckx MP. Preparing a business justification for going electronic. Radiol Manage. 2002;24(1):14–21.
85. Bergh B. Enterprise imaging and multi-departmental PACS. Eur Radiol. 2006;16(12):2775–91.
86. Isaacs M, Lennerz JK, Yates S, Clermont W, Rossi J, Pfeifer JD. Implementation of whole slide imaging in surgical pathology: a value added approach. J Pathol Inform. 2011;2(1):39.
87. Ghaznavi F, Evans A, Madabhushi A, Feldman M. Digital imaging in pathology: whole-slide imaging and beyond. Annu Rev Pathol Mech Dis. 2013;8(1):331–59.
88. Business Wire. FDA Grants Breakthrough Designation to Paige.AI [Internet]. 2019 [cited 2020 Aug 18]. Available from: https://www.businesswire.com/news/home/20190307005205/en/FDA-Grants-Breakthrough-Designation-Paige.AI.
89. Topol EJ. High-performance medicine: the convergence of human and artificial intelligence. Nat Med. 2019;25(1):44–56.
90. Acs B, Rimm DL. Not just digital pathology, intelligent digital pathology. JAMA Oncol. 2018;4(3):403–4.
91. Niazi MKK, Parwani AV, Gurcan MN. Digital pathology and artificial intelligence. Lancet Oncol. 2019;20(5):e253–61.
92. Tizhoosh HR, Pantanowitz L. Artificial intelligence and digital pathology: challenges and opportunities. J Pathol Inform. 2018;9(1):38.
93. Definitions of the SI units: The twenty SI prefixes [Internet]. [cited 2020 Aug 18]. Available from: https://physics.nist.gov/cuu/Units/prefixes.html.
94. Seibert J. Archiving, Chapter 2: Medical Image Data Characteristics [Internet]. SIIM.org. [cited 2020 Aug 18]. Available from: https://siim.org/page/archiving_chapter2.

95. Philips. Pathology Remote Viewing IT requirements [Internet]. 2015 [cited 2020 Aug 18]. Available from: http://incenter.medical.philips.com/doclib/enc/fetch/2000/4504/577242/577260/593280/593786/452220726501_Pathology_Remote_viewing.pdf%3Fnodeid%3D11281278%26vernum%3D-2.
96. Alba D, Kang C. So We're Working From Home. Can the Internet Handle It? The New York Times [Internet]. 2020 Mar 16 [cited 2020 Aug 18]; Available from: https://www.nytimes.com/2020/03/16/technology/coronavirus-working-from-home-internet.html.
97. Gibson D. Hot, Warm and Cold Data Find a Home With Storage Groups [Internet]. 2012 [cited 2020 Aug 13]. Available from: https://ibmsystemsmag.com/Power-Systems/09/2012/storage-groups-hot-warm-cold.
98. Stansberry M. Explaining the Uptime Institute's Tier Classification System [Internet]. Uptime Institute Blog. 2014 [cited 2020 Aug 18]. Available from: https://journal.uptimeinstitute.com/explaining-uptime-institutes-tier-classification-system/.
99. Computer Security Resource Center. Disaster recovery plan (DRP), NIST [Internet]. [cited 2020 Aug 18]. Available from: https://csrc.nist.gov/glossary/term/disaster_recovery_plan.
100. College of American Pathologists. Anatomic Pathology Checklist. CAP Accreditation Program. College of American Pathologists. 2020.
101. Balis UGJ, Williams CL, Cheng J, Parwani A, McClintock DS. Whole-slide Imaging: thinking twice before hitting the delete key. AJSP Rev Rep. 2018;23(6):249–50.

Whole Slide Imaging: Applications

Sambit K. Mohanty and Anil V. Parwani

Introduction

Over the last 5 years, the concept and landscape of digital pathology has been revolutionized as new powerful and affordable scanners along with assisted technologic advancement, and mass- or cloud-based storage technologies have appeared in the market. The practice of pathology has been particularly impacted by the widespread use of whole slide imaging (WSI) [1–8]. The impact of the technology has resulted in many different applications including utility in education, research, and clinical arenas [9]. Pathologists have begun to realize the importance of digitized images rather than static images and have started the transition from viewing glass slides under the microscope to the computer monitor. Additionally, the virtual slides can be navigated and annotated seamlessly as glass slides using viewer software with many different tools and annotation capabilities [10, 11].

Two scanners have now received regulatory clearance of WSI for primary diagnosis in the United States leading to easing of some barriers to adoption of digital pathology, and others are in the pipeline. However, there are still some challenges to the widespread adoption [12]. Implementation of WSI remains a difficult prospect for many institutions, especially those with the stakeholders unfamiliar with the technologies necessary to implement a system or who cannot effectively communicate to executive leadership and sponsor the benefits of a technology that may lack clear and immediate reimbursement opportunity [13]. Adding to the abovementioned issues, there are several technical and logistic hindrances and barriers need to

S. K. Mohanty (✉)
Department of Pathology and Laboratory Medicine, Advanced Medical Research Institute, Bhubaneswar, Odisha, India

A. V. Parwani
Department of Pathology, College of Medicine, The Ohio State University Wexner Medical School, Columbus, OH, USA

A. V. Parwani (ed.), *Whole Slide Imaging*,
https://doi.org/10.1007/978-3-030-83332-9_3

be addressed before WSI platform becomes a widely accepted modality in the practice of pathology. For example, current scanning technology does not satisfactorily accommodate thick smears and three-dimensional cell groups in cytopathology [14, 15].

WSI can be categorized as bright-field, fluorescent, and multispectral. Some scanners can accommodate more than one modality, for example, enabling both bright-field and fluorescent scanning. Bright-field scanning emulates standard bright-field microscopy and is the most common and cost-effective approach. Fluorescent scanning is akin to fluorescent microscopy and is used to digitize fluorescently labeled slides (i.e., fluorescent immunohistochemistry [IHC], fluorescent in situ hybridization). Fluorescent scanners always capture images as tiles [16]. Multispectral imaging captures spectral information across the spectrum of light. It can be applied to both the bright-field and fluorescent settings [17]. Methods of focusing along the z-axis of a slide vary from focusing every individual tile or focusing on selected tiles to using a series of focus points [16].

Whole slide imaging offers an opportunity to expand the set of tools available to users to include digital annotation, rapid navigation/magnification, and computer-assisted viewing and analysis [18]. Typically, the intended use dictates the preferred method by which users will access whole slide images. For example, when whole slide images are used for educational purposes, instructors often need access to a dedicated image viewer that enables them to annotate images so that trainees can quickly identify and navigate to regions of interest in the slide [18]. Similarly, the use of WSI to support clinical diagnostics is often aided by the ability to view images in association with the patient's clinical history, or alongside other slides or images that may have been acquired from the same patient (e.g., serial sections, IHC, gross photos, radiology) [19, 20]. Some image viewing software supports advanced viewing tools, enabling users to simultaneously view multiple images in a single frame or overlay different stains from serial sections. Many WSI systems include image viewing software that can be installed locally on user computers. Other vendors offer this ability as part of a larger software suite residing on network servers, enabling users to view whole slide images in their web browsers [20]. For users who wish to apply image analysis algorithms to whole slide images, some of the viewers provided by vendors are packaged with algorithms that can detect cells, compute positive staining, perform regional segmentation, or perform nuclear segmentation in H&E images [21]. Viewers often support the ability to annotate images, save regions of interest, take snapshots of selected regions, and export images to other formats. For users who require more sophisticated image analysis algorithms than their vendor provides, a number of software solutions have hit the market with exceptional capabilities. These can often be integrated into a department's workflow in a seamless manner, providing on-demand image analysis in conjunction with whole slide viewing [18, 21, 22].

Regulation and Validation

In the United States, federal regulations set forth in the Food, Drug, and Cosmetic Act of 1938 and the Medical Device Amendments of 1976 provide the FDA with limited authority over medical devices. Some of these devices are subject to premarket review through 510(k) premarket notification process or premarket approval application (PMA). These US federal regulations pertain primarily to manufacturers of whole slide digital imaging systems and potentially also to laboratories that incorporate WSI in diagnostic services [11, 23, 24]. The FDA convened a panel hearing in October 2009 that focused on how best to regulate WSI systems that are to be used for primary diagnosis in surgical pathology [23, 25–27]. While WSI systems are clearly medical devices subject to FDA regulation, there are a number of open issues the FDA will need to address before the regulatory environment is clarified, and this is an ongoing issue. Some key milestones have been reached such as the approval of two systems for primary diagnosis use [25, 28]. Table 1 lists some of the specific validation issues raised by WSI. Evaluators must consider a range of issues that include sample size and statistical power, separating pathologist performance issues from device performance issues; the scope of cases to include in a challenge set, whether the set should be "enriched" with difficult cases; washout (time interval before asking a pathologist to review the same diagnostic material); the time it takes pathologists to become facile with WSI instruments; and the setting in which validation is assessed [5, 24, 28–35]. Table 2 lists some key considerations for WSI validation. Table 3 lists key clinical benefits of WSI.

Applications of Whole Slide Imaging

Healthcare facilities are witnessing tremendous digitization efforts with inclusion of digital imaging in medical specialities such as radiology connected to hospital information systems, laboratory information systems, picture archiving, and

Table 1 Issues to be considered while validating whole slide imaging for routine diagnostic application

1	Separating the device from the practitioner
2	Pathologist experience (in practice and with the device)
3	Washout and validation setting
4	Types of data generated
5	Measuring accuracy
6	Measuring bias
7	Measuring precision (intra-rater, inter-rater, and inter-instrument)
8	Sample size
9	Generalization of the observations

Table 2 Preferences for whole slide imaging validation for routine diagnostic application

1	Measure intra-observer bias and precision
2	Use general pathologists with defined device experience
3	Utilize high-quality display
4	Enrich the case sample (stack with difficult cases)
5	Washout period >2 weeks
6	Analyze each parameter separately (e.g., tumor type, tumor grade, etc.)
7	80% power to detect 10% difference in bias or precision
8	Generalize to all specimens except hematology, cytology, and dermatopathology

Table 3 Key clinical benefits of whole slide imaging

1	Whole slide imaging of selected or all slides from the cases submitted for consultation
2	Directly enhances patient care through the availability, portability, and permanence of the images for patient care conferences, e.g., tumor board
3	Provision of a quality assurance function
4	Whole slide imaging of slides that will be destroyed by ancillary testing
5	Whole slide imaging of slides that will be sent out to another institution
6	Whole slide imaging of medicolegal cases
7	Whole slide imaging of cases for digital image analysis for further study or biomarker validation

communication systems. Pathology laboratories equipped with WSI facility would fall into place well in such a setting with varied applications in diagnosis, education, and research [11, 20, 25, 28, 31, 36].

WSI in Education, Tumor Boards, Presentations, Quality Assurance, and Research

WSI has gained tremendous acceptance for education, at the tumor boards, and for presentations, research, and quality assurance (QA) [6, 8, 10, 20, 30, 37–52]. Digitized slides are more interactive than glass slides, easy to share anywhere at any time, and can help standardize training and research material. The successful use of WSI in undergraduate medical education and pathology resident and fellow training has been highlighted by several authors [48–54] including the creation of digital slide teaching sets [10, 42]. Unlike glass slide teaching sets, digital slides will not fade, break, or disappear. Digital slides also offer the ability to standardize images, permit annotation, and can provide a wide case range for trainees, including rare cases [53, 54]. Digital teaching sets that can be accessed on a server over a network are available to multiple users and can be developed to contain test modules for trainees. Not surprisingly, many medical schools are abandoning the light microscope.

Collaboration among students is easier with WSI, and this technology supports the creation of a virtual slide laboratory in medical schools. WSI also allows one to track how users view, pan, and zoom around a WSI [18, 55–57]. This function has been shown to be particularly helpful with respect to tutoring and assessing trainees, as well as for the development of image processing tools. WSI can also facilitate preparation and conduct of tumor boards through obviating the need of a multi-headed microscope or microscope with projection attachment or acquisition of multiple static images of a case [40, 42, 43]. It also had a positive impact on pathologists presenting cases at tumor boards in several institutions. This is because WSI offers higher quality images with annotation and greater educational value for clinicians, involves less preparation time than photographing cases, and permits real-time flexibility (e.g., easy to add on cases, perform side-by-side viewing, and give access to the entire slide which allows one to answer "on-the-spot" questions) [13]. WSI has also permeated into other areas such as E-education, virtual workshops, and for proficiency testing [58]. The use of this technology in QA programs in surgical pathology and cytopathology can help in cost cutting and overcoming transportation difficulties, as also minimizing the potential second reviewer bias by hiding the initial diagnosis [15, 19, 49, 59, 60]. Studies have also demonstrated the ease of same-day QA reviews with >90% diagnostic agreement. Thus, WSI collections can also be employed for pathology examinations and proficiency testing. For instance, the American Board of Pathology utilized 25 virtual slides along with 120 static digital images during a computer-based anatomic pathology examination. Online WSI resources such as CAP Virtual Slide Box, Digital Pathology Association-hosted repository, and the Cancer Digital Slide Archive offer virtual slide sets for training and learning purposes. Virtual slides are also being used in pathology conferences and meetings to promote interactive learning and provide ease of visualization of multiple images of different stains in conjunction with relevant clinical material [18]. WSI has attracted the attention of biotechnology and pharmaceutical companies because of the opportunity to understand spatial relationship of various biological phenotypes and assistance in development of immunohistochemistry-based biomarkers that can be utilized further in translational research studies. In conjunction with tissue microarrays, WSI with image analysis tools allows the researchers to assess and score the biomarkers across all specimens quickly and objectively. In instances of possible biomarker heterogeneity, fluorescent WSI or multispectral imaging facilitates multiplexed analysis and supports further biomarker or drug discovery. This technology can also be employed in development of oncologic biomarker strategies with augmented throughput and quantitative accuracy, hence supporting drug discovery. Since advanced WSI scanners can function with transmitted light as well as fluorescent modes, their range of applications in research is radical. Electronic publication of textbooks and articles in scientific journals has also opened new panoramas of scientific communication [61]. Utilization of WSI-generated high-quality virtual images has proven to be the single most upgrade for pathology journals, thus empowering the readers to be involved in a scientifically based diagnostic approach to the lesion described [8].

WSI in Primary Frozen Section/Intraoperative Consultation/ Diagnosis

WSI in recent years has been effectively utilized by several groups for telepathology, including primary frozen section diagnosis and secondary/tertiary teleconsultation [1, 10, 30, 40, 46, 56, 62–68]. The advantages include access to an entire digitized slide or even an entire case (set of slides), automated scanning, the high resolution of images available for review, rapid interpretation time, and the ability of teleconferencing.

An example of using WSI in intraoperative consultation is described below. The University Health Network (UHN) in Ontario, Canada, has extensive experience using WSI for telepathology, particularly in frozen section assessment [26, 40].

UHN is a multi-site academic institution comprising the Princess Margaret Hospital (PMH), Toronto Western Hospital (TWH), and Toronto General Hospital (TGH) which houses UHN's consolidated pathology department. TWH has no on-site pathologist and is located approximately one mile to the west of TGH. It is also the only UHN site where neurosurgery is performed, generating up to ten frozen sections in a typical week [29]. By sending a single pathologist to TWH to cover this small volume of frozen sections, most of which come from neurosurgery, created several challenges including delays in regular case sign-out at TGH, delays in carrying out academic responsibilities at TGH, and no possibility of consulting with colleagues on difficult frozen sections. The latter issue created the risk of compromised diagnostic accuracy and/or unnecessarily deferred frozen section diagnoses. Telepathology was identified as a viable solution to these challenges and has been in use at UHN for over 7 years [26, 29, 40].

At UHN, a team that consisted of a pathologist, a senior histotechnologist, and an information technology (IT) support person was formed in 2003 to select a digital pathology vendor, validate the system to be used for frozen section diagnosis, train new users, and carry out due diligence that included consultation with the medical malpractice insurance provider, development of a protocol for approval by UHN's Medical Advisory Committee, and engagement of the surgeons at TWH. After an 18-month development period, the system went live in November of 2004 initially using a robotic microscope (Leica TPS2, Leica Microsystems) for making frozen section diagnoses at TWH in the absence of an on-site pathologist. Since October 2006, UHN pathologists have used WSI to make over 1800 primary frozen section diagnoses in the absence of an on-site pathologist. WSI has provided diagnostic accuracy that is equivalent to that experienced with light microscopy and facilitates the reporting of single block frozen sections with total TATs in the range of 14–16 min. They have experienced a 5% deferral rate with at least two pathologists reviewing the case before a deferred diagnosis is given, a quality measure that is not possible with a lone on-site pathologist reporting frozen sections by light microscopy [29, 40].

Several factors have contributed to the success of the UHN program including a well-defined clinical application in the form of a small volume of neuropathology frozen sections, an uncomplicated frozen section workflow where most cases involve single pieces of tissue <10 mm in size, an implementation period of approximately 18 months that allowed all team members to build confidence in the system, and a team approach involving pathologists, histotechnologists, IT support staff, vendors, and surgeons committed to making the program work. It has been the UHN experience that consistently high-quality frozen section slides produced by a skilled histotechnologist are an absolute requirement in order to have image quality that is sufficient to allow reliable frozen section diagnoses to be made via WSI. System failure, requiring a pathologist to travel from TGH to TWH to report a frozen section, has occurred on six occasions (0.3% of cases) with a 15-min delay in TAT for the affected cases [65].

A high concordance rate between WSI-based frozen section and permanent section diagnosis or on-site interpretation has been demonstrated in several studies [11, 14, 69, 70]. However, further studies on a range of pathologies from various organ systems are required to validate the utility and limitations of WSI. Successful implementation requires effective planning and communication, a willingness to adjust old routines without compromising quality, and histotechnologists who are able to provide consistently high-quality frozen section slides [26, 71–75].

WSI in Routine Pathological Diagnosis

WSI is increasingly being used in the day-to-day practice of surgical pathology, particularly for teleconsultation [12, 21, 30, 76–82]. Digitized slides have been used for certain quality assurance practices, such as obtaining second opinions. However, the question on most pathologists' minds is whether WSI will be utilized for making routine pathologic diagnoses, ushering in the era of the "slideless" laboratory. This has been a particularly important challenge during the COVID-19 pandemic [43, 69, 83]. The adoption of digital pathology has been slower than the adoption of digital images in radiology [21, 76, 84, 85]. This is partly related to the fact that pathology digital data is acquired in a slightly different manner from that in radiology. Although both disciplines require an imaging modality to collect primary data, in radiology, images begin as *digital* data, whereas pathology images have to be converted from an *analog* substrate into a digital format [84, 85]. Other differences between radiology and pathology digital imaging are the picture archiving systems (i.e., Picture Archiving and Communication System or PACS) and associated standards (e.g., Digital Imaging and Communications in Medicine or DICOM) available for radiology, larger file size, and associated metadata of pathology digital image files and workflow efficiencies in radiology [33, 36]. Some of the barriers to the adoption of digital pathology images are related to the performance, workflow efficiency, infrastructure, integration with other software, and exposure to digital images [85]. Despite significant increases in technology, current adoption of WSI in the clinical space has been slower and limited largely to niche practices or in academic settings [1, 10, 86].

The general pathology laboratory at Kalmar County Hospital in Kalmar, Sweden, is unique in that for around 2 years they have been digitizing all of their glass slides [2, 87]. They scan around 60,000 histopathology slides per year, and over 75% of their histopathology diagnostic work is performed using digital pathology. Their impetus to go "slideless" was related to ergonomics as well as the need to network with colleagues in a country where there was a shortage of pathologists. Essential requirements for their success included full integration with the digital pathology system and laboratory information system (LIS), reliable scanning, running the slide scanner continually with limited use of lab personnel, and good image quality. Obtaining consultations on their difficult cases in a timely manner was greatly facilitated through digital slide sharing and conferencing [11]. More institutions are following suit; for example, at the Ohio State University, routine use of WSI is increasing in adoption, and several pathologists have transitioned to a digital sign-out [43]. Several other institutes are implementing a digital sign-out process [2, 11, 60, 87–89].

Rendering routine pathologic diagnoses using WSI is feasible if the images truly represent an accurate digital reproduction of the scanned glass slide which can be saved, archived, reviewed, and later retrieved without degradation of the image [90–92]. Moreover, apart from integration with the LIS, the routine use of WSI in pathology laboratories will require seamless connectivity over broadband networks, efficient workstations, cost-effective storage solutions, and standards-based informatics transactions for integrating information with WSI [66, 78, 93]. It is difficult to think of WSI for diagnostic purposes without considering the rest of the electronic medical record. It seems unlikely that pathologists will render diagnoses without access to additional medical information [94]. One of the reasons for reported discrepancies between digital and glass slide diagnoses is attributed to inadequate clinical data, apart from other factors such as image quality, missed tissue on the digital slide, and the pathologists' lack of experience using a WSI system [95]. It was demonstrated in one telepathology study using a virtual slide system that the correct diagnosis was made in 66% of cases without clinical data provided compared to a correct diagnosis of 76% with clinical data provided [95, 96]. Therefore, in order for WSI to become an accepted diagnostic modality, the provision of adequate medical information (e.g., gross pathology description, prior pathology reports, clinical history, imaging and other relevant laboratory parameters, etc.) will need to be weaved into the imaging system [86, 97, 98]. Additional concerns that have yet to be satisfactorily addressed relate to malpractice and liability issues, as well as reimbursement for technical services related to producing the WSI [78, 98, 99].

Digital slides offer several advantages over glass slide review in terms of fidelity of the diagnostic material, portability, ease of sharing and retrieval of archival images, and ability to make use of computer-aided diagnostic tools (e.g., image algorithms) [1, 9, 11, 73, 100–102]. Image analysis tools can automate or quantify with greater consistency and accuracy than light microscopy [103, 104]. WSI has also permitted new business models of care in pathology [12]. One such example is the virtual IHC service provided by large national laboratories. After the remote reference laboratory performs technical staining and slide scanning services, the referring pathologist is provided with full access to these IHC slides for their interpretation or referral to a teleconsultant [10]. This has allowed some pathology practices to recapture a portion of the reimbursement for professional interpretation services that has previously been diminished by these business practices [13]. In the near future, the adoption of standards, validation guidelines, automation of workflow, creation of new revenue streams, and nuances of clinical digital practice will likely dictate a new standard of care for primary pathologic interpretations [14, 29, 30, 45, 105–107].

WSI and Immunohistochemistry and Electron Microscopy

WSI offers advantages in enhancing objectivity in the interpretation of IHC used in tumor diagnosis, prognosis, and evaluation of biomarkers for targeted therapy [63, 82, 101, 108]. A concordance of 90% or greater between WSI and glass slides of HER2/neu expression in breast cancer has been reported [101]. Application of automated image analysis with algorithm-based scoring for the prognostic markers can assist in improving the scoring protocols and thereby enhance the efficacy of targeted therapies [101]. Also in electron microscopy, virtual ultrathin slide allows the pathologists to navigate the slide in their office while noting the exact location of the specific features. Apart from this, WSI technology can be valuable for obtaining consultation on ultrathin sections from experts located in higher centers [109].

WSI and Cytopathology The role of WSI and adoption in cytopathology continues to increase [15, 110–113]. There are some understandable obstacles such as the inherent complexity of scanning, higher scanning time, and storage costs. The scanning of cytology smear is difficult as well as complex because of its three-dimensional character [111]. Consequently, it is essential to integrate z-stacking or multiplane scanning feature into the systems intended for use in cytopathology [113, 114]. The z-stacking can be avoided by multiplane scanning and use of the best focused image at each tile into the final file. Alternative approach that has been recently attempted includes the conversion of z-stacks of images into video frames and storing the stack as a high-efficiency video coding file(s). Subsequent video compression has demonstrated to exceed the JPEG compression with comparable image quality [115]. There have been a few studies on the use of WSI in cytopathology. A comparison of conventional glass slides and WSI in 10 cervical and 20 non-gynecologic cytology cases showed similar diagnostic concordance between the two modalities among the reviewing cytopathologists [116, 117].

Another recent study comparing WSI with glass slides of thin-layer cervical specimens demonstrated 95.3% concordance rates, paving the way for WSI use in routine cytologic diagnosis [112]. Wright et al., in their study, evaluated the efficiency of WSI in cervicovaginal cytology and highlighted issues such as a lack of familiarity with the technology, difficulty for the WSI in detecting few abnormal cells in the smears, problems with hyperchromatic nuclei, dark and crowded groups of cells, and massive image file size leading to increased duration of scanning. Another issue that is probably unique and intrinsic to cytology is the inability of the whole slide scanners to scan the edges of the coverslip [118]. The quality of WSI images when applied to cytology smears is fraught with certain problems that are not encountered in the histology sections, such as (a) presence of dense overlapping tissue fragments making it difficult for scanners to focus on the cells, (b) red cell contamination of the smear and/or background acellular material(s) leading the scanner to focus on red cells and/or the background material rather than the cells of interest, (c) smears with scant cellularity making z-stacking difficult, and (d) need to remove the screening marks/dots before scanning (for which keeping a photographic record of the diagnostic screening marks is recommended) [119]. Papanicolaou- and H&E-stained smears, due to their wet fixation, often have cells in multiple planes and thus require z-scanning to obtain a crisp and high-quality image. On the other hand, air-dried Romanowsky-stained smears can be scanned with only x and y-axes, as air drying flattens the cells thus minimizing the requirement of z-stacking [119, 120].

The need of WSI in cytopathology is immense. Given the ongoing need for a cytological diagnosis, the trend may possibly increase in future as minimally invasive procedures to obtain material for genetic/molecular analysis are used [117]. Furthermore, there will be shortage of suitably trained cytopathologists. All these most likely increase the need for WSI in cytology. Intuitively, the possibility to scan whole slides and to organize them in structured databases accessible via the Internet would represent a powerful educational resource. Every glass slide, particularly in cytopathology, is "unique and not repeatable." The examples of rare cases can be shared without the risk of stain fading or loss or breakage of slide(s). It is increasingly obvious that digital scanning can provide a more standardized setting for testing and assessing, as experienced by some National External Quality Assurance Schemes in the British National Health System. Moreover cytology cases are often unique, and it is very difficult to provide multiple sets of exactly similar cytological preparations, typically aspiration cytology rather than exfoliative cytology. A selected list of websites, with public or restricted access, including cytopathology teaching resources, is as follows:

- http://www.bsccp.org.uk/, http://www.eurocytology.eu, http://www.cytest.eu/, http://www.cytology-asc.com/, http://www.cytology-iac.org/http://www.cytologyiac.org/educationalresources/virtual-slide-library, http://www.cytologystuff.com/,http://www.cytopathology.org/, http://www.cytology.cloud/gk/,
- http://www.papsociety.org/index.html, http://www.tasteproject.eu/, http://www.uscap.org/, http://www.viewsiq.com, https://bethesda.soc.wisc.edu/
- http://nih.techriver.net/, http://icytology.wordpress.com/, http://pathhsw5m54.ucsf.edu/introduction.html, http://pathorama.ch/, http://screening.iarc.fr/, http://www.virtualpathology.leeds.ac.uk/slides/, http://137.189.150.85/cytopathology/

WSI in Artificial Intelligence

Education

WSI is already used for teaching at conferences, virtual workshops, presentations, and tumor boards [25, 49, 91, 121]. Equipped with whole slide imaging, artificial intelligence (AI) tools can help further training of the next generation of pathologists by providing on-demand, standardized, and interactive digital slides that can be shared with multiple users anywhere, at any time [4, 122, 123]. Additionally, AI tools can provide automated annotations in the form of quizzes for trainees. With the help of these interactive tools, trainees can view, pan, and zoom enhanced digital slides, which can provide tutoring in real time and in a dynamic teaching environment. For the purpose of generating synthetic images, researchers extracted individual and clustered nuclei that were both positively and negatively stained from real whole slide imaging images and systematically placed the extracted nuclei clumps on an image canvas – cut-and-paste approach. These images were evaluated by trained pathologists in the task of estimating the ratio of positive to total number of nuclei. The resulting concordance correlation coefficients between the pathologist and the true ratio range from 0.86 to 0.95 [103].

In the follow-up study, the conditional Generative Adversarial Networks approach was used. This method included two main components: the generator and the discriminator. Although the generator tries to create fake stained images, the discriminator tries to catch these fake images, each getting better at generating and detecting fake stained images in an iterative manner. The main idea is to force the generator to learn the underlying distribution of the images from the training data. The accuracy of five experts (three pathologists and two image analysts) in distinguishing between 15 real and 15 synthetic images was only 47.3% (±SD 8.5%). Generation of numerous synthetic histopathology images could be useful for educational purposes because it will give pathology trainees the opportunity to test their skills. Additionally, these approaches can be very useful for quality control and understanding the perceptual and cognitive challenges that pathologists face [9, 103].

Quality Assurance

The development of automated, high-speed, and high-resolution WSI has a substantial effect on QA. Digitized slides that are readily available to pathologists in the LIS or on the intranet can be used for several QA tasks, including teleconsultation, gauging inter-observer and intra-observer variance, proficiency testing, and archiving of slides [24, 37, 124–126]. For example, the CAP optionally sends WS images in addition to glass slides of certain proficiency testing cases. AI can have an important role in QA. By providing feedback manually or with intelligent deep learning and AI tools, a pathologist has the potential to keep improving on his or her performance. AI can be used as a supplement to these manual digital reviews in routine diagnostic workflow or as a complement to the more formal quality reviews that are part of a pathology laboratory's quality management process. AI can also provide a quality check on the diagnosis rendered by a pathologist by applying automated diagnostic algorithms prospectively or retrospectively. These methods can continue to serve as patient safety mechanisms to improve the quality of diagnosis and to prevent error [9].

Pathological Diagnosis

Rendering routine pathological diagnoses using WSI is a feasible approach. Several studies have shown a range of concordance from 89% to 99% when comparing diagnostic interpretation using digital slides to diagnoses rendered using glass slides and a conventional light microscope [1, 4, 10, 17, 22, 35, 58, 66, 92, 127, 128]. The range is wide and encompasses multiple organ systems and different types of specimen preparations. AI could improve on current solutions by detecting of out-of-focus areas and improving color standardization [68, 129]. The quality of images produced by WSI scanners has a direct influence on the readers' performance and their reliability of diagnosis. Most modern scanners come equipped with autofocus optics system to select focal planes to accurately capture the three-dimensional tissue morphology similar to a two-dimensional digital image [10]. To account for varying thickness of tissue sections, autofocus optics systems determine a set of focus points at different focal planes. From these focal planes, scanners capture images to produce sharp tissue representation. However, WSI scanners could still produce digital images with out-of-focus areas if the autofocus optics system erroneously selects focus points that lie in a different plane than the proper height of the tissue. A naive solution would be to add several extra focus points, but that would be impractical because it would cause long delays in slide scanning [10, 17]. AI provides a better alternative by automatically identifying out-of-focus regions and allowing WSI scanners to add a few extra focal points to those regions. AI achieves this by either feature engineering or via a representation learning approach. Lopez and colleagues have adopted a feature engineering approach by handcrafting texture features from gray-level co-occurrence matrices and gradient information. These features were used in conjunction with decision trees to classify 200 × 200 pixel-sized regions as focused or blurred. Unfortunately, the method is only sensitive to a high level of blurriness, and it requires modifying program parameters to adapt it to images acquired at different resolutions. Another approach called DeepFocus [130], based on representation learning, automatically discovers features from the images to identify blurry regions. Because the DeepFocus program automatically learns features at different levels of abstraction, it can generalize to different types of tissues and even to color variations due to different types of staining, H&E and IHC. Standardization of the color displayed by digital slides is important for the accuracy of AI. Color variations in digital slides are often produced because of different lots or manufacturers of staining reagents, variations in thickness of tissue sections, difference in staining protocols, and disparity in scanning characteristics. These variations often impose obstacles to the diagnosis and prognosis done by humans, as well as by machines. Moreover, these variations are one of the main hurdles in generalization of the machine learning algorithms to multiple sites. For this reason, the absence of color normalization in an AI pipeline could negatively affect the performance of machine learning algorithms. Despite all these challenges, the future looks at a world where AI algorithms will play a major role in pathology diagnosis, either by prescreening cases, by finding rare events in histology slides/images, or by helping with the multiple aspects of the complex diagnostic process [103].

Image Analysis

Image analysis tools can automate and quantify with greater consistency and accuracy than light microscopy [101, 131, 132]. Computer-aided diagnosis is widely used for ER, PR, and HER2/neu assessments in breast cancer [133, 134], Ki67 assessment in neuroendocrine neoplasms [135, 136], and PD-L1 as immune checkpoint molecules in various solid organ malignancies, as well as multiple other clinical and research stains. The reliability of these methods requires the standardization of the image acquisition step. The development of WSI has facilitated large growth in numerous researchers and companies seeking to use computer-aided diagnoses to analyze whole-stain imaging and to develop new software tools to assist pathologists. AI methods aid in enabling the regions of interest selection [137–139]. Nuclear segmentation in WSI enables extraction of high-quality features for nuclear morphometrics and other analysis in computational pathology [103]. For this reason, automatic nuclei segmentation is among the most studied problems in AI. In general, these algorithms estimate a probability map of the nuclear and nonnuclear (two-class) regions on the basis of learned nuclear appearances and rely on complex methods after processing to obtain the final nuclear shapes and separation between touching nuclei [140]. For example, Song and colleagues have used a multiscale convolutional network to generate a nuclear probability map. This map was subjected to graph partitioning to segment individual nuclei from the image. Moreover, these methods also do not generalize if the training and test images belong to different organs. To overcome these issues, there is a growing trend to train the nuclei segmentation methods on images taken from different organs. Kumar and colleagues have created a well-annotated database consisting of 30 whole slide images of digitized tissue samples from several organs. The slides were taken from the publically available database the Cancer Genome Atlas. The images were generated at 18 different hospitals, which add to the diversity of this dataset in terms of variation in slide preparation protocols among laboratories. Over 21,000 nuclei were manually annotated to train a deep learning algorithm. Unlike former methods, a nuclei segmentation as a three-class problem was created. They considered the nuclei edges as a third class when generating the tertiary probability map. This map was subjected to region growing to segment the individual nuclei [141].

During most pathological analysis, pathologists are interested in identifying a subset of nuclei in a particular anatomical region. For example, in T1 bladder cancer [123], pathologists are interested in identifying the tumor nuclei within the lamina propria. Similarly, in breast and neuroendocrine tumors, the pathologists are interested in the ratio of Ki67 tumor positive nuclei to total tumor nuclei within the hotspots. In follicular lymphoma, the analysis is limited to only the presence of centroblasts within the neoplastic follicles. For these reasons, there is an increasing interest in developing AI algorithms that can identify a subset of cells within a certain anatomical region. Also, whole slide is partitioned into superpixels on the basis of similarity at some magnification. Superpixels are grouped into anatomical regions (specifically epithelium) on the basis of graph clustering. Finally, each cluster is classified as ductal carcinoma in situ or benign or normal on the basis of features extracted by deep learning [138, 142, 143].

Caveats and Challenges of WSI

In order to integrate WSI into routine clinical pathology practice, an infrastructure needs to be developed in the pathology department [9, 11, 43, 60, 69, 71, 117]. This infrastructure consists of (i) hardware for scanning slides and storing the scanned images, transmission of the images to pathologists, and the interfaces necessary to display the images and report interpretations and (ii) software to facilitate the workflow of the image movement, display, and reporting of the results. Following development of the internal infrastructure, the addition of remote teleconsultation requires that other features be considered in the system. These include security of protected patient information, process validation, as well as regulatory, medicolegal, and billing issues all to be added to the software overlay. Additionally, it is prudent to acknowledge that many unresolved issues, as outlined below, still need to be addressed before WSI finds its place in routine application across the wide specialty of pathology [11, 40].

Cost

The cost of procurement, implementation, and operational costs of WSI may be prohibitive, especially for small pathology laboratories due to huge initial cost of the scanners and additional hidden costs of training of staff and pathologists, technical support, digital slide storage systems, and regulatory or licensing costs [1, 10]. Technological support for telepathology further compounds these costs. A recently published cost-benefit analysis at a large-volume academic center with slides in excess of 1.5 million showed a projected $1.3 million savings over a 5-year period [60]. However, the same analysis needs to be undertaken for smaller laboratories and low-resource settings.

Technological Issues

While considering the implementation of WSI, it must be kept in mind that the WSI images would be only as good as the original glass slide. Scanning the whole slide/smear is a tedious and time-consuming process at present. Scanning times can vary from 1 to 5 min for a small biopsy to 5–20 min for a surgical specimen and 3–5 min for a liquid-based cytology smear [68]. This time can further go up to hour(s) for multiplane or z-stacked scanning. Another limitation with currently available scanners is the requirement of massive data storage capacity. Scanning at × 40 magnification of a 1-mm^2 area results in a file size of 48 megabytes. Hence, majority of the WSI systems incorporate image compression algorithms (JPEG, JPEG 2000, and LZW) to reduce the file size. However, image compression introduces image artifacts. Some scanners offer the ability of multi-resolution representation (pyramid representation) where the field of view on the screen is inversely proportional to the magnification being viewed [10]. Majority of the WSI systems utilize a content management system (CMS) with specific programming in order to display the virtual slides in a consistent and specific manner [10]. Currently, there are vendor-dependent limitations with WSI systems. Some vendors use proprietary modules with limited scope of cross-browser compatibility or seamless execution on multiple devices.

Professional Barriers

Unlike radiology where digital systems obviate the need of making films, WSI in pathology does not reduce the laboratory's workload since glass slides still need to be prepared to be scanned. However, WSI does allow for streamlined navigation of the slides at various magnifications without the fear of accidentally breaking a slide at the microscope. The current WSI systems allow for batch-wise scanning of slides, thus improving the efficiency of the laboratory [10, 27, 144].

Other commonly encountered issues include available bandwidth of the network at the pathologists' workplace, security issues related to information technology, and installation of compatible browsers. However, with progress in information technology, the systems shall continue to be upgraded for improved speed and compatibility with browsers [69].

The FDA approval of WSI in primary surgical pathology diagnosis does open up the issue of legal implications for the reporting pathologists, as discussed earlier. The relevant regulatory agencies (such as CLIA) need to put forth their guidelines in light of the expected changes with adoption of WSI by pathologists.

Regulatory Issues

Since the FDA has accorded its approval for use of WSI scanner in surgical pathology practice in 2018, significant to tread towards this goal. At the same time, validation of WSI for introduction into the surgical pathology practice has recommendation of the CAP. Regulations also need to be put in place regarding the archiving, retrieval, and access rights of the virtual slide library so formed [23, 27, 144].

Conclusions

This is an exciting era in diagnostic pathology. The use of whole slide scanning combined with computational pathology is an area which is heralding rapid technologic development with multiple innovations and applications knocking on the door. This coupled with the promise of artificial intelligence, pathology is poised for new discoveries and solutions [4, 101]. Despite the advantages and claims of its non-inferiority compared with conventional microscopy, the adoption of this technique has been slow even in the developed nations. However, rapid strides have been taken to overcome several of the barriers referred to in this chapter. Some of these impediments may be overcome by collaborations between a reference laboratory equipped with a WSI system and smaller laboratories, through a hub-and-spoke model. Apart from the technical and cost-related issues, regulatory and validation requirements also need to be adequately addressed, especially for the developing nations. Nevertheless, WSI provide a unique opportunity for pathologists to guide its evolution, standardization, and implementation by playing a key role in defining/refining guidelines, designing the resource specific digital pathology laboratories, and propagating standardized educational modules to train the next generation of virtual pathologists.

Some key advancements to enhance adoption include the following:

1. Availability of high-resolution three-dimensional imaging, especially for tumors, would improve the use of this technology with correlation between radiologic imaging and WSI.
2. Multispectral imaging, when applied to WSI, would offer the ability to characterize chromatic properties and support color-based classification and multi-labeling studies [68].
3. Adoption of Digital Imaging and Communications in Medicine (DICOM) standards by the WSI vendors would allow vendor-neutral interoperability [33].
4. Refinement of artificial intelligence and machine learning algorithms would allow the pathologists contribute in a larger role in improving patient management and outcomes [40].

Overall, WSI technology is now mature and ready for prime time. There are many established applications of WSI as outlined in this chapter. WSI combined with the use of AI tools will usher in a new era of renewed adoption and widespread use of these tools for clinical diagnostics. Applications of artificial intelligence and machine learning techniques such as deep neural networks may be trained to not only recognize specific patterns on a whole slide image of an H&E slide, but in addition AI tools may also help in the interpretation of features in the tissue that are predictive and/or prognostic and advance the care of the patient.

References

1. Parwani AV. Next generation diagnostic pathology: use of digital pathology and artificial intelligence tools to augment a pathological diagnosis. Diagn Pathol. 2019;14:138.
2. Thorstenson S, Molin J, Lundstrom C. Implementation of large-scale routine diagnostics using whole slide imaging in Sweden: digital pathology experiences 2006-2013. J Pathol Inform. 2014;5:14.
3. Pantanowitz L, Sharma A, Carter AB, et al. Twenty years of digital pathology: an overview of the road travelled, what is on the horizon, and the emergence of vendor-neutral archives. J Pathol Inform. 2018;9:40.
4. Parwani AV. Digital pathology enhances cancer diagnostics. MLO Med Lab Obs. 2017;49:25.
5. Ordi J, Castillo P, Saco A, et al. Validation of whole slide imaging in the primary diagnosis of gynaecological pathology in a University Hospital. J Clin Pathol. 2015;68:33–9.
6. Saco A, Bombi JA, Garcia A, et al. Current status of whole-slide imaging in education. Pathobiology. 2016;83:79–88.
7. Borowsky AD, Glassy EF, Wallace WD, et al. Digital whole slide imaging compared with light microscopy for primary diagnosis in surgical pathology. Arch Pathol Lab Med. 2020;144:1245–53.
8. Glassy EF. Rebooting the pathology journal: learning in the age of digital pathology. Arch Pathol Lab Med. 2014;138:728–9.
9. Parwani AV, Amin MB. Convergence of digital pathology and artificial intelligence tools in anatomic pathology practice: current landscape and future directions. Adv Anat Pathol. 2020;27:221–6.
10. Zarella MD, Bowman D, Aeffner F, et al. A practical guide to whole slide imaging: a white paper from the digital pathology association. Arch Pathol Lab Med. 2019;143:222–34.
11. Hanna MG, Parwani A, Sirintrapun SJ. Whole slide imaging: technology and applications. Adv Anat Pathol. 2020;27:251–9.
12. Parwani A. Overcoming barriers to digital pathology. MLO Med Lab Obs. 2016;48:38.
13. Ho J, Ahlers SM, Stratman C, et al. Can digital pathology result in cost savings? A financial projection for digital pathology implementation at a large integrated health care organization. J Pathol Inform. 2014;5:33.
14. Farris AB, Cohen C, Rogers TE, Smith GH. Whole slide imaging for analytical anatomic pathology and telepathology: practical applications today, promises, and perils. Arch Pathol Lab Med. 2017;141:542–50.
15. Cucoranu IC, Parwani AV, Pantanowitz L. Digital whole slide imaging in cytology. Arch Pathol Lab Med. 2014;138:300.
16. Indu M, Rathy R, Binu MP. "Slide less pathology": fairy tale or reality? J Oral Maxillofac Pathol. 2016;20:284–8.
17. Higgins C. Applications and challenges of digital pathology and whole slide imaging. Biotech Histochem. 2015;90:341–7.
18. Pantanowitz L, Szymas J, Yagi Y, Wilbur D. Whole slide imaging for educational purposes. J Pathol Inform. 2012;3:46.
19. Pantanowitz L, Wiley CA, Demetris A, et al. Experience with multimodality telepathology at the University of Pittsburgh Medical Center. J Pathol Inform. 2012;3:45.
20. Park S, Pantanowitz L, Parwani AV. Digital imaging in pathology. Clin Lab Med. 2012;32:557–84.
21. Isaacs M, Lennerz JK, Yates S, et al. Implementation of whole slide imaging in surgical pathology: a value added approach. J Pathol Inform. 2011;2:39.

22. Saco A, Diaz A, Hernandez M, et al. Validation of whole-slide imaging in the primary diagnosis of liver biopsies in a University Hospital. Dig Liver Dis. 2017;49:1240–6.
23. Parwani AV, Hassell L, Glassy E, Pantanowitz L. Regulatory barriers surrounding the use of whole slide imaging in the United States of America. J Pathol Inform. 2014;5:38.
24. Ho J, Aridor O, Glinski DW, et al. Needs and workflow assessment prior to implementation of a digital pathology infrastructure for the US Air Force Medical Service. J Pathol Inform. 2013;4:32.
25. Evans AJ, Bauer TW, Bui MM, et al. US Food and Drug Administration Approval of whole slide imaging for primary diagnosis: a key milestone is reached and new questions are raised. Arch Pathol Lab Med. 2018;142:1383–7.
26. Evans AJ, Kiehl TR, Croul S. Frequently asked questions concerning the use of whole-slide imaging telepathology for neuropathology frozen sections. Semin Diagn Pathol. 2010;27:160–6.
27. Abels E, Pantanowitz L. Current state of the regulatory trajectory for whole slide imaging devices in the USA. J Pathol Inform. 2017;8:23.
28. Pantanowitz L, Sinard JH, Henricks WH, et al. Validating whole slide imaging for diagnostic purposes in pathology: guideline from the College of American Pathologists Pathology and Laboratory Quality Center. Arch Pathol Lab Med. 2013;137:1710–22.
29. Evans AJ, Vajpeyi R, Henry M, Chetty R. Establishment of a remote diagnostic histopathology service using whole slide imaging (digital pathology). J Clin Pathol. 2021;74(7):421–4.
30. Romero Lauro G, Cable W, Lesniak A, et al. Digital pathology consultations-a new era in digital imaging, challenges and practical applications. J Digit Imaging. 2013;26:668–77.
31. Hanna MG, Reuter VE, Ardon O, et al. Validation of a digital pathology system including remote review during the COVID-19 pandemic. Mod Pathol. 2020;33(11):2115–27.
32. Jukic DM, Drogowski LM, Martina J, Parwani AV. Clinical examination and validation of primary diagnosis in anatomic pathology using whole slide digital images. Arch Pathol Lab Med. 2011;135:372–8.
33. Clunie D, Hosseinzadeh D, Wintell M, et al. Digital imaging and communications in medicine whole slide imaging connectathon at digital pathology association pathology visions 2017. J Pathol Inform. 2018;9:6.
34. Yagi Y. Color standardization and optimization in whole slide imaging. Diagn Pathol. 2011; 6 Suppl 1: S15.
35. Wack K, Drogowski L, Treloar M, et al. A multisite validation of whole slide imaging for primary diagnosis using standardized data collection and analysis. J Pathol Inform. 2016;7:49.
36. Singh R, Chubb L, Pantanowitz L, Parwani A. Standardization in digital pathology: supplement 145 of the DICOM standards. J Pathol Inform. 2011;2:23.
37. Ho J, Parwani AV, Jukic DM, et al. Use of whole slide imaging in surgical pathology quality assurance: design and pilot validation studies. Hum Pathol. 2006;37:322–31.
38. Hartman DJ. Whole-slide imaging: clinical workflows and primary diagnosis. Adv Anat Pathol. 2020;27:236–40.
39. Hartman DJ, Parwani AV, Cable B, et al. Pocket pathologist: a mobile application for rapid diagnostic surgical pathology consultation. J Pathol Inform. 2014;5:10.
40. Volynskaya Z, Evans AJ, Asa SL. Clinical applications of whole-slide imaging in anatomic pathology. Adv Anat Pathol. 2017;24:215–21.
41. Pantanowitz L, Parwani AV, Khalbuss WE. Digital imaging for cytopathology: are we there yet? Cytopathology. 2011;22:73–4.
42. Li L, Dangott BJ, Parwani AV. Development and use of a genitourinary pathology digital teaching set for trainee education. J Pathol Inform. 2010;1:2.
43. Scarl RT, Parwani A, Yearsley M. From glass-time to screen-time. Arch Pathol Laeb Med. 2021;145:644.
44. Singh A, Monroe R. Diagnosis for digital pathology. MLO Med Lab Obs. 2009;41:28–9.
45. Yoshida H, Yokota H, Singh R, et al. Meeting report: the international workshop on harmonization and standardization of digital pathology image, held on April 4, 2019 in Tokyo. Pathobiology. 2019;86:322–4.

46. Girolami I, Parwani A, Barresi V, et al. The landscape of digital pathology in transplantation: from the beginning to the virtual E-slide. J Pathol Inform. 2019;10:21.
47. Rhoads DD, Habib-Bein NF, Hariri RS, et al. Comparison of the diagnostic utility of digital pathology systems for telemicrobiology. J Pathol Inform. 2016;7:10.
48. Rohde GK, Ozolek JA, Parwani AV, Pantanowitz L. Carnegie Mellon University bioimaging day 2014: Challenges and opportunities in digital pathology. J Pathol Inform. 2014;5:32.
49. Evans AJ, Salama ME, Henricks WH, Pantanowitz L. Implementation of whole slide imaging for clinical purposes: issues to consider from the perspective of early adopters. Arch Pathol Lab Med. 2017;141:944–59.
50. Lee BC, Hsieh ST, Chang YL, et al. A web-based virtual microscopy platform for improving academic performance in histology and pathology laboratory courses: a pilot study. Anat Sci Educ. 2020;13:743–58.
51. Arnold MA, Chenever E, Baker PB, et al. The College of American Pathologists guidelines for whole slide imaging validation are feasible for pediatric pathology: a pediatric pathology practice experience. Pediatr Dev Pathol. 2015;18:109–16.
52. Chen YK, Hsue SS, Lin DC, et al. An application of virtual microscopy in the teaching of an oral and maxillofacial pathology laboratory course. Oral Surg Oral Med Oral Pathol Oral Radiol Endod. 2008;105:342–7.
53. Fraggetta F, Yagi Y, Garcia-Rojo M, et al. The importance of eSlide macro images for primary diagnosis with whole slide imaging. J Pathol Inform. 2018;9:46.
54. Guo H, Birsa J, Farahani N, et al. Digital pathology and anatomic pathology laboratory information system integration to support digital pathology sign-out. J Pathol Inform. 2016;7:23.
55. Krupinski EA, Silverstein LD, Hashmi SF, et al. Observer performance using virtual pathology slides: impact of LCD color reproduction accuracy. J Digit Imaging. 2012;25:738–43.
56. Pantanowitz L, Valenstein PN, Evans AJ, et al. Review of the current state of whole slide imaging in pathology. J Pathol Inform. 2011;2:36.
57. Bruch LA, De Young BR, Kreiter CD, et al. Competency assessment of residents in surgical pathology using virtual microscopy. Hum Pathol. 2009;40:1122–8.
58. Girolami I, Pantanowitz L, Marletta S, et al. Diagnostic concordance between whole slide imaging and conventional light microscopy in cytopathology: a systematic review. Cancer Cytopathol. 2020;128:17–28.
59. Eccher A, Brunelli M, Pantanowitz L, et al. Innovation in transplantation: the digital era. J Pathol Inform. 2018;9:33.
60. Hanna MG, Reuter VE, Hameed MR, et al. Whole slide imaging equivalency and efficiency study: experience at a large academic center. Mod Pathol. 2019;32:916–28.
61. Kayser K, Ogilvie R, Borkenfeld S, Kayser G. E-education in pathology including certification of e-institutions. Diagn Pathol. 2011; 6 Suppl 1: S11.
62. Wilbur DC, Madi K, Colvin RB, et al. Whole-slide imaging digital pathology as a platform for teleconsultation: a pilot study using paired subspecialist correlations. Arch Pathol Lab Med. 2009;133:1949–53.
63. Parwani AV. Preface. Pathology informatics. Surg Pathol Clin. 2015;8:xi–xii.
64. Pantanowitz L, Dickinson K, Evans AJ, et al. ATA clinical guidelines for telepathology. Telemed J E Health. 2014;20:1049–56.
65. Evans AJ, Depeiza N, Allen SG, et al. Use of whole slide imaging (WSI) for distance teaching. J Clin Pathol. 2021;74(7):425–8.
66. Camparo P, Egevad L, Algaba F, et al. Utility of whole slide imaging and virtual microscopy in prostate pathology. APMIS. 2012;120:298–304.
67. Al Habeeb A, Evans A, Ghazarian D. Virtual microscopy using whole-slide imaging as an enabler for teledermatopathology: a paired consultant validation study. J Pathol Inform. 2012;3:2.
68. Ghaznavi F, Evans A, Madabhushi A, Feldman M. Digital imaging in pathology: whole-slide imaging and beyond. Annu Rev Pathol. 2013;8:331–59.
69. Williams BJ, Fraggetta F, Hanna MG, et al. The future of pathology: what can we learn from the COVID-19 pandemic? J Pathol Inform. 2020;11:15.

70. Afework A, Beynon MD, Bustamante F, et al. Digital dynamic telepathology–the Virtual Microscope. Proc AMIA Symp. 1998:912–6.
71. Park S, Pantanowitz L, Parwani AV, et al. Workflow organization in pathology. Clin Lab Med. 2012;32:601–22.
72. Pantanowitz L, Dickinson K, Evans AJ, et al. American Telemedicine Association clinical guidelines for telepathology. J Pathol Inform. 2014;5:39.
73. Pantanowitz L, McHugh J, Cable W, et al. Imaging file management to support international telepathology. J Pathol Inform. 2015;6:17.
74. Tetu B. The Canadian Association of Pathology guidelines for establishing a diagnostic telepathology service using whole-slide imaging. Ann Pathol. 2014;34:256–7.
75. Zhao C, Wu T, Ding X, et al. International telepathology consultation: three years of experience between the University of Pittsburgh Medical Center and KingMed Diagnostics in China. J Pathol Inform. 2015;6:63.
76. Montalto MC. Pathology RE-imagined: the history of digital radiology and the future of anatomic pathology. Arch Pathol Lab Med. 2008;132:764–5.
77. Montalto MC. An industry perspective: an update on the adoption of whole slide imaging. J Pathol Inform. 2016;7:18.
78. Weinstein RS, Graham AR, Richter LC, et al. Overview of telepathology, virtual microscopy, and whole slide imaging: prospects for the future. Hum Pathol. 2009;40:1057–69.
79. Weinstein RS, Descour MR, Liang C, et al. Telepathology overview: from concept to implementation. Hum Pathol. 2001;32:1283–99.
80. Lopez AM, Graham AR, Barker GP, et al. Virtual slide telepathology enables an innovative telehealth rapid breast care clinic. Hum Pathol. 2009;40:1082–91.
81. Feldman MD. Beyond morphology: whole slide imaging, computer-aided detection, and other techniques. Arch Pathol Lab Med. 2008;132:758–63.
82. Aeffner F, Zarella MD, Buchbinder N, et al. Introduction to digital image analysis in whole-slide imaging: a white paper from the digital pathology association. J Pathol Inform. 2019;10:9.
83. Mindiola Romero AE, Black CC, Jackson CR. Overcoming Educational challenges and impact of COVID-19 in a pathology residency program. Acad Pathol. 2021;8:2374289521994235.
84. Hipp JD, Fernandez A, Compton CC, Balis UJ. Why a pathology image should not be considered as a radiology image. J Pathol Inform. 2011;2:26.
85. Patterson ES, Rayo M, Gill C, Gurcan MN. Barriers and facilitators to adoption of soft copy interpretation from the user perspective: lessons learned from filmless radiology for slideless pathology. J Pathol Inform. 2011;2:1.
86. Iyengar JN. Whole slide imaging: the futurescape of histopathology. Indian J Pathol Microbiol. 2021;64:8–13.
87. Lundstrom C, Thorstenson S, Waltersson M, et al. Summary of 2(nd) Nordic symposium on digital pathology. J Pathol Inform. 2015;6:5.
88. Jantti T, Luhtala S, Maenpaa J, Staff S. Characterization of immunoreactivity with whole-slide imaging and digital analysis in high-grade serous ovarian cancer. Tumour Biol. 2020;42:1010428320971404.
89. Cornish TC, Swapp RE, Kaplan KJ. Whole-slide imaging: routine pathologic diagnosis. Adv Anat Pathol. 2012;19:152–9.
90. Ammendola S, Bariani E, Eccher A, et al. The histopathological diagnosis of atypical meningioma: glass slide versus whole slide imaging for grading assessment. Virchows Arch. 2021;478:747–56.
91. Rao V, Subramanian P, Sali AP, et al. Validation of Whole Slide Imaging for primary surgical pathology diagnosis of prostate biopsies. Indian J Pathol Microbiol. 2021;64:78–83.
92. Mukhopadhyay S, Feldman MD, Abels E, et al. Whole slide imaging versus microscopy for primary diagnosis in surgical pathology: a multicenter blinded randomized noninferiority study of 1992 cases (Pivotal Study). Am J Surg Pathol. 2018;42:39–52.

93. Graham AR, Bhattacharyya AK, Scott KM, et al. Virtual slide telepathology for an academic teaching hospital surgical pathology quality assurance program. Hum Pathol. 2009;40:1129–36.
94. Khushi M, Edwards G, de Marcos DA, et al. Open source tools for management and archiving of digital microscopy data to allow integration with patient pathology and treatment information. Diagn Pathol. 2013;8:22.
95. Daniel C, Rojo MG, Klossa J, et al. Standardizing the use of whole slide images in digital pathology. Comput Med Imaging Graph. 2011;35:496–505.
96. Jara-Lazaro AR, Thamboo TP, Teh M, Tan PH. Digital pathology: exploring its applications in diagnostic surgical pathology practice. Pathology. 2010;42:512–8.
97. Blum AE, Murphy GF, Lee JJ. Digital dermatopathology: the time is now. J Cutan Pathol. 2021;48:469–71.
98. Chordia TD, Vikey A, Choudhary AB, et al. Current status and future trends in telepathology and digital pathology. J Oral Maxillofac Pathol. 2016;20:178–82.
99. Farahani N, Pantanowitz L. Overview of telepathology. Surg Pathol Clin. 2015;8:223–31.
100. Abels E, Pantanowitz L, Aeffner F, et al. Computational pathology definitions, best practices, and recommendations for regulatory guidance: a white paper from the Digital Pathology Association. J Pathol. 2019;249:286–94.
101. Lara H, Li Z, Abels E et al. Quantitative image analysis for tissue biomarker use: a white paper from the digital pathology association. Appl Immunohistochem Mol Morphol. 2021.
102. Kim D, Pantanowitz L, Schuffler P, et al. (Re) Defining the high-power field for digital pathology. J Pathol Inform. 2020;11:33.
103. Niazi MKK, Parwani AV, Gurcan MN. Digital pathology and artificial intelligence. Lancet Oncol. 2019;20:e253–61.
104. Turner OC, Aeffner F, Bangari DS, et al. Society of Toxicologic Pathology Digital Pathology and Image Analysis Special Interest Group Article*: Opinion on the application of artificial intelligence and machine learning to digital toxicologic pathology. Toxicol Pathol. 2020;48:277–94.
105. McClintock DS, Lee RE, Gilbertson JR. Using computerized workflow simulations to assess the feasibility of whole slide imaging full adoption in a high-volume histology laboratory. Anal Cell Pathol (Amst). 2012;35:57–64.
106. Hassell LA, Parwani AV, Weiss L, et al. Challenges and opportunities in the adoption of College of American Pathologists checklists in electronic format: perspectives and experience of Reporting Pathology Protocols Project (RPP2) participant laboratories. Arch Pathol Lab Med. 2010;134:1152–9.
107. Thrall MJ, Wimmer JL, Schwartz MR. Validation of multiple whole slide imaging scanners based on the guideline from the College of American Pathologists Pathology and Laboratory Quality Center. Arch Pathol Lab Med. 2015;139:656–64.
108. Fine JL, Grzybicki DM, Silowash R, et al. Evaluation of whole slide image immunohistochemistry interpretation in challenging prostate needle biopsies. Hum Pathol. 2008;39:564–72.
109. Lee KC, Mak LS. Virtual electron microscopy: a simple implementation creating a new paradigm in ultrastructural examination. Int J Surg Pathol. 2011;19:570–5.
110. Lee RE, McClintock DS, Laver NM, Yagi Y. Evaluation and optimization for liquid-based preparation cytology in whole slide imaging. J Pathol Inform. 2011;2:46.
111. Khalbuss WE, Pantanowitz L, Parwani AV. Digital imaging in cytopathology. Pathol Res Int. 2011;2011:264683.
112. Bongaerts O, Clevers C, Debets M, et al. Conventional microscopical versus digital whole-slide imaging-based diagnosis of thin-layer cervical specimens: a validation study. J Pathol Inform. 2018;9:29.
113. Hanna MG, Pantanowitz L. Why is digital pathology in cytopathology lagging behind surgical pathology? Cancer Cytopathol. 2017;125:519–20.
114. Mosquera-Zamudio A, Hanna MG, Parra-Medina R, et al. Advantage of Z-stacking for teleconsultation between the USA and Colombia. Diagn Cytopathol. 2019;47:35–40.

115. Zarella MD, Jakubowski J. Video compression to support the expansion of whole-slide imaging into cytology. J Med Imaging (Bellingham). 2019;6:047502.
116. Hanna MG, Monaco SE, Cuda J, et al. Comparison of glass slides and various digital-slide modalities for cytopathology screening and interpretation. Cancer Cytopathol. 2017;125:701–9.
117. Hanna MG, Pantanowitz L. Feasibility of using the Omnyx digital pathology system for cytology practice. J Am Soc Cytopathol. 2019;8:182–9.
118. Wright AM, Smith D, Dhurandhar B, et al. Digital slide imaging in cervicovaginal cytology: a pilot study. Arch Pathol Lab Med. 2013;137:618–24.
119. Van Es SL, Greaves J, Gay S, et al. Constant quest for quality: digital cytopathology. J Pathol Inform. 2018;9:13.
120. Van Es SL, White V, Ross J, et al. Digital cytopathology: a constant evolution (Comments on Capitanio et al. digital cytology: a short review of technical and methodological approaches and applications). Cytopathology. 2019;30:262–3.
121. Amin W, Srintrapun SJ, Parwani AV. Automated whole slide imaging. Expert Opin Med Diagn. 2008;2:1173–81.
122. Somanchi S, Neill DB, Parwani AV. Discovering anomalous patterns in large digital pathology images. Stat Med. 2018;37:3599–615.
123. Niazi MKK, Yazgan E, Tavolara TE, et al. Semantic segmentation to identify bladder layers from H&E images. Diagn Pathol. 2020;15:87.
124. Lam AK, Leung M. Whole-slide imaging of esophageal squamous cell carcinoma. Methods Mol Biol. 2020;2129:107–17.
125. Hanna MG, Pantanowitz L, Evans AJ. Overview of contemporary guidelines in digital pathology: what is available in 2015 and what still needs to be addressed? J Clin Pathol. 2015;68:499–505.
126. Bauer TW, Schoenfield L, Slaw RJ, et al. Validation of whole slide imaging for primary diagnosis in surgical pathology. Arch Pathol Lab Med. 2013;137:518–24.
127. Amin S, Mori T, Itoh T. A validation study of whole slide imaging for primary diagnosis of lymphoma. Pathol Int. 2019;69:341–9.
128. Yu H, Gao F, Jiang L, Ma S. Development of a whole slide imaging system on smartphones and evaluation with frozen section samples. JMIR Mhealth Uhealth. 2017;5:e132.
129. Wang S, Yang DM, Rong R, et al. Artificial intelligence in lung cancer pathology image analysis. Cancers (Basel). 2019;11:1673.
130. Senaras C, Niazi MKK, Lozanski G, Gurcan MN. DeepFocus: Detection of out-of-focus regions in whole slide digital images using deep learning. PLoS One. 2018;13:e0205387.
131. Slodkowska J, Rojo MG. Digital pathology in personalized cancer therapy. Folia Histochem Cytobiol. 2011;49:570–8.
132. Bera K, Schalper KA, Rimm DL, et al. Artificial intelligence in digital pathology – new tools for diagnosis and precision oncology. Nat Rev Clin Oncol. 2019;16:703–15.
133. Yamada M, Saito A, Yamamoto Y, et al. Quantitative nucleic features are effective for discrimination of intraductal proliferative lesions of the breast. J Pathol Inform. 2016;7:1.
134. Li AC, Zhao J, Zhao C, et al. Quantitative digital imaging analysis of HER2 immunohistochemistry predicts the response to anti-HER2 neoadjuvant chemotherapy in HER2-positive breast carcinoma. Breast Cancer Res Treat. 2020;180:321–9.
135. Feng M, Deng Y, Yang L, et al. Automated quantitative analysis of Ki-67 staining and HE images recognition and registration based on whole tissue sections in breast carcinoma. Diagn Pathol. 2020;15:65.
136. Volynskaya Z, Mete O, Pakbaz S, et al. Ki67 quantitative interpretation: insights using image analysis. J Pathol Inform. 2019;10:8.
137. Mercan E, Mehta S, Bartlett J, et al. Assessment of machine learning of breast pathology structures for automated differentiation of breast cancer and high-risk proliferative lesions. JAMA Netw Open. 2019;2:e198777.
138. Komura D, Ishikawa S. Machine learning approaches for pathologic diagnosis. Virchows Arch. 2019;475:131–8.

139. Chang HY, Jung CK, Woo JI, et al. Artificial intelligence in pathology. J Pathol Transl Med. 2019;53:1–12.
140. Colling R, Pitman H, Oien K, et al. Artificial intelligence in digital pathology: a roadmap to routine use in clinical practice. J Pathol. 2019;249:143–50.
141. Kumar A, Prateek M. Localization of nuclei in breast cancer using whole slide imaging system supported by morphological features and shape formulas. Cancer Manag Res. 2020;12:4573–83.
142. Mahmood T, Arsalan M, Owais M, et al. Artificial intelligence-based mitosis detection in breast cancer histopathology images using faster R-CNN and deep CNNs. J Clin Med. 2020;9
143. Komura D, Ishikawa S. Machine learning methods for histopathological image analysis. Comput Struct Biotechnol J. 2018;16:34–42.
144. Griffin J, Treanor D. Digital pathology in clinical use: where are we now and what is holding us back? Histopathology. 2017;70:134–45.

Developing a Clinical Workflow That Fits Your Needs

Douglas J. Hartman

The process of evaluating the adoption digital pathology for a practice can be a daunting task. Besides the change management, the process depends on the available budget and departmental structure. These factors can influence and be influenced by different clinical uses of digital pathology that will be desired. In this manuscript, I will describe the different levels of adoption and associated equipment that can be of interest. Based on my personal discussions, it seems that there are many different structures to pathology departments across the United States and the world, and hopefully this will aid in the process.

Remote Access

One of the first uses for digital pathology was for remote access to physical slides. Performing remote diagnosis was piloted by Massachusetts General Hospital with the Logan International Airport Medical Station and reported out in 1974 [1]. Of course with the current COVID-19 pandemic, it is easy to see the advances that telediagnosis has made since then. Although many different diagnoses were made, some peripheral blood smears were diagnosed at the time, and this has been described as the first use of remote telepathology. The value that this remote access represents is allowing expertise to be shared across geographic locations. In this first example, it was 2.7 miles away from Massachusetts General Hospital, but it could also simply be across a sprawling medical campus [1]. At a basic level, this extends the areas that could be covered by a pathology department. In the past we have requested the material to be centralized within our departments, but this technology allows pathology to

D. J. Hartman (✉)
University of Pittsburgh Medical Center, Department of Pathology, Pittsburgh, PA, USA

Department of Anatomic Pathology, University of Pittsburgh Medical Center, Pittsburgh, PA, USA
e-mail: hartmandj@upmc.edu

A. V. Parwani (ed.), *Whole Slide Imaging*,
https://doi.org/10.1007/978-3-030-83332-9_4

decentralize to where care is being delivered to patients. This de-centralization process allows pathology to become more valuable for the delivery of timely patient care. Although placing a physical person from the pathology department in those locations would be an alternative solution, this is neither efficient nor cost-effective. The cost of technology to facilitate this type of process is relatively minimal, and these costs fall within the operational budgets of most pathology departments. The most frequently described use case relates to support for frozen section/intraoperative consultations. Numerous papers have described different institutional experiences with performing remote intraoperative consultations [2–7]. Sophisticated devices have evolved for these uses. The more recent models have incorporated both the ability to remotely control the movement of the slide and the ability to make a whole slide image from the slide (so-called hybrid scanners). These scanners generally have a low capacity for scanning slides between one and four slides at a single time. This type of remote access can even be performed with the use of "smartphones" [8]. A recent meta-analysis of studies using telepathology has been published summarizing the described experiences within the literature [9].

Although related, the use of telecytology has also been expanding. The remote cytology use case is somewhat different than intraoperative consultations because it generally involves a viewing/streaming experience rather than the user who is distant controlling the navigation. The nature of cytology (i.e., having cytotechnicians and having three-dimensional slide preps) facilitates this different workflow. Several articles have described the uses for telecytology [10–14]. The clinical decisions for intraoperative assessment generally revolve around the diagnosis as well as decisions by the surgical team while the clinical decisions for telecytology revolve around the diagnosis and the adequacy of the specimen. Cytology is a rapid relatively diffuse method that can be applied for the diagnostic workup for patients while frozen section/intraoperative consultations occur in a more limited setting (i.e., operating rooms). Therefore, the geographic demands for remote telecytology are greater than that for intraoperative consultation.

The financial calculation for these types of remote access will depend on your departmental structure. If you are within a large integrated hospital, this remote access can facilitate an investment in subspecialty expertise. One single site within the integrated system may not be able to support solely a subspecialist but by combining all of the sites there is justification through the volume of work across the multiple sites. More and more clinical work is being shifted from a hospital-based environment to outpatient clinics. As this occurs, the demand to support remote cytology evaluation will increase in order to reduce unsatisfactory specimens. Fortunately, the implementation of a system for remote access is relatively low, and the efficiencies gained/cost reduced generally justify the purchase costs.

Slide Archival

A more broad/expansive use case for digital pathology is for archival access to prior cases. This use case refers to the scanning of slides once the clinical case has already been signed out. Since this use case does not involve delaying/interrupting the sign-out process, the time demands are reduced for this process (i.e., outside the boundaries of clinical care delivery). One benefit of this use case is that a department could potentially reduce/nearly eliminate the need to pull old slides for review/comparison. This work is routinely performed by the operational staff within a pathology department. When a pathology department has an archive of their prior cases, these images can be accessed nearly instantaneously. That represents both a savings in time to review and labor costs to go and find the slides. There are many reasons that a prior case might be pulled for review – these include (a) second opinion, (b) legal case, (c) comparison to current case, (d) tumor board review, (e) educational, or (f) research studies. With the creation of a digital slide, these multiple stakeholders can all have access to the slides without being concern for loss or damage of the slides. Although not mandatory, being able to connect these archival slides to the original clinical case generates more value from this use case. To this end, barcode-labeled slides allow for connection to the clinical archive and then therefore add more value to what is contained with the digital slides (the clinical outcome/data for that patient). Using barcode labels for slide identification has been demonstrated to promote better quality within the clinical lab [15]; it is an efficient method to connect archival slides to the clinical cases.

The numerous potential reasons each represent a risk that a physical slide may be damaged or lost. Pathology departments are aware of this risk, and therefore they have created systems to mitigate these risks to the best of their abilities, but those systems have not eliminated the risk. Particularly at an academic medical center, the number of reasons for retrieval tends to be more. However, a department may use these demands/risks as a rationale for the cost of this use case. This use case will generally require some sort of system of filing/storage (server-based or cloud-based). Additionally, the scanning device that would be used for this use case will generally scan large volumes of slides (on the order of 100 s of slides per day). With having a storage system, there are associated IT support people that are necessary as well as technicians that will be needed to load the slides into the scanners. These costs can approach a million to several millions of dollars, so consideration of the use cases is an important aspect of the evaluation process. An example deployment is described by Huisman and others [16]. Fortunately some of the costs can replace existing costs within a departmental budget related to the use cases.

It can be helpful to reach to other stakeholders within your institution to see if the costs of creating a system could be shared – this will generally occur at an academic institution. There is a large amount of morphologic data that can be derived from digital slides, and having access to large repositories has great value both for researchers within the department of pathology who may not perform diagnostic work and for researchers in other departments. One analogy to consider is with paraffin blocks. Prior to the late 1990s, these were retained for similar reasons to those mentioned above for slides. However, with the introduction of the ability to extract DNA from paraffin blocks, the blocks took on a new value. This value can be seen in the Cancer Genome Atlas project that has provided digital images to pair with much of the DNA and protein data that was generated [17, 18]. Storage of the images may be an area where sharing can be facilitated within a large hospital system predominantly with a radiology department. Many authors have compared the journey of pathology into digital to the journey that was undertaken by radiology in the 1990s. Radiology uses systems to store their images, and these systems can be used to store pathology images. Some vendors have taken to labeling one system for all images within a hospital/health system as enterprise imaging/vendor neutral archives [19, 20]. Another tool that an archival system can help with is potential collaboration with software development companies or research grant applications. It is important to clearly define expectations and deliverables when embarking on collaborative projects.

Primary Diagnosis/Facilitate Clinical Sign Out

Another use case for digital pathology is to use digital pathology to facilitate clinical diagnostic sign out. The primary focus for this has been toward primary diagnostic sign out and has been focused on vendors obtaining clearance from the US Food and Drug Administration to market whole slide scanners for primary diagnosis. The first approval occurred in April of 2017, and a second vendor has since been approved [21]. Numerous non-inferiority studies have been published comparing digital slides to glass slides [22–26].

The consolidation of technical services to a single site may generate efficiencies within an integrated hospital system. Adopting digital pathology can facilitate some of these consolidations. It is relatively common to pool testing (particularly complex testing). The clinical lab is experiencing an increasingly difficult time to recruit employees. By consolidating these technical services into a centralized location, this can reduce the competition for this valuable talent. This consolidation does represent some trade-offs (less proximity to the histology lab), but there will be gains in efficiency. Consolidation may facilitate multiple daily shifts within the lab and also gives greater flexibility for employee hours. The distance/time between this lab and the pathologists can be reduced by adopting digital pathology.

Besides the consolidation of technical services, a large pathology department can pool their specimens in order to justify the hiring of subspecialty pathologists. With digital pathology, these cases can be seamlessly shared for diagnostic sign out by the subspecialist. Although still controversial, there is a general trend toward more subspecialty training and subspecialty sign-out practice [27–33]. At a minimum, certain types of pathology have been recognized to need specialty sign out – neuropathology, renal pathology, transplant pathology, hematopathology, and others. Depending on the practice, there may be a low volume of these specimens such that it makes business sense to contract for these services in an ad hoc fashion (i.e., consultation). Digital pathology could facilitate more rapid turnaround of these cases because the transport time could be eliminated. The delivery of pathology services has been changing in recent years with a trend toward consolidation of practices [34–39]. The current COVID-19 pandemic is likely to add more pressure to smaller practices as the financial impacts start to make their way thru hospitals/healthcare systems.

The COVID-19 pandemic has had major impacts on how medical care and pathology practice was performed at this current time. It is unclear how long these changes will be in place or what the long-term impact to the practice of pathology will be. Besides the relaxation of the requirements for clinical pathology lab tests, there was also a relaxing of the enforcement for the location delivery of anatomic pathology services (related to the CLIA license). The Digital Pathology Association at the time of this publication is surveying members about their experience during this extraordinary time period [40]. There will likely be many lessons learned thru this testing "by fire."

Moving to a primary diagnostic sign-out method may generate additional cost saving thru the transitioning of pathologists to a work from home behavior. Several corporate entities have already stated that they will be moving forward with work from home as they emerge from this pandemic crisis. It is unclear if this can fully be done within the hospital environment, but some degree of work from home is likely to be adopted in pathology departments as a result of these events.

When considering using a digital pathology system for clinical work, proper validation of the system must be performed. Guidelines to perform this have been published from the College of American Pathologists [41]. Briefly, at least 60 hematoxylin and eosin cases should be compared in the digital system to glass slides diagnoses. Additional validations for special stains and immunostains should also be performed (20 cases for each type are recommended). Evaluation of the user experiences have been described, and review of these methods can be helpful to determine how a pathology department should proceed [42].

Image Analysis

The use of image analysis (particularly for breast cancer biomarkers estrogen receptor, progesterone receptor, and Her2) has been around for more than 10 years [43–45]. The early process required a lot of manual manipulation, but the process of image analysis has advanced since then, and there have been many aspects of automated image analysis that have been improved as well as multiple image analysis methods [45–49]. A recent whitepaper from the Digital Pathology Association described aspects of image analysis [50].

The first goals in image analysis were providing a more reproducible way of analyzing an immunohistochemical stains. The easiest target to perform technically was to analyze nuclear expression of a marker. For breast cancer, Ki-67, progesterone receptor and estrogen receptor immunostains are nuclear markers. Nuclear analysis is easier since one nucleus equals one cell and the distribution of the immunostain is more concentrated. Although the analysis of a nuclear marker is more reproducible, there are some situations where it falters. For Ki-67, this can stain the tumor markers but can also stain infiltrating immune cells, and so recent studies have begun to exclude non-tumor cells within the analysis [49]. Nuclear assessment guidelines generally separate cancers into high expression or low expression. This dichotomous separation reduces the interobserver variability, and so it has slowed adoption of digital image analysis.

The next image analysis method that was developed was the assessment of membranous positivity. The marker that this was most related to was Her2. The analysis of this marker was accelerated by the fact that a targeted therapy was developed for tumors with this marker. Membranous expression presents challenges in that determining the cells that are positive for the marker is a little more difficult (membranes are thin border around the cell, and the expression of the marker can be incomplete within the membrane). The completeness of the expression of the immunostain is a critical feature of interpreting the immunostain. For these reasons, this marker is more difficult to interpret analog methods and therefore is suitable for an automated method to analyze. For Her2, this was initially evaluated by fluorescence which is a technically more difficult test and less widely available when compared to immunostains. Image analysis for fluorescence was developed [51]. Also by having a second method, it was easier to validate the relevance of the evaluation of Her2 by immunostains.

More recently, image analysis for cytoplasmic markers (i.e., CD8) by immunostains has been reported [52–57]. This has taken on greater relevance in the era of immune-based therapies [58–62]. This image analysis method is more complex because enumerating the cells can be more difficult when there is cytoplasmic expression (separation of one cell from another) and the immunostaining pattern is more diffuse than it occurs with either nuclear or membranous expression patterns.

The future of image analysis will likely perform tasks that cannot be easily accomplished with routine microscopy – for instance, the "vascularity" or a lesion or the proximity of immune cells to tumor cells. Since these tasks cannot be easily accomplished by routine evaluation under a microscope, validation of the value of the proposed analysis is critical for adoption. Since digital analysis will be the only method to perform this analysis, only departments that have adopted some form of digital pathology will be able to offer this for their patients.

Several of the image algorithms have received regulatory clearance, mostly in reference to breast biomarkers. Many of these clearances were obtained prior to the approval by the Food and Drug Administration for vendors to market digital pathology for primary diagnosis. Additionally, a specific CPT code was created for enhanced analysis of an immunostain by a digital/automated method, 88,361. The original analysis methods required the selection of a region of interest/field of view, and therefore sampling error within a tumor section had to be considered. More recent advances have allowed for larger areas to be analyzed by these image analysis algorithms. Additionally, web-based image analysis is even now available for use [63].

At the University of Pittsburgh Medical Center, we have created a dedicated laboratory to perform clinical reporting of image analysis (as we have for fluorescence in situ hybridization and solid tumor molecular evaluation). Deciding about whether there is a dedicated image analysis lab or if all pathologists will be responsible for reporting digital image analysis will need to be based on an individual department's assessment.

Artificial Intelligence/Machine Learning

Currently, one of the hottest topics in digital pathology is the promise/potential of machine learning/artificial intelligence [64]. This field is still relatively new in digital pathology, and as such there are still some things that are yet to be well established for this methodology (i.e., how to perform validation). The Food and Drug Administration has already approved some artificial intelligence/machine learning for use in medicine [65]. To date, there has not been any guidance about how artificial intelligence will be regulated.

These algorithms have been largely developed by computer scientists. The development of the algorithms has required having large data sets because the algorithms require many instances in order to develop rules for how to classify cases/morphology. The more diverse the spectrum of the entity that the algorithm is trying to classify, the more widely variable the training sets need to be. The development work can benefit from archival digital images that can be created in many pathology departments. This represents a potential opportunity for a pathology department to save on the acquisition costs for this technology. Public challenges have been created to encourage the use of a universal set of images (raw data) so that it is easier to determine the value of the algorithms [66]. Although there are a lot of possible tasks that might be amenable to artificial intelligence/machine learning, if they always use different training conditions, it will be difficult to compare the usefulness of the algorithms. One of the more well-publicized artificial intelligence challenges was the CAMELYON challenge [67]. This challenge presented the task of identifying a focus of metastasis within lymph nodes. The first year (CAMELYON 16) used patches or regions of interest while the following year (CAMELYON 17) used whole slide images of tissue sections [67]. As you can see from this example, the initial year was a relatively limited task while the follow-up year required the algorithms to be able to identify the focus within a much larger digital area [67].

There remains resistance to the adoption of this technology, because it still is (a) relatively novel, (b) related to its regulation/validation, and (c) out of concern that this may represent a potential replacement of pathologists. The discipline of radiology has been digital for several decades, and there is still relatively limited application of machine learning/artificial intelligence to replace radiologists. Some authors have suggested that artificial intelligence by itself may be inferior to artificial intelligence together with a radiologist in an optimal use, so-called centaur radiologists [68, 69].

The infrastructure that is necessary to efficiently train the algorithms are expensive and have been rapidly changing/advancing. As greater adoption of the methodology occurs broadly within the medical field, resources are likely to be available within an environment to run these algorithms. However, at the current time, this field remains at the cutting edge with the limited evidence about how the ultimate solutions will be used in diagnostic pathology.

External Consultation

Another use for digital pathology has been for external consultation. Several institutions have described their experience with international consultation using digital pathology [70–76]. This setup has sometimes been referred to as "in-sourcing" and can represent a positive revenue for a department. There can be challenges related to establishing these relationships.

When setting up an international consultation relationship, it is important to have a personal connection between the sending and receiving sites. This personal connection can help to facilitate the design and navigate the challenges that arise when you are sending digital images along a large distance, across time zones, and across languages.

Education

Besides the education of housestaff, a pathology department often has the responsibility of teaching in the early years of medical school. Reform within the medical school teaching curricula have reduced the role of didactic lectures and therefore the exposure of medical students to the field of pathology [77]. The evaluation of pathology material in the medical school curriculum has migrated to a digital format [78]. The reduced emphasis on pathology has generated deficiencies in exiting medical students [79]. We have piloted some efforts to integrate pathology education alongside the clinical rotations for pediatric rotations during the clinical years of medical school [80]. This lack of exposure to the role of pathology in the delivery of medical care is regretful and may be a contributing factor to a decreased interest in medical students entering the field of pathology [81, 82]. These educational responsibilities are often minimally reimbursed to the pathology department but are still expected from the pathology department. Although there may not be direct costs that can be applied to the cost of the system, efficiencies gained by repurposing digital material represent true convenience and value for members within pathology. Utilizing digital material to teach housestaff may also represent a valuable asset because digital slides have a reduced degradation over time as glass slides experience. In contrast to the simple exposure of cases as they come through a clinical service, digital case collections offer the ability to demonstrate the wide variety of morphologic spectrums that can often be seen with exposure to many cases. Historically, the only way to obtain this knowledge was to review teaching sets or to review many thousands of cases over time. Digital material can concentrate these morphologic variations into a condensed experience and therefore more efficiently transfer knowledge from one generation of pathologists to the next. Besides the education of housestaff, these digital materials can also be used for educating other pathologists. Creating digital sets represent a truly freeing and liberating effect to the morphologic features that are present on glass slides. From a content creator perspective, digital slides represent efficient methods to create content in a simplified fashion.

Stakeholder Engagement

Adopting any level of digital pathology clinical workflow will require an alteration in the behavior of both the technical staff and physicians. The process to institute these changes can have a positive impact on the daily work of those within your department as well as in the delivery of care for your patients. Frequent engagement with pertinent stakeholders can create ownership from them about the process beginning with the choice of adoption and continuing to implementation.

Some possible stakeholders include the administrative leadership of the department, the technical staff, the information technology staff, possibly research stakeholders/cancer centers, and or billing/purchasing staff. The more stakeholders that are engaged, the broader the use cases and therefore the greater return on investment for a deployed system. However, the broader the use cases, the size of the purchase will increase. Designating a person to lead this effort can help to make it a successful exercise. The responsibilities for this designated person will depend on the size of the overall project and the number of areas that will be impacted by the project.

Selecting a System/Use Cases

The process of investing in equipment for a pathology department is important for the future success of the department. Thoughtfully evaluating the competing demands for the departmental resources is an important part of the process. As with all technology projects, it is critical to be aware of the market for that technology, how mature the technology is, and what adoption will provide to the department. Recent studies have suggested that there is a pending shortage of pathologists within the United States market and this has been compounded by a reduction to exposure to the pathology discipline referenced in one of the prior sections [83]. The medical education environment in the United States has converted to a nearly entire digital pathology experience. However, since the diagnostic work in the majority of pathology departments is still performed by using physical slides, very few pathologists are being trained during their critical formative years to use digital pathology and the tools. The lack of familiarity and comfort with digital pathology impedes even the partial adoption. Even though pathology departments are regarded as cost centers, this has not prevented them from developing novel testing modalities (most notably molecular testing in recent years). Having a component of your department's strategic mission address plans for the use/adoption of digital pathology even in a minimal fashion will benefit the long-term goals of the department. The recent COVID-19 pandemic clearly demonstrates that those who are prepared can rapidly change and utilize this technology. At our department, we were able to begin using digital pathology for primary sign out within a few weeks of the crisis appearing in the cities within the United States, but this was principally due to the prior efforts to deploy digital pathology technology. It can be helpful to speak with other pathology departments and share experience with how they view digital pathology within their strategic mission.

Conclusion

Investing in a digital pathology solution can be particularly challenging especially for someone unfamiliar with the technology. The technology has evolved from a relatively new product to a mature solution (especially in regard to remote access). However, ignoring digital pathology and not addressing it within the strategic plans for a pathology department can potentially be detrimental to the future success of the department. The adoption of digital pathology does not require a large budget and can be done in a step-wise fashion in order to accommodate most budgets. Engagement of stakeholders early and often can facilitate a successful utilization of this technology for the benefit of the department. There is promise within both image analysis and artificial intelligence that suggests that the adoption of digital pathology may become a necessity for the practice of pathology rather than a luxury. Evaluating the relative importance of different competing values within your individual pathology practice will inform the selection process.

References

1. Murphy RL Jr, Bird KT. Telediagnosis: a new community health resource. Observations on the feasibility of telediagnosis based on 1000 patient transactions. Am J Public Health. 1974;64(2):113–9.
2. Pantanowitz L, et al. Experience with multimodality telepathology at the University of Pittsburgh Medical Center. J Pathol Inform. 2012;3:45.
3. Kaplan KJ, et al. Use of robotic telepathology for frozen-section diagnosis: a retrospective trial of a telepathology system for intraoperative consultation. Mod Pathol. 2002;15(11):1197–204.
4. Weinstein RS, et al. Overview of telepathology, virtual microscopy, and whole slide imaging: prospects for the future. Hum Pathol. 2009;40(8):1057–69.
5. Ghosh A, Brown GT, Fontelo P. Telepathology at the Armed Forces Institute of Pathology: a retrospective review of consultations from 1996 to 1997. Arch Pathol Lab Med. 2018;142(2):248–52.
6. Farahani N, Pantanowitz L. Overview of telepathology. Surg Pathol Clin. 2015;8(2):223–31.
7. Dietz RL, et al. Review of the use of telepathology for intraoperative consultation. Expert Rev Med Devices. 2018;15(12):883–90.
8. Ekong D, et al. Evaluation of android smartphones for telepathology. J Pathol Inform. 2017;8:16.
9. Dietz RL, Hartman DJ, Pantanowitz L. Systematic review of the use of telepathology during intraoperative consultation. Am J Clin Pathol. 2020;153(2):198–209.
10. Collins BT. Telepathology in cytopathology: challenges and opportunities. Acta Cytol. 2013;57(3):221–32.
11. Khurana KK. Telecytology and its evolving role in cytopathology. Diagn Cytopathol. 2012;40(6):498–502.
12. Archondakis S, et al. Telecytology: a tool for quality assessment and improvement in the evaluation of thyroid fine-needle aspiration specimens. Telemed J E Health. 2009;15(7):713–7.
13. Monaco SE, et al. Assessing competency for remote telecytology rapid on-site evaluation using pre-recorded dynamic video streaming. Cytopathology. 2019;31:411.
14. Monaco SE, et al. Telecytology implementation: deployment of telecytology for rapid on-site evaluations at an Academic Medical Center. Diagn Cytopathol. 2019;47(3):206–13.
15. Heher YK, et al. Achieving high reliability in histology: an improvement series to reduce errors. Am J Clin Pathol. 2016;146(5):554–60.

16. Huisman A, et al. Creation of a fully digital pathology slide archive by high-volume tissue slide scanning. Hum Pathol. 2010;41(5):751–7.
17. Finn WG. Diagnostic pathology and laboratory medicine in the age of "omics": a paper from the 2006 William Beaumont Hospital Symposium on Molecular Pathology. J Mol Diagn. 2007;9(4):431–6.
18. Gutman DA, et al. The digital slide archive: a software platform for management, integration, and analysis of histology for cancer research. Cancer Res. 2017;77(21):e75–8.
19. Pantanowitz L, et al. Twenty years of digital pathology: an overview of the road travelled, what is on the horizon, and the emergence of vendor-neutral archives. J Pathol Inform. 2018;9:40.
20. Marques Godinho T, et al. An efficient architecture to support digital pathology in standard medical imaging repositories. J Biomed Inform. 2017;71:190–7.
21. Evans AJ, et al. US Food and Drug Administration approval of whole slide imaging for primary diagnosis: a key milestone is reached and new questions are raised. Arch Pathol Lab Med. 2018;142(11):1383–7.
22. Mills AM, et al. Diagnostic efficiency in digital pathology: a comparison of optical versus digital assessment in 510 surgical pathology cases. Am J Surg Pathol. 2018;42(1):53–9.
23. Jen KY, et al. Reliability of whole slide images as a diagnostic modality for renal allograft biopsies. Hum Pathol. 2013;44(5):888–94.
24. Kent MN, et al. Diagnostic accuracy of virtual pathology vs traditional microscopy in a large dermatopathology study. JAMA Dermatol. 2017;153(12):1285–91.
25. Glatz-Krieger K, et al. Factors to keep in mind when introducing virtual microscopy. Virchows Arch. 2006;448(3):248–55.
26. Hanna MG, et al. Comparison of glass slides and various digital-slide modalities for cytopathology screening and interpretation. Cancer Cytopathol. 2017;125(9):701–9.
27. Sarewitz SJ. Subspecialization in community pathology practice. Arch Pathol Lab Med. 2014;138(7):871–2.
28. Huber AR, et al. Accuracy of vascular invasion reporting in hepatocellular carcinoma before and after implementation of subspecialty surgical pathology sign-out. Indian J Pathol Microbiol. 2017;60(4):501–4.
29. Iezzoni JC, et al. Selective pathology fellowships: diverse, innovative, and valuable subspecialty training. Arch Pathol Lab Med. 2014;138(4):518–25.
30. Sharma M, et al. Effects of subspecialty signout and group consensus on the diagnosis of microscopic colitis. Virchows Arch. 2019;475(5):573–8.
31. Leong AS, Braye S, Bhagwandeen B. Diagnostic 'errors' in anatomical pathology: relevance to Australian laboratories. Pathology. 2006;38(6):490–7.
32. Manion E, Cohen MB, Weydert J. Mandatory second opinion in surgical pathology referral material: clinical consequences of major disagreements. Am J Surg Pathol. 2008;32(5):732–7.
33. Strosberg C, et al. Second opinion reviews for cancer diagnoses in anatomic pathology: a comprehensive cancer center's experience. Anticancer Res. 2018;38(5):2989–94.
34. Satta G, Edmonstone J. Consolidation of pathology services in England: have savings been achieved? BMC Health Serv Res. 2018;18(1):862.
35. Gu J, Taylor CR. Practicing pathology in the era of big data and personalized medicine. Appl Immunohistochem Mol Morphol. 2014;22(1):1–9.
36. Wood JP. Legal issues for pathologists. Adv Anat Pathol. 2011;18(6):466–72.
37. Martin SA, Styer PE. Assessing performance, productivity, and staffing needs in pathology groups: observations from the College of American Pathologists PathFocus pathology practice activity and staffing program. Arch Pathol Lab Med. 2006;130(9):1263–8.
38. Johnson P. Branding an anatomic pathology practice to build revenue. Clin Leadersh Manag Rev. 2004;18(4):220–5.
39. Chorneyko K, et al. Canada's pathology. CMAJ. 2008;178(12):1523–6.
40. Digital Pathology Association Survey for Digital Pathology. May 22, 2020]; Available from: https://vr2.verticalresponse.com/emails/46179488376453?contact_id=46179491246273&sk=aXYQB2JgqjBIJQGhRANUF5NkdMNR7i4qbu1NmWr7QH9g=/aHR0cHM6Ly92cjIudm-

VydGljYWxyZXNwb25zZS5jb20vZW1haWxzLzQ2MTc5NDg4Mzc2NDUzP2NvbnRhY3RfaWQ9NDYxNzk0OTEyNDYyNzM=/3088BgyqSse7WoOHcuEdmw==.
41. Pantanowitz L, et al. Validating whole slide imaging for diagnostic purposes in pathology: guideline from the College of American Pathologists Pathology and Laboratory Quality Center. Arch Pathol Lab Med. 2013;137(12):1710–22.
42. Hanna MG, et al. Whole slide imaging equivalency and efficiency study: experience at a large academic center. Mod Pathol. 2019;32(7):916–28.
43. Vrekoussis T, et al. Image analysis of breast cancer immunohistochemistry-stained sections using ImageJ: an RGB-based model. Anticancer Res. 2009;29(12):4995–8.
44. Laurinavicius A, et al. Immunohistochemistry profiles of breast ductal carcinoma: factor analysis of digital image analysis data. Diagn Pathol. 2012;7:27.
45. Mofidi R, et al. Objective measurement of breast cancer oestrogen receptor status through digital image analysis. Eur J Surg Oncol. 2003;29(1):20–4.
46. Lopez C, et al. Digital image analysis in breast cancer: an example of an automated methodology and the effects of image compression. Stud Health Technol Inform. 2012;179:155–71.
47. Brugmann A, et al. Digital image analysis of membrane connectivity is a robust measure of HER2 immunostains. Breast Cancer Res Treat. 2012;132(1):41–9.
48. Koopman T, et al. What is the added value of digital image analysis of HER2 immunohistochemistry in breast cancer in clinical practice? A study with multiple platforms. Histopathology. 2019;74(6):917–24.
49. Bankhead P, et al. Integrated tumor identification and automated scoring minimizes pathologist involvement and provides new insights to key biomarkers in breast cancer. Lab Investig. 2018;98(1):15–26.
50. Aeffner F, et al. Introduction to digital image analysis in whole-slide imaging: a white paper from the digital pathology association. J Pathol Inform. 2019;10:9.
51. Theodosiou Z, et al. Evaluation of FISH image analysis system on assessing HER2 amplification in breast carcinoma cases. Breast. 2008;17(1):80–4.
52. Hartman DJ, et al. Utility of CD8 score by automated quantitative image analysis in head and neck squamous cell carcinoma. Oral Oncol. 2018;86:278–87.
53. Hartman DJ, et al. Automated quantitation of CD8-positive T cells predicts prognosis in colonic adenocarcinoma with mucinous, signet ring cell, or medullary differentiation independent of mismatch repair protein status. Am J Surg Pathol. 2020;44:991.
54. Monaco SE, et al. Quantitative image analysis for CD8 score in lung small biopsies and cytology cell-blocks. Cytopathology. 2020;31:393.
55. Galon J, Fridman WH, Pages F. The adaptive immunologic microenvironment in colorectal cancer: a novel perspective. Cancer Res. 2007;67(5):1883–6.
56. Pages F, et al. Immune infiltration in human tumors: a prognostic factor that should not be ignored. Oncogene. 2010;29(8):1093–102.
57. Galon J, et al. Type, density, and location of immune cells within human colorectal tumors predict clinical outcome. Science. 2006;313(5795):1960–4.
58. Klebanoff CA, Gattinoni L, Restifo NP. CD8+ T-cell memory in tumor immunology and immunotherapy. Immunol Rev. 2006;211:214–24.
59. Indar A, et al. Current concepts in immunotherapy for the treatment of colorectal cancer. J R Coll Surg Edinb. 2002;47(2):458–74.
60. Taube JM, et al. Implications of the tumor immune microenvironment for staging and therapeutics. Mod Pathol. 2018;31(2):214–34.
61. Schalper KA, et al. Objective measurement and clinical significance of TILs in non-small cell lung cancer. J Natl Cancer Inst. 2015;107(3):dju435.
62. Jackson SR, Yuan J, Teague RM. Targeting CD8+ T-cell tolerance for cancer immunotherapy. Immunotherapy. 2014;6(7):833–52.
63. Yeo MK, et al. Clinical usefulness of the free web-based image analysis application ImmunoRatio for assessment of Ki-67 labelling index in breast cancer. J Clin Pathol. 2017;70(8):715–9.

64. Niazi MKK, Parwani AV, Gurcan MN. Digital pathology and artificial intelligence. Lancet Oncol. 2019;20(5):e253–61.
65. FDA permits marketing of artificial intelligence-based device to detect certain diabetes-related eye problems. October 22, 2019]; Available from: https://www.fda.gov/newsevents/newsroom/pressannouncements/ucm604357.htm.
66. Hartman DJ, et al. Value of public challenges for the development of pathology deep learning algorithms. J Pathol Inform. 2020;11:7.
67. Litjens G, et al. 1399 H&E-stained sentinel lymph node sections of breast cancer patients: the CAMELYON dataset. Gigascience. 2018;7(6):giy065.
68. Choy G, et al. Current applications and future impact of machine learning in radiology. Radiology. 2018;288(2):318–28.
69. Dreyer KJ, Geis JR. When machines think: radiology's next frontier. Radiology. 2017;285(3):713–8.
70. Jara-Lazaro AR, et al. Digital pathology: exploring its applications in diagnostic surgical pathology practice. Pathology. 2010;42(6):512–8.
71. Romero Lauro G, et al. Digital pathology consultations-a new era in digital imaging, challenges and practical applications. J Digit Imaging. 2013;26(4):668–77.
72. Baidoshvili A, et al. Validation of a whole-slide image-based teleconsultation network. Histopathology. 2018;73(5):777–83.
73. Mosquera-Zamudio A, et al. Advantage of Z-stacking for teleconsultation between the USA and Colombia. Diagn Cytopathol. 2019;47(1):35–40.
74. Wilbur DC, et al. Whole-slide imaging digital pathology as a platform for teleconsultation: a pilot study using paired subspecialist correlations. Arch Pathol Lab Med. 2009;133(12):1949–53.
75. Nahal A, et al. Setting up an ePathology service at Cleveland Clinic Abu Dhabi: joint collaboration with Cleveland Clinic, United States. Arch Pathol Lab Med. 2018;142(10):1216–22.
76. Zhao C, et al. International telepathology consultation: three years of experience between the University of Pittsburgh Medical Center and KingMed Diagnostics in China. J Pathol Inform. 2015;6:63.
77. Humphreys H, et al. Pathology in Irish medical education. J Clin Pathol. 2020;73(1):47–50.
78. Dee FR. Virtual microscopy in pathology education. Hum Pathol. 2009;40(8):1112–21.
79. Ford J, Pambrun C. Exit competencies in pathology and laboratory medicine for graduating medical students: the Canadian approach. Hum Pathol. 2015;46(5):637–42.
80. Chen CP, et al. Improving medical students' understanding of pediatric diseases through an innovative and tailored web-based digital pathology program with philips pathology tutor (Formerly PathXL). J Pathol Inform. 2019;10:18.
81. Jajosky RP, et al. Fewer seniors from United States allopathic medical schools are filling pathology residency positions in the Main Residency Match, 2008-2017. Hum Pathol. 2018;73:26–32.
82. Magid MS, Cambor CL. The integration of pathology into the clinical years of undergraduate medical education: a survey and review of the literature. Hum Pathol. 2012;43(4):567–76.
83. Metter DM, et al. Trends in the US and Canadian pathologist workforces from 2007 to 2017. JAMA Netw Open. 2019;2(5):e194337.

Whole Slide Imaging: Applications in Education

Matthew G. Hanna, Rajendra Singh, and Anil V. Parwani

Introduction

Education is one of the three primary focuses of all academic hospitals besides clinical care and research. Education in pathology departments is traditionally conducted over multi-head microscopes with glass slides or through PowerPoint-like presentations with static images in conferences. While this format has stood the test of time, it is becoming increasingly outdated and has many limitations. Pathology over the last 10 years has been transitioning to a digital format with digital whole slide scanners able to produce high-quality whole slide images (WSI) that can be viewed on any display device [3–8]. This has revolutionized pathology, especially pathology education. Education with WSI provides numerous advantages over glass slides. Use of WSI also allows building of various software programs that allow easy integrations into online learning resources and provide ready-access tools for education to a larger audience [1, 2, 9, 10].

Multiple studies have shown the superiority of WSI in education [11]. The traditional pathology glass slides for teaching purposes can only be shared among a limited number of simultaneously viewing pathologists, with the same field of view. Another factor that enables digital pathology longevity is due to glass slide staining deterioration over time. In contrast, the WSI slides can easily be shared with an infinite number of users anywhere, and pathologists can view at the same time or asynchronously. Identifying diagnostic areas of interest using conventional microscope glass slides relies on crude techniques like pen-marking or ink dotting

M. G. Hanna
Memorial Sloan Kettering Cancer Center, Department of Pathology, New York, NY, USA

R. Singh (✉)
Northwell Health, Department of Pathology, New York, NY, USA

A. V. Parwani
Department of Pathology, College of Medicine, The Ohio State University Wexner Medical School, Columbus, OH, USA

A. V. Parwani (ed.), *Whole Slide Imaging*,
https://doi.org/10.1007/978-3-030-83332-9_5

utilizing a marker and manually coordinating under the microscope eyepiece that can only be navigated by a single user at one time. Digital pathology enables virtual, hideable annotations (geometric shapes, arrows, texts, etc.) that can be easily placed and viewed by all users at the same time. This has now become even easier with cloud services being accessible from anywhere and the decreasing cost of digital storage space. Unwieldy costs have been considered one of the obstacles to implementing and using WSI. Each digital slide can consume hundreds of megabytes up to several gigabytes of storage space. At a large scale, this can easily occupy terabytes or petabytes of storage space. Each year, the costs of cloud storage have become more affordable and continue to keep decreasing in the future. Besides, retrieving cases from the cloud is much easier and faster than from physical warehouses transferring glass slides and can result in cost savings [12]. Training materials can be more objective, and images may be made available by hyperlinks to the file servers [8] that can be hosted on local on-premise or cloud servers. The cost of digital pathology in education can be considered reasonable if accounting for costs to buy additional/replace brightfield microscopes, off-site glass slides maintenance storage costs, and space constraints; a computer monitor can replace a large multi-headed scope (Fig. 1).

For the easy adoption of digital pathology in education, it is critical for tools to allow minimum disruption to the workflow and should simulate current teaching techniques that have stood the test of time. We will discuss a roadmap on how this

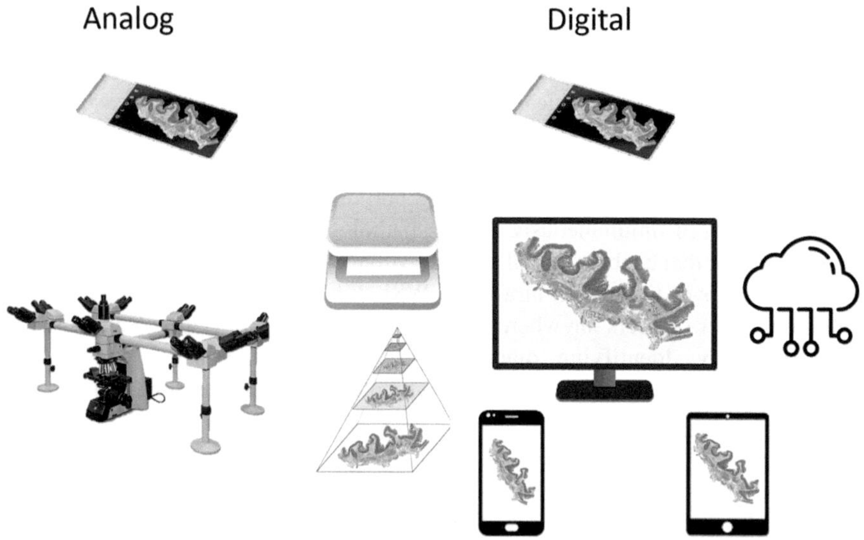

Fig. 1 Educational workflow for pathology, analog, and digital. Analog or conventional pathology education is done at the microscope, with a maximum number of participants based on the number of microscope eyepieces available. Usually even the largest multi-headed microscopes can accommodate less than 30 simultaneous participants. The digital workflow includes creating a digitized version of the glass slide through a whole slide scanner, which can then be displayed on display devices through local or cloud availability

could be easily done and help turn every department into an educational powerhouse not only for all its trainees but also for the entire world.

Building a Workflow for Enhancing Education

Most departments have scheduled weekly conferences either over a multi-headed scope or in conference rooms. Digital pathology can truly enhance both of these learning experiences. WSI can be shared with residents to preview the slides. Current software tools allow easy integration of WSI with PowerPoints combining conference room teaching and teaching over multi-head scopes. These conferences can be transmitted live using screen sharing software allowing trainees to attend conferences from anywhere. There is also no limit to the number of people that can be taught through these conferences. Trainees can review the presentations after the conference, thus helping in better retention. Preview, review, and post review of WSI make education very powerful when academic centers start using digital pathology.

Current WSI viewers provide the ability to pre-annotate areas of interest, annotate during presentations, pull out other WSI for comparison side by side, simultaneously open radiology images, hyperlink slides to references, and rotate slides for good orientation (Fig. 2). All these features enhance the teaching and learning experience of pathology. Medical school students can be tested using polls with provided choices and linked to special features on slides like types of cells, organisms, etc. Software programs also allow integration of WSI into multiple choice questions or short answer questions which can be used to test residents and fellows and also used

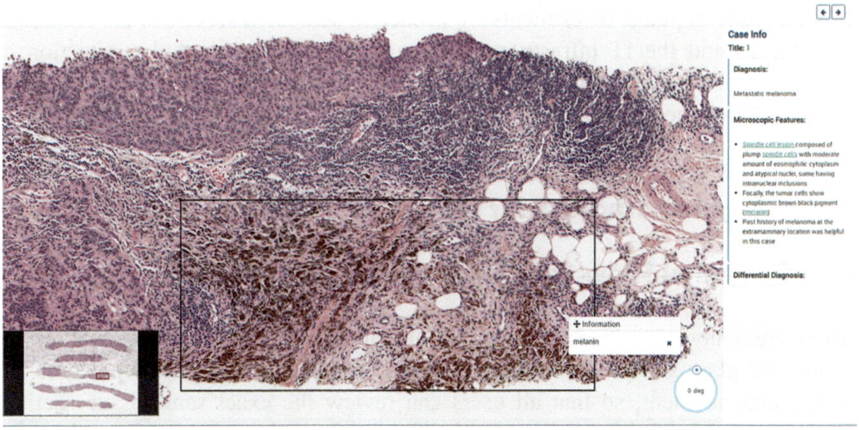

Fig. 2 Web-based educational platforms. Interactive web-based modules can be developed for teaching and presenting pathology content. Custom content development can be added to display diagnoses, microscopic descriptions, gross images, radiology, differential diagnoses, etc. Hyperlinking of diagnostic foci creates a dynamic learning experience that can be made available to any user with internet access

as pre and post assessments tools for conferences. Using WSI with such software will also facilitate CME for practicing pathologists and allow them to maintain license requirements without leaving their offices or homes. Statistical models and graphs can provide visual assessment of trainee progress over periods of time and help easy documentation of effectiveness of training programs.

Current residents and pathologists are tuned into social media. Adding questions of the day or allowing previewing of slides before conferences using social media platforms will allow better use of time spent on social media platforms, keep current generation engaged, and increase reach of education. Digital pathology can truly transform how education is conducted at scale using WSI and various software programs [8, 12].

Challenges and Barriers

One of the main limitations in the current scenario is that for web-based digital pathology education platforms, the slow download speeds of the very large digital images. This can be frustrating and without internet connectivity is impossible. Local digital WSIs can be navigated on vendor-specific applications; however, with the lack of a standard file format, this requires a separate local computer application for each vendors' scanner digital images. While there has been progress to standardize a WSI file format, the lack of interoperability between scanning vendors is a significant limitation for a seamless multi-vendor digital pathology educational experience. The act of converting the glass slide to a digital WSI is also time-consuming as this is an added step in the process. This often includes taking time to de-identify glass slide teaching sets for digitization. These extra steps in the process require justification for additional investments if existing hardware or infrastructure is not already in place. Investments are needed in dedicated servers or cloud storage capabilities and the IT infrastructure. Significant concerns include protection of PHI, interobserver variability of diagnosis on publically available WSI resources, and associated medico-legal implications.

Use of Digital Pathology for Education: Advantages

How Do Digital Slides Enhance Pathology Education

There are many advantages to using digital pathology over the conventional microscope and glass slides. Digital images can be standardized, with the potential for image enhancement, so that all users can review the exact same tissue section. Digital pathology can establish standardization as each user will view the exact same image and field of view as the other users and not different level sections where small foci of interest may be lost. This variability in slide section may not be identical that can lead to discrepancies in examination of trainees. Glass slides are also prone to fading, breakage, and loss over time. The quality of a digital image can be maintained in perpetuity. Another benefit of digital pathology is that rare cases of

Table 1 Comparison of digital pathology and glass microscopy

Digital pathology	Glass microscopy
Standardized images Image quality maintained over time Multiple images viewed at one time Multiple annotations with clinical metadata Rare cases can be stored and shared easily Cost-effective over time	Staining variability over time Tissue sections may lose foci of interest Requires ink markings that can only be seen by one user at a time Requires microscope and glass slide (physical space) Maintenance of glass slides and microscope is more time-consuming during presentations/lectures to organize/switch between slides

glass slides cannot be duplicated and made available for the trainees. Pathology trainees can benefit from a standardized education program such that the material would be presented to all trainees alike [5] (Table 1).

Advantages with Presentations, Conferences, Tumor Boards, and Social Media

Digital pathology has now been used across medical schools, pathology training programs, veterinary schools, and dental schools [7, 13]. Open-access and private whole slide image repositories are available to provide pathologists familiarity with navigating digital images, as well as for an educational experience [14]. These repositories are curated for specific subspecialty use cases or can be used for proficiency testing. Several pathology professional societies also provide a "case of the month" to introduce pathologists and pathology trainees to digital images as well as providing a novel democratized educational experience. Case-based teaching becomes readily available and simple to collate in a digital workflow compared to the traditional glass slide teaching sets that are prone to fading, breakage, or losing slides altogether. Digital pathology enables an unprecedented convenience for pathology education using WSI. Most web-based educational software also can be deployed on mobile devices and are readily available [15]. This has been shown to enhance pathologist remote learning [16]. Platforms also exist to combine presentations using digital images with other multimedia and presentation documents for a seamless experience. Inclusion of WSI in presentations can replace a multi-headed scope training session and add benefits of integrating radiology images, gross dissection videos, or other clinical metadata. For multidisciplinary conferences, presenting pathology findings in a digital workflow adds a modern approach to pathology presentations and also minimizes the time to collect data for presentations [17]. Academic centers where multiple medical domain specialties meet to discuss challenging patient cases through medical presentations are crucial for patient management and discussion. Digital slides can be compared side by side, which is not possible on a conventional microscope. Digital pathology can help facilitate pathology presentations and also have the entire WSI or patient case available to be displayed to the audience instead of just a static image of one region of

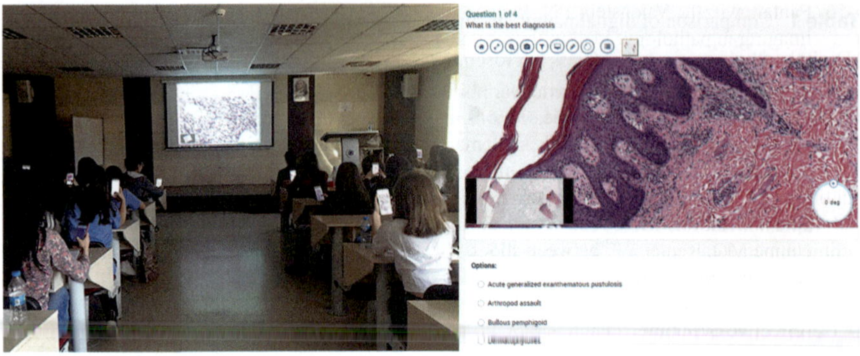

Fig. 3 Classroom setting. Digital pathology being used in a classroom for synchronous and asynchronous educational teaching of pathology. Individual users can navigate the digital slides included in their curricula. Examinations using digital pathology can also be developed to assess user performance

interest [13, 18]. These conferences can also be managed much easier for remote participants using a digital workflow (Fig. 3).

As newfound technology continues to outpace prior years, additional e-learning solutions for conferences have and will become available. Remote or in-person conference participation can also further be accomplished using digital pathology. This virtual learning environment provides a more flexible and cost-effective platform for pathology educational experiences. Many annual national and international conferences offer microscope slide sessions and are increasingly offering digital services through use of WSI. Digital pathology use in conferences can facilitate remote access without the need of shipping or duplicating glass slides through recuts. Digital workflows can also support virtual assessments with live polling for conference attendees. Previewing of digital material can also be possible prior to possible conference travel, and the digital environment offers significant adaptability. This also allows conference attendees the use of tablet or mobile devices [2] (Fig. 4).

Digital Pathology and Social Media

Social media use has increased across the globe for transmitting information across various platforms. Digital pathology and educational opportunities have taken advantage of the ease of access and ready accessibility of social media platforms. Recommendations on sharing patient pathology have been published and help guide the pathologist community when posting pathology images [19]. The social media community have exponentially surged, with numerous groups for each subspecialty, board review, or even rare or exotic diagnostic categories. Sharing cases can be for educational purposes with enthusiastic social media members providing succinct and well-summarized content in this new educational delivery model.

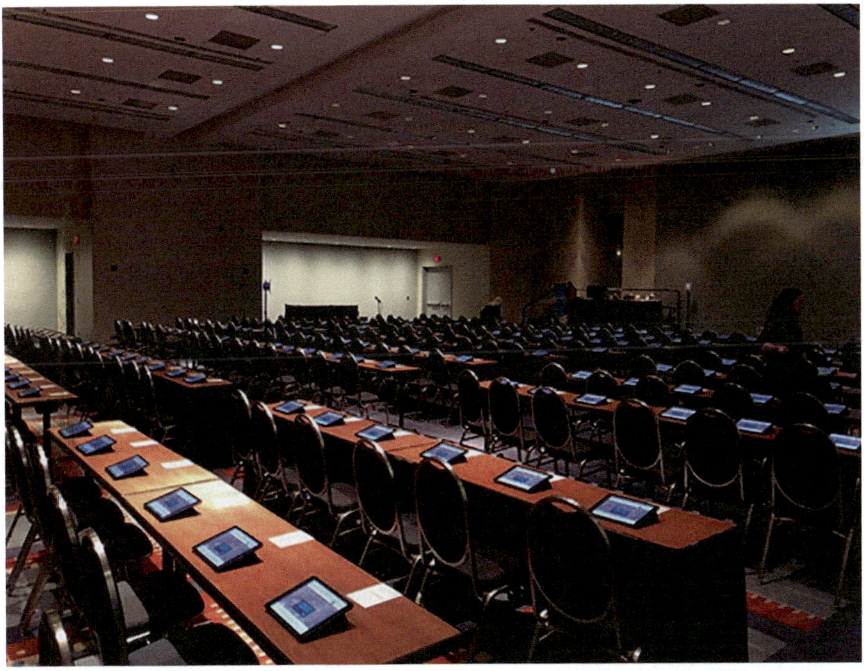

Fig. 4 Conferences. Digital pathology can be used for live or remote multidisciplinary meetings or national/international conferences. The digital pathology presentations can be structured to include digital slides in unison with other content for a complete digital learning experience

Future of Pathology Education Using Digital Slides

The future of pathology education using digital slides is bright but challenged by the current generation to establish its foundation. Pathology education typically starts in medical schools. The findings from a survey of pathology chairs did not show a significant difference between the United States Medical Licensing Examination STEP exam pathology scores from institutions with or without microscopes in their curricula [20]. The authors stated "a possible conclusion is that the microscope is now irrelevant for teaching pathology to medical students" [20]. Fast-forward over a decade, medical schools no longer use microscopes to teach pathology in the current era. In pathology training programs, in the United States, the majority still use conventional microscopy for clinical purposes, but many are implementing or using digital pathology for educational purposes [21, 22]. As massive pathology image archives become available, pathology education may become democratized, and rare diagnostic cases will be able to be viewed within a moment's notice rather than being kept in a treasure box in a pathologist's office [22, 23]. These resources will be available to pathologists to use for teaching, trainee learning, and conference presentations and will become the new norm as adoption continues to increase.

Digital pathology is also increasingly being used during the American Board of Pathology certification exam [24]. Pathology trainees will need to be well-versed with navigating digital images to be prepared for this exam but more importantly to prepare them for their future clinical practice in the years to come [6, 25].

References

1. Romer DJ, Suster S. Use of virtual microscopy for didactic live-audience presentation in anatomic pathology. Ann Diagn Pathol. 2003;7:67–72.
2. Al Janabi S, Huisman A, Van Diest PJ. Digital pathology: current status and future perspectives. Histopathology. 2012;61:1–9.
3. Iyengar JN. Whole slide imaging: the futurescape of histopathology. Indian J Pathol Microbiol. 2021;64:8–13.
4. Hartman DJ. Mobile technology for the practice of pathology. Adv Anat Pathol. 2016;23:118–24.
5. Pantanowitz L, Szymas J, Yagi Y, Wilbur D. Whole slide imaging for educational purposes. J Pathol Inform. 2012;3:46.
6. Donnelly AD, Mukherjee MS, Lyden ER, Radio SJ. Virtual microscopy in cytotechnology education: application of knowledge from virtual to glass. Cytojournal. 2012;9:12.
7. Huisman A. Digital pathology for education. Stud Health Technol Inform. 2012;179:68–71.
8. Park S, Pantanowitz L, Parwani AV. Digital imaging in pathology. Clin Lab Med. 2012;32:557–84.
9. Brachtel E, Yagi Y. Digital imaging in pathology--current applications and challenges. J Biophotonics. 2012;5:327–35.
10. Garcia RM. State of the art and trends for digital pathology. Stud Health Technol Inform. 2012;179:15–28.
11. Downing SW. A multimedia-based histology laboratory course: elimination of the traditional microscope laboratory. Medinfo 1995; 8 Pt 2: 1695.
12. Hanna MG, Parwani A, Sirintrapun SJ. Whole slide imaging: technology and applications. Adv Anat Pathol. 2020;27:251–9.
13. Saco A, Bombi JA, Garcia A, et al. Current status of whole-slide imaging in education. Pathobiology. 2016;83:79–88.
14. DPA. Digital Pathology Association whole-slide image repository. 2021.
15. Hanna MG, Parwani AV, Pantanowitz L, et al. Smartphone applications: a contemporary resource for dermatopathology. J Pathol Inform. 2015;6:44.
16. Kayser K, Ogilvie R, Borkenfeld S, Kayser G. E-education in pathology including certification of e-institutions. Diagn Pathol 2011; 6 Suppl 1: S11.
17. Arnold CW, Wallace WD, Chen S, et al. RadPath: a web-based system for integrating and correlating radiology and pathology findings during cancer diagnosis. Acad Radiol. 2016;23:90–100.
18. Yin F, Han G, Bui MM, et al. Educational value of digital whole slides accompanying published online pathology journal articles: a multi-institutional study. Arch Pathol Lab Med. 2016;140:694–7.
19. Crane GM, Gardner JM. Pathology image-sharing on social media: recommendations for protecting privacy while motivating education. AMA J Ethics. 2016;18:817–25.
20. Taylor CR, DeYoung BR, Cohen MB. Pathology education: quo vadis? Hum Pathol. 2008;39:1555–61.
21. Brochhausen C, Winther HB, Hundt C, et al. A virtual microscope for academic medical education: the pate project. Interact J Med Res. 2015;4:e11.
22. Boyce BF. Whole slide imaging: uses and limitations for surgical pathology and teaching. Biotech Histochem. 2015;90:321–30.

23. Li L, Dangott BJ, Parwani AV. Development and use of a genitourinary pathology digital teaching set for trainee education. J Pathol Inform. 2010;1:2.
24. Pathology TABo. Anatomic pathology description of examination.
25. Hassell LA, Fung KM, Chaser B. Digital slides and ACGME resident competencies in anatomic pathology: an altered paradigm for acquisition and assessment. J Pathol Inform. 2011;2:27.

Suggested Readings

Blake CA, Lavoie HA, Millette CF. Teaching medical histology at the University of South Carolina school of medicine: Transition to virtual slides and virtual microscopes. Anat Rec B New Anat. 2003;275:196–206.
Boutonnat J, Paulin C, Faure C, Colle PE, Ronot X, Seigneurin D. A pilot study in two French medical schools for teaching histology using virtual microscopy. Morphologie. 2006;90:21–5.
Foster K. Medical education in the digital age: Digital whole slide imaging as an e-learning tool. J Pathol Inform. 2010;1:14.
Goldberg HR, Dintzis R. The positive impact of team-based virtual microscopy on student learning in physiology and histology. Adv Physiol Educ. 2007;31:261–5.
Harris T, Leaven T, Heidger P, Kreiter C, Duncan J, Dick F. Comparison of a virtual microscope laboratory to a regular microscope laboratory for teaching histology. Anat Rec. 2001;265:10–4.
Monaco SE, Kant P, Carter G, Trucco G, KanbourShakir A, Elishaev E. A “Virtual Slide Box” using whole slide imaging for reproductive pathology education for medical students. Mod Pathol. 2011;24:132A.

Whole Slide Imaging and Primary Diagnosis

Bethany Jill Williams and Darren Treanor

Introduction

Digital pathology is a transformative technology with the potential to revolutionise the way in which diagnostic histopathology services are delivered. Of all the use cases for whole slide images, replacement of the conventional light microscope with a digital microscopy system for routine assessment is one of the most ambitious, fundamentally changing the way in which pathologists perform and manage their daily diagnoses. WSI primary diagnosis has been implemented and documented for all or part of the departmental workload by a number of pioneering institutions across the globe, including Linköping in Sweden [1]; Toronto, Canada [2]; Leeds, United Kingdom [3]; and Utrecht, Netherlands [4].

B. J. Williams
Leeds Teaching Hospitals NHS Trust, Department of Histopathology, Leeds, UK

University of Leeds, Leeds, UK

D. Treanor (✉)
Leeds Teaching Hospitals NHS Trust, Department of Histopathology, Leeds, UK

University of Leeds, Leeds, UK

Department of Clinical Pathology, and Department of Clinical and Experimental Medicine, Linköping University, Linköping, Sweden

Center for Medical Image Science and Visualization (CMIV), Linköping University, Linköping, Sweden
e-mail: darrentreanor@nhs.net

A. V. Parwani (ed.), *Whole Slide Imaging*,
https://doi.org/10.1007/978-3-030-83332-9_6

Benefits of Large-Scale Digitisation for Primary Diagnosis

Large-scale digitisation of the glass slide output of a clinical laboratory is a significant and ambitious undertaking, but this effort should be weighed against potential benefits. The benefits of primary WSI diagnosis versus conventional diagnosis can be broadly divided into four categories – efficiency and workflow improvements, service quality improvements, workforce optimisation and patient safety improvements [5].

Efficiency and Workflow

The flexibility and agility of digital pathology systems allow for a number of *improvements* to the diagnostic workflow, including the ability to manipulate workload allocations by pushing and pulling of cases to respond to fluctuations in workload or case mix in a department. Rapid case tracking, archiving and retrieval and faster case transfer times between the laboratory and primary pathologist and the pathologist and internal or external second opinion pathologists should streamline turnaround times and diagnostic pathways.

Service Quality

Improved information sharing and collaboration, in particular streamlined double reporting and rapid access to second opinion, can lead to better quality diagnosis, and accuracy and convenience of the recording of cancer staging parameters could drive up the quality and reproducibility of cancer dataset reporting. Digital slides are a prerequisite for the use of augmented intelligence and computer-aided diagnostic algorithms, which are likely to play an increasing role in supporting the pathologist over the next few years.

Workforce Optimisation

Improvements in workforce factors are some of the key benefits service managers seek to capitalise on in a digital deployment. The innate flexibility of the digital diagnosis offers the potential for diverse and appealing patterns of work, freeing the diagnostician from geographical and temporal constraints on where and when they work. Digital reporting can enable optimisation of the workforce, supporting those that work less than full time to maximise the hours they can offer and providing an incentive for those considering retirement to continue to offer their services on more flexible terms. Working arrangements more conducive to "work-life balance" are likely to appeal to the next generation of pathologists and drive recruitment of medical graduates into the specialty.

Patient Safety

Finally, we should consider patient safety – the cornerstone of clinical decision-making. Use of an integrated digital pathology system offers obvious advantages, with paperless transmission of digital slides directly to the pathologist lessening the possibility of a misidentification or transposition error at multiple points in the diagnostic workflow. Furthermore, digital slides offer a readily portable, instantaneously transmissible diagnostic substrate which is not subject to the physical limitations frailties and risks of glass slides and their transport.

Timely adoption of digital pathology may allow managers more flexibility to deliver diagnostic pathology services to a population whilst enabling pathologists to enjoy the workflow and diagnostic quality benefits of digital reporting.

The Evidence Base for Primary Diagnosis

A systematic review of digital pathology accuracy synthesising data from 38 peer-reviewed validation studies found a mean concordance of whole slide imaging diagnosis and conventional light microscopy diagnosis of 92.4%, compared with a concordance rate of 93.7% for repeat light microscopy review of cases [6]. Given the acknowledged inter- and intra-observer variability in histopathological diagnosis, this statistic is very encouraging. A more recent review analysed in depth the small number of instances of WSI: glass diagnostic discordance [7]. In this study, 8069 documented instances of WSI and glass slide comparison were found, and amongst these were 335 instances of diagnostic discordance: 4% of all WSI: glass comparisons. The majority of these discordances represented areas of appreciable diagnostic difficulty and recognised inter-observer variation, such as the difference between two adjacent cancer grades. The largest single non-inferiority study of diagnostic discordance utilising whole slide imaging versus standard light microscopy, which included 1992 cases, found a major discordance rate with the reference standard diagnosis of 4.9% for WSI and 4.6% for standard light microscopy [8].

Technical Considerations

Complete digitisation of standard clinical microscopy workflows requires the creation of an end-to-end WSI system in which digitisation of slides does not significantly impede the flow of cases from the laboratory to the diagnostician.

IT Considerations

Any large-scale laboratory digitisation requires adequate budgeting for IT requirements including storage, network capability upgrades, hardware procurement and systems integration.

Integration Is Key

In order to fully realise the efficiencies of WSI workflows, a number of IT systems need to be coordinated and integrated. The key elements of this system are likely to include a laboratory information system (LIS), specimen tracking system, slide management software and slide viewing software. Uni- or bidirectional interfaces may need to be constructed between these elements to ensure efficient flow of data between systems. Fully functional integration will allow the institution to benefit from a smoother transition to digital workflow, without reliance of manual data entry. It also allows for improved case tracking capabilities, faster notification of case availability and simplified workflows for pathologists and laboratory staff.

Barcoding and Tracking

For a large laboratory, where high quantities of slides are being scanned, the combination of barcoding and a slide tracking system is essential to avoid workflow and diagnostic disruption. The combination of case and slide information in a barcoded slide label allows for slides to be scanned in any order, split across multiple scanners, and for cases to be automatically organised and managed without need for human intervention. Barcodes also reduce the need for manual data entry during the scanning process and help improve patient safety by reducing the likelihood of misidentification and transposition errors. Real-time tracking of specimens and cases is possible, and your laboratory can access valuable operational and management information that can be used to optimise performance and efficiency.

IT Network and Storage Capacity

An adequate IT infrastructure is vital for successful digital implementation. This must be capable of supporting network demands and have sufficient digital slide data storage capacity. The department needs to consider the number of slides that will be scanned at different equivalent magnifications, the image compression used and the overall growth year on year. Experience from Leeds Teaching Hospitals NHS Trust indicates that on average, a standard format slide scanned at 40× equivalent magnification produces between 1 and 2GB of data, dependent on the size of the tissue sample [3]. This equates to approximately 1 terabyte of data per day in our 100% digital laboratory.

Scanned image retention time will be one of the key factors that impacts on storage requirements. Ideally, images should form part of the permanent diagnostic record for the patient, but compromises may need to be made. Physical or cloud-based solutions can be implemented, and older cases could be archived onto cheaper storage.

In terms of network, there are two main aspects to consider – connectivity between scanners and image servers and network performance for the total number of pathologists/viewers when running at full capacity. WSI generation is likely to generate continuous high traffic, so a dedicated connection between scanners and the image server is recommended. Overnight scanning can reduce network load during the day.

Pathologist Interface for Primary Diagnosis

The digital pathology workstation and the key hardware components that constitute it contribute much to the pathologists overall satisfaction with digital pathology. Here, there are two key considerations – the display screen and input devices.

Whilst it is likely that the majority of diagnostic work can be accomplished safely on a standard desktop display screen (3–4MP), certain cases, particularly those involving appreciation of high-power nuclear detail, may be assessed more confidently using a high-resolution, high-contrast, medical-grade display.

Digital pathology allows for a great deal of flexibility in terms of input device selection. Pathologists can trial and feedback on a range of devices, including a range of high-performance mice, joysticks, trackpads and keyboard shortcuts, and should find a device, or combination of devices, that allows easy, ergonomic navigation of slides.

Laboratory Considerations

Non-standard Slide Formats

When selecting a scanner, and designing scanning workflows, it is important to consider the scope of glass slides which your department produces. Large "mega-block" slides are used by many departments to capture crucial cancer metrics and demonstrate anatomical relationships, particularly in prostate and breast pathology. These can be scanned on scanners with special capacity to do so, creating very useful images, but these images take much longer to capture than a standard format glass slide (as much as 10× longer at 40× equivalent magnification and 5× longer at 20× equivalent magnification). If you wish to make use of WSIs of these large format slides, you will need to purchase a compatible scanner and consider the extra time and storage required for these images.

Scanning Magnification

The majority of commercially available scanners can capture images at 20× (0.50 microns per pixel) or 40× (0.25 microns per pixel) equivalent magnification. Images captured at 20× can be used to make a confident diagnosis in the majority of cases, but there is marked improvement in the ability to make difficult and borderline diagnoses using images captured at 40× [7]. Identifying and grading dysplasia, identifying and categorising granulocytes and identifying microorganisms can all be accomplished with greater accuracy and confidence on images captured at 40×, and for this reason, routine scanning at 40× of all diagnostic specimens is recommended for primary diagnosis. Alternatively, departments may elect to routinely scan at 20×, with reflex 40× scanning on pathologist request, but this is likely to disrupt workflows in the laboratory, and critical detail may be missed on 20× scans.

Primary Diagnosis Validation and Training

It is important that pathologists have a period of meaningful training to validate their personal use of the technology. Any histopathology department will usually house a mixture of enthusiasts and sceptics, and we all differ in our skills and confidence with IT. A pathologist needs to reach a state where they are confident in their competence using the WSI reporting system and the validity of their digital diagnosis. A number of approaches are possible, but a successful training and validation procedure should result in the following:

- Pathologists that are confident in their abilities and their limitations with digital diagnosis.
- Pathologists that are familiar with their hardware and software and can recognise and report performance issues.
- A department with a shared understanding and investment in the digital pathology system.
- A department that can develop bespoke ways of using digital to improve its outputs, workflows and working environment.

The College of American Pathologists guidelines advises that a minimum of 60 cases per use case should be viewed on digital and glass, with a washout period of at least 2 weeks between reads, and diagnostic concordance rate observed [9]. The Royal College of Pathologists recommends a protocol combining a brief period of hardware and software familiarisation, followed by focussed training using cases relevant to the pathologists workload which test potential “pitfalls” of digital diagnosis, and a period of dual reporting, with initial digital assessment followed by a safety check on glass slides [10]. Table 1 summarises the phases of this validation protocol. Use of the protocol for the validation of a cohort of breast pathologists resulted in an observed clinical concordance rate of 98.8% [11], whilst a cohort of neuropathologists observed 98.1% concordance [12].

Table 1 Summary of the Royal College of Pathologists endorsed validation protocol for digital primary diagnosis

Phase	Overview
Training	One-to-one formalised training in digital microscope use Observed practice with feedback
Validation training cases	Training set of approx. 20 challenging and informative cases relevant to the pathologists scope of work Participant views digital slides, makes notes on diagnosis and immediately checks corresponding glass slides, noting any difference in opinion Allows identification and mitigation of pitfalls
Validation-live reporting	All cases scanned prospectively Diagnosis made on digital slides with reconciliation with glass slides prior to sign out Pathologist aims to complete approx. 2 months whole time equivalent workload in this way Difficulties reported and discussed Library of problematic cases assembled and viewed with group
Summary and recommendations	Validation document produced with each pathologist documenting concordance/discordance Recommendations made for scope of digital practice/further training

General and Specific Training Points for Primary Digital Diagnosis

Experience from Leeds Teaching Hospitals NHS Trust in training and validating more than 30 consultants in primary digital diagnosis has identified a number of key areas where novice digital pathologists can experience difficulty. This experience is documented in a practical guide to digital pathology published in 2019 [13]. Diagnosis of all types of case is possible on the digital microscope, but confident and efficient sign out of all cases will take time and experience. "Safety nets" such as the use of adjunct immunohistochemistry, or glass slide deferral in particular circumstances, or for particular types of case can be utilised and should not be viewed as "failure" of the digital system. As a pathologists digital reporting experience grows, they will find the proportion of cases they are comfortable to sign increases.

Detection of Small Diagnostic and Prognostic Objects

The smooth and efficient navigation of digital cases, both between slides in a multi-slide case and within a slide that requires a high-magnification search, can be problematic. The initial low-magnification, whole slide image displayed on the computer screen can provide a fantastic "spot diagnosis" of a predominantly architecture-based diagnosis, e.g. adenomatous polyp and fibroadenoma, but it can also provide false reassurance. One of the commonest diagnostic discordances that can occur when a novice starts digital diagnostic training is missing a small diagnostic or prognostic object [7]. Examples of this include missing a metastasis or micrometastasis in a sentinel lymph node case or failing to identify a single focus of cryptitis in a multi-slide colonic biopsy series.

It is vitally important that pathologists have sufficient time to adapt and develop their own navigation strategies on the digital microscope. The tried and tested "lawnmower" technique to ensure complete high-power coverage of a slide on the light microscope is difficult to replicate on the digital microscope. Judicious use of whole slide and whole case thumbnails can aid navigation of a digital case, and features such as indicators that warn pathologists of missed slides/regions of slides can help, particularly in the early stages of digital training.

Dysplasia

The diagnosis and grading of dysplasia on the digital microscope is a recurrent theme in the WSI discordance literature and is a potential pitfall for the new digital pathologist. There are two areas of concern here: diagnostic issues at "low power" and "high power". Discordance can result from a failure to detect a focal region of dysplasia on the initial low-power assessment of epithelium (e.g. in a cervical biopsy). This type of problem is discussed above. The other issue implicated in the misdiagnosis/grading of digital dysplasia relates to the rendering of nuclear detail on digital scans, with some authors implicating poor focus, exacerbated by compression artefact and the limited dynamic range of the WSI. There is a definite learning curve for digital dysplasia assessment, and a validation procedure involving direct comparison of a pathologists digital and glass assessment of dysplasia cases can help the pathologist reconcile their digital and glass dysplasia identification and grading. Routine use of 40x scans for diagnostic biopsies and a high-contrast, high-resolution, medical-grade display can also improve confidence in diagnosis of tricky or borderline cases.

Mitotic Figure Counting

Accurate identification and counting of mitoses is another recurrent theme in the digital pathology discordance literature. In the absence of z-stacking, pathologists have to rely on an image captured at a single best plane of focus and cannot adjust this to focus through the depth of the nucleus for chromatin assessment. Similarly to assessment of dysplasia, there is a learning curve for digital mitotic counting. In cases of uncertainty, where the mitotic count on digital is at a critical cut-off level, which would affect overall grading and treatment for a patient, a confirmatory glass slide check should be encouraged. Mitotic counting is an area where artificial intelligence and computer-assisted diagnosis could assist the digital pathologist in the near future.

Table 2 Items/features documented as having different appearance on glass slides and WSI

Item or feature
Eosinophils
Neutrophils
Mast cells
Amyloid
Weddelite calcification
Mucin

Specific Diagnostic Items and Features

Examination of the literature highlights a number of diagnostic/prognostic items and features which may have a subtly different appearance on a WSI (see Table 2). Many of these items share common features: they are often eosinophilic, refractile entities. Other items of particular note include the weddelite form of calcification in breast biopsy specimens and amyloid. Both entities can be viewed on standard WSI images, but experience from validation studies suggests there is a learning curve for confident recognition on the digital slide.

Potential Pitfalls

The following table (Table 3) summarises some of the potential pitfalls of digital diagnosis in different diagnostic subspecialties, as evidenced by the validation literature and practical experience of validation. These potential pitfalls should form the basis of digital primary diagnostic training.

Continuing Surveillance and Audit

Following introduction of digital primary diagnosis, data should be collected routinely on:

- Frequency and root cause of poor quality/out of focus/artefact containing WSI.
- Frequency and details of instances when pathologists defer to glass slides.

WSI diagnosis can be audited in a similar way to existing departmental glass slide diagnostic audit, with a random sample representing a proportion of the diagnostic workload reviewed by a second pathologist.

Table 3 Summary of potential pitfalls of digital diagnosis in different subspecialties

Histopathology subspecialty	Potential pitfalls
General	Identification and grading of dysplasia
	Identification of lymph node metastasis and micrometastasis
	Identification and quantification of mitotic figures
	Identification of granulation tissue
	Identification of microorganisms
Breast	Identifying and grading of nuclear atypia
	Identifying microinvasion/lymphovascular space invasion
	Identification of lobular carcinoma
	Grading invasive cancers (mitotic count component)
	Identification of weddelite calcification
	Identification of sentinel node metastasis/micrometastasis
Skin and soft tissue	Identification and grading of squamous dysplasia
	Microorganism detection
	Granulomatous inflammation
	Melanocytic lesions
	Granulocyte identification and differentiation
	Identification of sentinel node metastasis
	Identification of amyloid
	Identification of lymphoproliferative disease/malignancy
Endocrine	Identification of granulomata
	Identification of lymph node metastasis
	Identification of amyloid in medullary carcinoma of thyroid
	Classification of thyroid neoplasms – Identification of cellular papillary features
	Identification of mitoses/atypical mitoses
Genitourinary	Identification and grading of urothelial dysplasia
	Identification of microorganisms
	Identification of granulomatous inflammation
	Identification/classification of inflammatory cells (granulocyte typing)
	Identification of amyloid
	Identification of lymphoproliferative disease/malignancy
	Grading renal carcinoma (nuclear features)
Gastrointestinal	Identification and grading of oesophageal dysplasia
	Identification of focal activity in inflammatory bowel disease
	Identification of eosinophils in oesophageal biopsies
	Identification of granulomata
	Identification of microorganisms – Particularly helicobacter pylori
Gynaecological	Identifying and grading cervical dysplasia
	Identifying metastasis/micrometastasis
	Assessing endometrial atypia
	Identifying mitotic figures (particularly in soft tissue uterine lesions)
	Identifying mucin

Table 3 (continued)

Histopathology subspecialty	Potential pitfalls
Head and neck	Identification and grading of squamous dysplasia
	Identification of microorganisms, including fungal forms
	Identification of granulomata
	Identification and typing of inflammatory cells
Hepatobiliary/ pancreatic	Interpretation of liver special stains
	Identification of dysplastic epithelium (especially gall bladder)
	Identification and typing of inflammatory cells
	Identification of granulomata
Cardiothoracic	Identification of dysplasia/malignancy in small biopsy specimens
	Identification of microorganisms including mycobacteria
	Identification of granulomatous inflammation
	Identification of micrometastasis/malignant cells in lymph node EBUS specimens
	Identification and classification of granulocytes in interstitial lung disease
Neuropathology	Identification of eosinophilic granular bodies
	Identification of necrosis
	Interpretation of nuclear detail
	Identification of mitotic figures
Placenta	Identification and classification of granulocytes
	Identification of nucleated red blood cells

Conclusion

Over the last 30 years, whole slide imaging has evolved from a niche technology to an accessible, "mainstream" diagnostic tool, with the potential to improve the working environment of pathologists and the service we deliver to our patients and clinician colleagues. As use of digital for primary diagnosis expands, and professional experience of the interpretation of digital diagnostic images expands, we are opening the door to the next generation of histological diagnosis – where the skilled digital pathologist is supported by augmented intelligence applications and computer-assisted diagnosis to optimise the quality and efficiency of the pathologist's final report. Automated triaging of cases, selection of regions of interest, interpretation of immunohistochemistry and quantification of prognostic and diagnostic features would allow the pathologist to devote more time to the intellectual and interpretive aspects of diagnosis, bringing together AI metrics, their personal interpretation of the histology and their professional understanding of the entire clinicopathological scenario to provide the patient with the best possible information regarding their diagnosis and prognosis.

References

1. Thorstenston S, Molin J, Lundström C. Implementation of large-scale routine diagnostics using whole slide imaging in Sweden: digital pathology experiences 2006-2013. J Pathol Inform. 2014;5:14.
2. Tetu B, Evans A. Canadian licensure for the use of digital pathology for routine diagnoses: one more step toward a new era of pathology practice without borders. Arch Pathol Lab Med. 2014;138(3):302–4.
3. Williams BJ, Treanor D. The Leeds guide to digital pathology. Leeds teaching hospitals NHS trust and the University of Leeds, United Kingdom Available at http://www.virtualpathology.leeds.ac.uk/research/clinical/docs/2018/pdfs/18778_Leeds%20Guide%20to%20Digital%20Pathology_Brochure_A4_final_hi.pdf.
4. Stathonikos N, Veta M, Huisman A, van Diest PJ. Going fully digital: perspective of a Dutch academic pathology lab. J Pathol Inform. 2013;4:15.
5. Williams BJ, Bottoms D, Treanor D. Future-proofing pathology. The case for clinical adoption of digital pathology. J Clin Path. 2017;70:1010–8.
6. Goacher E, Randell R, Williams BJ, Treanor D. The diagnostic concordance of whole slide imaging and light microscopy: a systematic review. Arch Pathol Lab Med. 2016;141(1):151–61.
7. Williams BJ, DaCosta P, Goacher E, Treanor D. A systematic analysis of discordant diagnoses in digital pathology compared with light microscopy. Arch Pathol Lab Med. 2017;141:1712–8.
8. Mukhopadhyay S, Feldman M, Abels E, et al. Whole slide imaging versus microscopy for primary diagnosis in surgical pathology. Am J Surg Pathol. 2018;42(1):39–52.
9. Validating whole slide imaging for diagnostic purposes in pathology. Guideline from the College of American Pathologists Pathology and Laboratory Quality Center. Arch Pathol Med. 2013;137;1710–22.
10. Royal College of Pathologists. Best practice recommendations for digital pathology. 2018. https://www.rcpath.org/resourceLibrary/best-practicerecommendations-for-implementing-digital-pathology-pdf.
11. Williams BJ, Hanby A, Millican-Slater R, Nijhawan A, Verghese E, Treanor D. Digital pathology for the primary diagnosis of breast histopathological specimens: an innovative validation and concordance study on digital pathology validation and training. Histopathology. 2018;72:662–71.
12. Williams BJ, Ismail A, Chakrabarty A, Treanor D. Experience and observations from a departmental digital pathology training programme, validation and deployment. J Clin Pathol. Published Online First: 05 March 2020. https://doi.org/10.1136/jclinpath-2019-206343
13. Williams BJ, Treanor D. Practical guide to training and validation for primary diagnosis with digital pathology. J Clin Pathol. 2019;73:418–22. https://doi.org/10.1136/jclinpath-2019-206319.

Whole Slide Imaging and Telepathology

Toby C. Cornish and David S. McClintock

Introduction to Telepathology

The word "telepathology" is derived from the Greek word *telo-*, meaning "distance," *patho-*, meaning "disease," and *-logy*, meaning "study" and literally means "the study of disease at a distance." Although the word itself had been used in the scientific literature to describe an entirely different phenomenon [1], the first identified use of the word "telepathology" in its current sense was by Dr. Ronald Weinstein in 1986 [2]. Dr. Weinstein defined telepathology as "the practice of pathology by visualizing an indirect image on a television screen rather than viewing a specimen directly through a microscope…." The term rapidly gained acceptance to describe the process of remote viewing and diagnosis of pathology specimens, replacing earlier terms such as "television microscopy," "telemicroscopy," "video microscopy," and "telediagnosis" [3–6].

At the time Dr. Weinstein coined the term robotically-controlled, video-enabled microscopes were the state of the art for telepathology, and he suggested that widespread adoption might follow in the next decade (the 1990s) [2]. In the interim, there have been a significant number of telepathology demonstrations, studies, and even some long-running clinical programs, but the percentage of pathologists practicing telepathology on a regular basis has remained rather small. The failure of telepathology to flourish using live video microscopy was at least in part due to intrinsic properties of the technology itself, but extrinsic factors were also at play. Implementation of early telepathology was restricted to specific sites due to the

T. C. Cornish (✉)
University of Colorado School of Medicine, Department of Pathology, Aurora, CO, USA
e-mail: toby.cornish@cuanschutz.edu

D. S. McClintock
University of Michigan, Department of Pathology, Ann Arbor, MI, USA
e-mail: dsmcclin@umich.edu

A. V. Parwani (ed.), *Whole Slide Imaging*,
https://doi.org/10.1007/978-3-030-83332-9_7

need for dedicated communications channels over which video signals could be sent. Prior to the widespread adoption of high-speed Internet, these signals were typically analog and required point-to-point connections such as closed circuits over dedicated cables, microwave beams, or satellite connections. None of these media were widely available, easily deployed or inexpensive, and this significantly limited the appeal of telepathology. Remotely-controlled robotic microscopes were likewise expensive, finicky, and highly-specialized instruments that few possessed.

Beyond these technical considerations, the failure of widespread adoption of telepathology can also be attributed to a lack of pressing use cases. Quite obviously, the prime motivation for implementing telepathology is a need to provide timely services that overcome geographic distances. The nature of pathology practices in the latter half of the twentieth century was predominantly that of separate and independent laboratories, with very few practices distributed over large geographic areas. The consolidation of healthcare practices into large networked systems has reawakened the demand for telepathology to the point where it is becoming a mainstream technology. Accelerating this transformation has been whole slide imaging (WSI), a technology that creates a single, high-magnification digital image ("whole slide image") from a standard histologic glass slide. Digitization of glass slides allows them to be transmitted and viewed in remote locations, making the technology an ideal enabler of telepathology services.

Definitions

Telepathology

At first blush, defining "telepathology" should be straightforward—as noted above, it is literally "the study of disease at a distance." However, the introduction of whole slide imaging has blurred the definition of what constitutes telepathology. In practice, whole slide images are stored on a server, and small portions of the image ("tiles") are forwarded over a network to a local viewer on a network-connected workstation. In this configuration, there is clearly some distance involved in the process of viewing whole slide images; however, the viewer experience should ideally be identical regardless of whether she is located next door or halfway around the world. The only difference is the length and topology of the network used to transmit the data packets. Indeed, the College of American Pathologists (CAP), in their Laboratory Accreditation Program Checklists, gives a definition of telepathology that does not even mention distance:

> **Telepathology** - The practice of pathology and cytology in which digitized or analog video, still image(s), or other data files are examined and an interpretation is rendered that is included in a formal diagnostic report in the patient record. It also includes the review of images by a cytotechnologist when a judgment of adequacy is recorded in the patient record [7]

One might therefore assert that "all WSI is telepathology" and be technically correct. Practically speaking, though, local serving and viewing of images should not routinely be classified as telepathology. To do so would rob the concept of telepathology from all meaning. Instead, most people would consider the crossing of a significant geographic, organizational, political, or infrastructural barrier as the sine qua non of telepathology. Despite this, there are a handful of entirely local use cases that clearly fall under the umbrella of telepathology. One prominent example is the practice of "telecytology" for remote on-site evaluation (ROSE), where the distance involved may simply be a few floors in a hospital [8]. Ultimately, while there really is no universal definition for when WSI use transitions from "pathology" to "telepathology," telepathology is probably best delineated by the underlying motivation for using WSI (i.e., primarily to overcome distance) more than the actual distance traversed.

Transmitting Site

In telepathology (and telemedicine in general), the term "transmitting site" can refer to one of two things depending on the context in which it is used. In a purely technical sense, the "transmitting site" is the site where WSIs are stored and from which they are served to the client viewer. In a medicolegal and regulatory sense, though, the "transmitting site" typically refers to the location where the patient is receiving medical care, such as the hospital or clinic where a biopsy or surgical resection is performed. The discrepancy between these two usages arises because the patient tissue and/or slides may be transported away from the original site where the patient received his/her care to one or more intermediary sites where they are processed and ultimately scanned into whole slide images. The whole slide images themselves may then be moved to a server at yet another site (such as a cloud server). When considering issues of a legal and regulatory nature, the transmitting site should always be considered as the location of the patient or procedure and *not* where the WSI files are stored or from which they are served.

Further complicating matters, the Centers for Medicare and Medicaid Services (CMS) rules on telemedicine use the concept of "originating site," which corresponds to the second definition of transmitting site given above. The CMS definition of originating site is "the location of an eligible Medicare beneficiary at the time the service furnished via a telecommunications system occurs" [9]. Many times, the transmitting site and originating site may be identical, but in other instances, they may differ. With regard to issues of medical practice (medical licensure, reimbursement, jurisdiction, etc.), originating site is the more applicable of the two.

Receiving Site

The "receiving site" is considerably more straightforward and refers to the location where the pathologist is viewing the whole slide images and rendering a diagnosis. CMS also refers to providers performing telehealth services as "distant site practitioners" [9].

Store and Forward

There has been considerable confusion about the term "store and forward" with regard to WSI. WSI technology is unquestionably a store and forward (asynchronous) form of communication. CMS defines store and forward as "asynchronous transmission of medical information to be reviewed at a later time by physician or practitioner at the distant site" and that it "may include, but [is] not limited to, video clips, still images, x-rays, MRIs, EKGs and EEGs, laboratory results, audio clips, and text" [10]. Store and forward technology contrasts with live (synchronous) technologies that use real-time, interactive transmission of data typically to provide services while the patient is present. While a user may experience remote viewing of whole slide images as an interactive experience, it is important to remember that whole slide images are, in fact, just very large high-resolution still images (see Chap. 2 for more details). Recognizing that WSI telepathology is a "store and forward" technology is important both for comparing it to other technologies and to understand the ramifications for CMS reimbursement of telemedicine services.

Primary Diagnosis

Primary diagnosis is defined as the rendering of a definitive diagnosis by the pathologist of record with the most direct responsibility to the patient. Traditionally, one can consider primary diagnosis as the process colloquially known as "signout" when reviewing glass slides produced by the primary pathologist's histology laboratory. With the De Novo granting of the first WSI system by the FDA in 2017, the term primary diagnosis now includes a pathologist rendering a definitive diagnosis on either glass or digital slides [11, 12].

Primary diagnosis by telepathology assumes that the pathologist of record is rendering a definitive diagnosis only through the use of telepathology and without the benefit of glass slides. An additional assumption is that the pathologist is located at some distance from the primary laboratory. For example, one does not perform primary diagnosis via telepathology simply by using WSI while on the premises of the primary CLIA-certified laboratory. Contrast this to a pathologist signing out cases at a remote, satellite site (i.e., separate CLIA); in this case, he/she would be performing primary diagnosis via telepathology. Overall, the distance requirement is arbitrary, with the emphasis on both the specific situation and tools used for diagnosis.

Secondary Diagnosis

Secondary diagnosis is defined as the rendering of a diagnosis by a separate (secondary) pathologist who is not the pathologist of record (i.e., not the primary pathologist). Cases submitted for secondary diagnosis take two principle forms: (1) a consultative ("true" consult) case, where the primary pathologist, clinician, or patient has requested an expert or confirming opinion on a case, and (2) a patient "transfer" case, where a patient is transferring care to a new hospital or clinical group and the pathologist has been asked for a formal second opinion (an "over-read") of the outside material to confirm the original diagnosis.

Unlike primary diagnosis, secondary diagnosis via telepathology can either be performed in a formal or informal manner. Formal secondary diagnosis via telepathology occurs when a formal consultative report is issued and the secondary pathologist bills for his or her services. However, when a formal report is not needed or desired, an informal consultation via telepathology can be performed between pathologists. This informal use of telepathology can be considered as a type of digital "curb-side" consultation and has proven to be one of the driving forces behind WSI telepathology, given this feature's inclusion into multiple vendor WSI image management systems (e.g., Philips, Leica, etc.). Whether secondary diagnosis is formal or informal significantly impacts legal, regulatory, and accreditation requirements.

Intraoperative Diagnosis

Intraoperative diagnosis refers to the formal rendering of a diagnosis on an intraoperative specimen that is immediately communicated, usually verbally, to the operating surgeon. Intraoperative diagnosis is commonly known as a "frozen section" diagnosis, in which the tissue is frozen, sectioned, and stained rapidly, but it can also take other forms, such as a direct smear, touch prep, or gross-only interpretation. In all cases, intraoperative diagnoses become part of the formal patient record, either at the time of surgery or as a section within the case's final diagnostic report.

An intraoperative diagnosis made via telepathology assumes that the glass slides created are not interpreted directly during the immediate intraoperative period. Instead, remote pathologists render their diagnoses using whole slide images (the frozen section slides are immediately scanned) or from live streaming video. Of note, even if the glass slides are reviewed prior to rendering the final primary diagnosis, as long as the immediate intraoperative period has ended, this is still considered to be an intraoperative diagnosis performed via telepathology.

A Brief History of Telepathology

The earliest form of telepathology was television microscopy, which was invented in 1951 by the Radio Corporation of America (RCA) [13]. Television microscopy allowed live microscopic imagery to be transmitted over long distances via closed circuit connections, point-to-point microwave connections, and broadcast airwaves. In practice, however, early television microscopy was primarily used for direct observation of samples and local sharing in classrooms or other educational settings [3]. Early applications of television microscopy for long-distance telepathology and diagnosis were rare.

One of the earliest examples of regular-performed telepathology was by Drs. Light and Krigman who reported on a closed-circuit television microscopy system that entered use in 1963 [14]. Light and Krigman worked at the US Army Edgewood Arsenal Chemical Research and Development Laboratories (now part of Aberdeen Proving Ground, Aberdeen, Maryland), and the system was "utilized in our laboratory… by working pathologists on a day-to-day basis." [14] This system was in use for several years and connected two buildings over a distance of around 4400 feet. This effort included what is likely the first telepathology concordance study, which showed only a 71% concordance between glass and television microscopy diagnosis. This less-than-stellar result was largely attributed to the use of black and white television and poor image quality [14].

Telecytology did not lag far behind, with cytopathology applications of television microscopy first described in 1965 by Drs. Weaver, Frost, and Nieburgs [15]. These applications included teaching with "various kinds of audiences [including] remote demonstration between offices, classrooms, [and] laboratories," as well as staff conferences, measurement, and diagnosis. Dr. John K. "Jack" Frost of Johns Hopkins Hospital noted that:

> Television microscopy with remote monitors and a two-way audio system offers a unique opportunity not available with other equipment. The fine resolution of the television microscope is able to be appreciated in seminar or conference rooms away from the examining pathologist [15].

In 1968, the first long-running telemedicine program was initiated in Boston, linking the medical station at Logan Airport with the Massachusetts General Hospital 2.7 miles distant [6, 16]. The telemedicine program ran until 1977 and incorporated remote peripheral blood smear and urine sediment analysis. The "telemicroscope" used in the program transmitted black and white television images via a microwave link directly connecting the two sites.

In the mid-1970s, NASA sponsored the Space Technology Applied to Rural Papago Advanced Health Care (STARPAHC) telemedicine program along with the Papago Tribe (now the Tohono O'odham Indian Nation) and Lockheed Corporation [17, 18]. The STARPAHC project used telemedicine technology, including dynamic telepathology, to provide medical care to the Papago Tribe of southern Arizona via microwave, VHF radio, and telephone. It was notably one of the first projects to use a color television camera for telepathology [19]. NASA operated STARPAHC from 1973 to 1977.

The practice of telepathology entered the mainstream in 1986 when Dr. Weinstein and others demonstrated a new robotic telepathology system [16, 20]. In this demonstration, pathologists located at the Communications Satellite Corporation headquarters in Washington, D.C. remotely-controlled a microscope at the William Beaumont Army Medical Center in El Paso, Texas some 1700 miles away [20]. The live microscopic imagery was transmitted back to Washington via a satellite link. In the opinion of many, this event ushered in the modern era of telepathology [21]. The key US patent for robotic telepathology was subsequently issued to Dr. Weinstein's company, Corabi International Telemetrics, Inc., in 1993 [22]. This patent expired in 2011.

For many years, robotic telepathology remained the dominant platform for telepathology, spawning a number of notable programs in the late 1980s and throughout the 1990s [23–28]. In the late 1990s, WSI emerged as a competing technology. Interestingly, like commercial robotic telepathology, commercial WSI also emerged from an imaging group at Rush University Medical Center in Chicago [21]. James W. Bacus founded Bacus Laboratories in 1994 and eventually marketed the BLISS

System, the first commercially available WSI slide scanner [29]. It is unclear from historical sources exactly when the BLISS system was first sold, but Bacus was granted two seminal patents for the system in 1997 and 1998 [30, 31].

While BLISS was the first commercial WSI system, it was not the first to appear in the literature. That distinction goes to a collaboration between The Johns Hopkins University and the University of Maryland [32]. This group was the first to apply the term "virtual microscope" to describe a client-server based system for reviewing fully-digitized slides (i.e., whole slide images). While their "virtual microscope" system had a rudimentary user interface, it supported many functions of modern WSI systems, including panning, zooming, and focusing through multiple captured focal planes (i.e., z-stacking). Notably, both the BLISS system and the "virtual microscope" permitted remote viewing of whole slide images over both local networks and the Internet [32].

WSI was not an overnight success for telepathology, and many review articles on telepathology from the late 1990s and early 2000s fail to acknowledge the existence of the technology [33–35]. WSI slowly revealed its utility as more vendors joined Bacus in the WSI market in the early 2000s. As WSI scanners and software improved, the installed base increased significantly, quickly eclipsing the number of robotic telepathology systems sold. WSI systems, frequently purchased for teaching, research, or image analysis purposes, found an additional application in telepathology, while most robotic telepathology systems remained narrowly-focused devices with few additional uses. The late 2000s saw the beginning of numerous new WSI-based telepathology programs and the conversion of some robotic telepathology programs to WSI [27, 36]. The increased interest in WSI telepathology is reflected by the surge of publications on the topic in the 2010s (Fig. 1). This trend

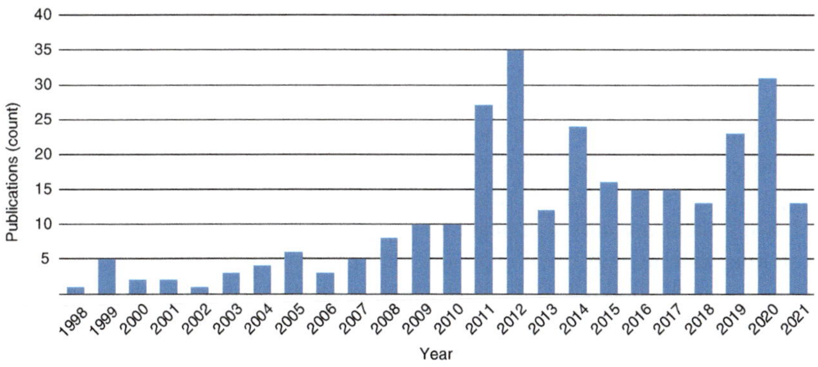

Fig. 1 WSI telepathology publications over time. The earliest publications were in the late 1990s and the number of publications per year peaked in 2012. The search string used in PubMed included a variety of synonyms for whole slide imaging: (wsi[All Fields] OR "whole slide image"[All Fields] OR "whole slide imaging"[All Fields] OR "virtual microscope"[All Fields] OR "virtual microscopy"[All Fields] OR "digital pathology"[All Fields]) AND ("telepathology"[MeSH Terms] OR "telepathology"[All Fields])

has continued to the present day, especially given the impact of the SARS-CoV-2 (COVID-19) global pandemic in the early 2020s, with numerous clinical validations and deployments of WSI for primary, secondary, and intraoperative diagnosis in programs around the world [37–41].

Drivers of Adoption for Telepathology

Interest in telepathology has been increasing over the last three decades as it has transitioned from a fringe curiosity to a mainstream technology. For many, the question has shifted from "why would I use telepathology?" to "why can't I use telepathology?" A large part of this is attributable to progressive improvement in the underlying technologies. WSI systems are undeniably more versatile than robotic microscopes. This versatility allows telepathology use cases to coexist with other use cases such as education and research. Additionally, today's WSI scanners are dramatically better than those of 20 years ago. Image quality, focus, and usability are much improved, and the time required to scan a typical slide at 20x has dropped from around 20 minutes 30 years ago to under 30 seconds today. Not to be outdone, dynamic telepathology systems have also benefited from updated technology. In fact, today there is a much larger market for, and more vendors of, dynamic and robotic telepathology systems than ever before. WSI telepathology and dynamic telepathology should no longer be considered competing technologies. Instead, they should be viewed as complementary technologies in a market where a rising tide lifts all boats. Combined, these technologies optimally cover a wide gamut of use cases.

While improvements in telepathology devices have been important, one cannot ignore the rise of the Internet, which provides a ubiquitous and universal transport medium for all types of digital telepathology. Prior to the Internet, analog video signals had to be broadcast over the airwaves or sent point-to-point via microwave links or closed-circuit television systems. None of these mediums were ideal for routine telepathology. Satellite communications solved some of these issues but did not become a ubiquitous solution. In contrast, approximately 66% of the world population now (circa 2021) has access to the Internet [42]. In North America and Europe, access rates are higher, approximately 94% and 88%, respectively [42]. And while there are still significant disparities in access between developed and developing nations, most major population centers in the developing world now have access to the Internet facilitated by high-speed fiber optic backbones and more ubiquitous mobile/cellular device usage.

Changes to the business and practice of medicine are also driving adoption of telepathology. In the United States in particular, the ongoing consolidation of hospitals and other healthcare facilities has created large, sprawling healthcare systems that are under continuous pressure to streamline care, optimize workflows, and control costs. Creation of large healthcare systems has resulted in significant laboratory consolidation and brought similar pressures on labs to reorganize and increase efficiency. Consolidation of private and corporate labs has had much the same result outside of health systems. While consolidation of clinical laboratory services is not necessarily easy, it is typically more straightforward. In contrast, anatomic pathologists are still required to staff on-site hospital services such as tumor boards, rapid on-site evaluation for FNAs, and frozen section services. When histology services are centralized, staffing smaller hospitals with pathologists can result in significant underutilization of pathologist time. By distributing cases for primary, secondary, or intraoperative diagnosis using telepathology, pathologist time can be better utilized by spending more time signing out and less time commuting and idling.

Telepathology as a Use Case for WSI

As previously mentioned, from both technical (i.e., the components of a WSI system) and experiential (slide review and signout) points of view, the pathologists' use of whole slide imaging is identical regardless of the distance involved. Given this parity, it makes sense that telepathology arose as one of the primary use cases for using whole slide imaging, especially considering the substantial costs, workflow changes, and practice adjustments required when one goes "fully digital" [43]. In fact, over the past decade, the application of WSI telepathology to secondary diagnosis and informal consultation has been considered by some to be whole slide imaging's most widely used application [43].

Numerous academic talks over the years have presented telepathology as either the primary or an immediate secondary justification for purchasing a WSI system. During these sessions, practicing pathologists have expressed their yearning for the (theoretical) freedom that a fully digital workflow would allow, with telepathology paving the way. While these situations have varied from the practical (e.g., digital signout from multiple office locations, the frozen section suite, or from home) to the exotically impractical (while on vacation, poolside, or even from the beach!), their overall intent has fueled interest in WSI telepathology. As the use of WSI for primary diagnosis matures, telepathology will continue to be a leading use case for WSI as pathologists realize the benefit of using fully digital assets, with distance barriers quickly breaking down. At some future point where digital slides are the norm and WSI is just a routine part of the anatomic pathology laboratory, one can imagine that the term "telepathology" will transition back to its original purpose, primarily reserved for histopathology applications where WSI is not feasible.

Comparison with Other Telepathology Modalities

WSI Versus Static Image Telepathology

In addition to WSI, there is another form of store and forward telepathology: static imaging. Consisting essentially of remotely-shared digital photomicrographs, static imaging predates WSI and is as old as microscope-attached digital cameras. Rather than being displaced by newer technologies like WSI, a resurgence in static image telepathology has accompanied the rise of high-quality smartphone cameras and the availability of eyepiece mounts adapters for them [44]. Compared to WSI telepathology, static imaging uses commonly available imaging devices and is far cheaper and easier to use. Static images are also about three orders of magnitude smaller than whole slide images and can be easily exchanged via email or other means, even over poor network connections in low-resource environments. The biggest drawback to static image telepathology is that the receiving pathologist is completely dependent on the transmitting pathologist's selection of fields and focus. Despite this fact, static imaging is very likely the predominant form of telepathology worldwide, and its advantages should not be disregarded.

WSI Versus Dynamic Telepathology

Dynamic telepathology entails the use of a live, real-time (synchronous) video feed from a camera mounted on a conventional microscope. This methodology retains all of the advantages of traditional microscopy, but requires a trained individual at the transmitting site to remotely operate the microscope. This individual typically receives verbal instructions and feedback from the pathologist at the receiving site. Compared to static imaging, dynamic imaging allows the entire slide or slides to be interrogated at any magnification to the satisfaction of the remote pathologist. In theory, this eliminates (or at least greatly reduces) sampling bias by the transmitting site. Dynamic telepathology sessions can also be initiated quickly since no photomicrography or slide scanning is required prior to review. This makes dynamic telepathology a viable technology for performing time-sensitive tasks such as intraoperative diagnosis or rapid on-site evaluation of fine needle aspiration material [8, 45]. The ability to focus through thicker material also makes dynamic telepathology appealing for these types of specimens. Dynamic telepathology is also favored for predominantly passive remote observation such as in consensus conferences and educational sessions.

The cost of the equipment to perform dynamic telepathology compares favorably to low-throughput, low-cost WSI scanners. A digital camera with an acceptably high resolution (at least 1080p) and frame rate (30 or 60 fps) can be attached to an existing microscope with an appropriate camera port. Efficient transport of live imagery requires video compression, and encryption of the video stream is also needed, especially if the imagery is transported over a public network (i.e., the Internet). Video transmission may be facilitated entirely by software, but some high-end solutions use hardware-based compression (i.e., codecs) and encryption to keep latency as low as possible. Latency remains the biggest challenge to usability in dynamic telepathology, and implementing a low-latency solution depends on the camera, computer hardware, codecs, software (viewer, remote conferencing, etc.), and transport medium (network) utilized.

WSI Versus Robotic Telepathology

Robotic telepathology builds on the dynamic telepathology paradigm but replaces the remote microscope operator with a fully motorized robotic microscope. Prior to the adoption of WSI for clinical use cases in the mid-2000s, robotic telepathology was the mainstay of telepathology services [23–28]. While many longstanding telepathology services continue to use robotic telepathology, others have switched to WSI [27, 28]. Robotic telepathology retains many of the advantages of non-robotic dynamic telepathology, including immediate availability and the ability to adjust focus dynamically. In contrast to WSI scanners, which are becoming more commonplace in clinical settings, dedicated robotic microscopes are generally on the decline.

Hybrid WSI Scanners

A "hybrid" WSI scanner combines the capabilities of a WSI scanner with the ability to perform robotic telepathology [36]. This modality has also been called "dual dynamic/WSI" telepathology [37]. The emergence of these devices has been significantly buoyed by the expiration of robotic telepathology patents from the late 1980s [22]. While many WSI scanners can be jury-rigged for remote operation via remote desktop software, few WSI scanners are optimal for robotic telepathology. Almost all general-purpose WSI scanners on the market are equipped with only a single high-power objective (either 20× or 40×) for digitizing a slide at high magnification. While it is technically possible to review an entire slide using only a high-power objective, this practice is inefficient, unintuitive, and frankly painful for the operator. Hybrid WSI scanners are distinguished by the presence of a full turret of objectives (Fig. 2), typically five in number, ranging from low (e.g., 2×) to high (e.g., 40×) magnification. Thus, the hybrid scanner replicates a typical pathologist's microscope without significant reduction in functionality. A second distinguishing feature of hybrid slide scanners is software designed specifically for live, remote operation.

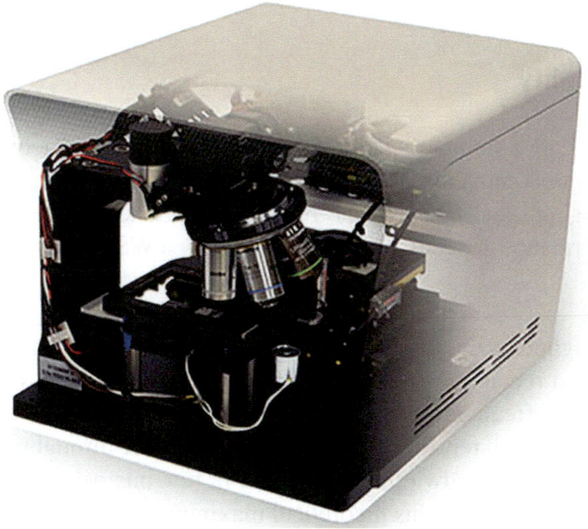

Fig. 2 An example of a hybrid slide scanner. This cut-away view of a hybrid slide scanner reveals a motorized turret with five objectives ranging from 2× to 40×. The full range of objective permits the scanner to be used for both dynamic robotic telepathology and WSI. (Photograph used with permission from Mikroscan, Inc. (Carlsbad, CA))

Hybrid scanners do have several drawbacks. They are typically low-capacity devices that use slide trays that hold between 2 and 6 slides. They are therefore not direct replacements for dedicated robotic microscopy platforms with high-capacity "slide hotels." For WSI use cases, their performance is adequate for low-volume applications, but they are neither as fast nor as feature-rich as general-purpose WSI scanners. They are, however, relatively inexpensive and offer significant value and versatility at their price point.

Technical Considerations for WSI Telepathology

General technical considerations for WSI will not be covered here as they are addressed elsewhere in this volume. We will highlight a few technical issues that are especially relevant to WSI telepathology.

The defining feature of telepathology is overcoming distance, which may range from a few hundred yards to thousands of miles depending on the particular use case. Indeed, the teleconsultation programs at UCLA and UPMC have used WSI to routinely perform secondary diagnosis on cases originating in China for nearly a decade [41, 46, 47]. While it is theoretically possible to perform telepathology between any two Internet-connected sites in the world, not all communication routes are created equally. Issues with network quality between the transmitting and receiving sites can render even the best WSI system essentially unusable. Thankfully, there are several approaches to implementing WSI telepathology that can overcome issues with network performance. As a result, there are very few (populated) geographic circumstances that will completely preclude using telepathology services.

Network Quality

Although there are a number of highly technical measures of network quality, the two measures predominantly affecting the end user experience in WSI telepathology are throughput and latency. The relative importance of these two aspects of network performance depends significantly on how a WSI system is deployed.

Throughput

Network throughput is the actual rate at which data can be transmitted between the transmitting and receiving sites. Throughput is closely related to bandwidth and the two terms are frequently used interchangeably; however, there is a significant distinction. Bandwidth represents the maximum possible throughput a network can theoretically deliver. Bandwidth is measured in raw bits per second (bps) of data transfer between points but this theoretical maximum is rarely achieved in practice because it does not account for communication protocols, retransmission (due to loss and errors), encryption, and other sources of overhead in transmission. Throughput, therefore, is a better term for describing the actual amount of data that can be delivered per unit of time.

There are no well-established minimums for throughput in WSI applications. Generally, though, network connections that are moving entire whole slide images (e.g., between the scanner and digital slide repository [DSR]) require considerably more throughput than those that are moving just image tiles (e.g., between the DSR and viewer client). While a connection of at least 1 Gbps would ensure no bottleneck when moving whole slide image files, a 100 Mbps connection between the DSR to the viewer client are likely more than sufficient [48]. Even a 2 Mbps connection may be usable for transferring image tiles provided that it has sufficiently low latency to deliver a good user experience [48].

Latency

Network latency is a measure of the delay between when the transmitting site sends a piece of information and when the receiving site receives the information. Increases in network latency significantly decrease the usability of "real-time" software such as video or audio streaming services. Likewise, increased latency also degrades WSI viewer responsiveness, sometimes to the point where it is virtually unusable. End users frequently refer to the resulting experience as "pixelation," and the actual defect is a delay in receiving higher resolution tiles to overlay the lower resolution tiles already displayed. This is a common user complaint in WSI.

Latency is a function of the distance the data is transmitted, the medium over which it is transmitted and any processing overhead occurring along its path. Latency has an absolute floor determined by the distance a signal is transmitted divided by the speed of light in that medium [49]. Signals in typical fiber optic cable propagate at 4.9 microseconds per km. A signal traveling halfway around the world on an ideal straight line path (20,038 km) would therefore take 98.2 milliseconds (ms) one way, with a round trip (request + response) time of 196 ms.

In practice, distance is only one contributing factor to latency, but it does account for an increasing proportion of total latency as distance increases. Other factors that influence latency are bandwidth utilization, intentional throttling and traffic shaping, the number of routers in the network route ("hops"), and other sources of delay due to intervening hardware and software. Latency may vary somewhat depending on the time of day, especially if portions of the route are highly congested.

Network latency between two endpoints can be measured by using the "ping" tool, which is widely available and can provide a measurement of round trip times for packets. Another tool, "traceroute," identifies the number of hops required in the route between two hosts. A third tool, "MTR," combines features of ping and traceroute with the added ability to visualize packet loss (which contributes to latency) in real time. These tools can be useful in both planning and troubleshooting WSI telepathology services.

It is important to note that image tiles slowly loading is not always due to network latency. The DSR itself is part of any round trip, and if demand on the server exceeds its ability to send tiles to all the requesting clients, requests for additional tiles will be queued until they can be sent. This phenomenon is not unique to WSI telepathology and can occur when servers connect to a large number of simultaneous clients regardless of the distance involved. Server load should be kept in mind when troubleshooting any issues that resemble intermittent network latency.

Network Firewalls

Information technology professionals can attest to the unexpected difficulties that may arise when moving data across the street, let alone around the world. Some of this difficulty arises from network firewalls, devices that live at the intersections of different networks and play a vital role in securing them against malicious attacks and unauthorized access. Firewalls are typically installed between an organization's private intranet and the public Internet and at the interface of directly connected but independent networks (e.g., a hospital and a university). It is common for network packets to traverse multiple firewalls on the way to their destination.

There is an ongoing "arms race" between cyberattack vectors and network security measures. Network firewalls are becoming increasingly sophisticated, and some current generation firewalls may implement a technology called deep packet inspection. Unlike earlier firewalls, which limited inspection to packet headers and were primarily concerned with blocking unauthorized traffic, deep packet inspection actually examines the content of every packet as it crosses the firewall. In the enterprise networking environment, deep packet inspection is very useful for identifying and blocking the transmission of malicious code such as viruses, trojans, and other malware. However, inspecting every packet crossing a firewall comes at the price of increased network latency. If whole slide image tile data is being sent across the firewall, the increased latency can result in poor image viewer performance (Fig. 3a). Latency is not an issue if entire whole slide images are being sent across the firewall (Fig. 3b); however, deep inspection of very large files (e.g., from 250 MB to 2GB) is time consuming and can impact overall network performance. For this reason, some network administrators choose to block large file transfers outright. This is obviously a problem when trying to transfer whole slide image files.

Mitigating issues with network firewalls usually requires adjustment of firewall settings to exempt or prioritize certain network traffic types or traffic exchanged between two or more known endpoints. Prior to initiating telepathology services across your organization's firewall, it is wise to consult with the network and cybersecurity teams managing your firewall and discuss options for optimizing the performance of telepathology solutions. Unintended changes made to firewall settings can also result in sudden, unexplained issues with telepathology systems. A failure to consider the firewall as a possible root cause of these issues can lead to hours of wasted troubleshooting and resultant downtime.

Approaches to Transmitting WSI Data for Telepathology

Today's end users are accustomed to effortless global web and mobile app experiences, but remain oblivious to the underlying technologies that make the access appear seamless. Much of this "magic" has to do with the use of content delivery networks (CDNs) and other forms of data caching that ensure websites appear responsive. A CDN is a system of geographically distributed servers that helps eliminate network latency and improves user experience. CDNs accomplish this by

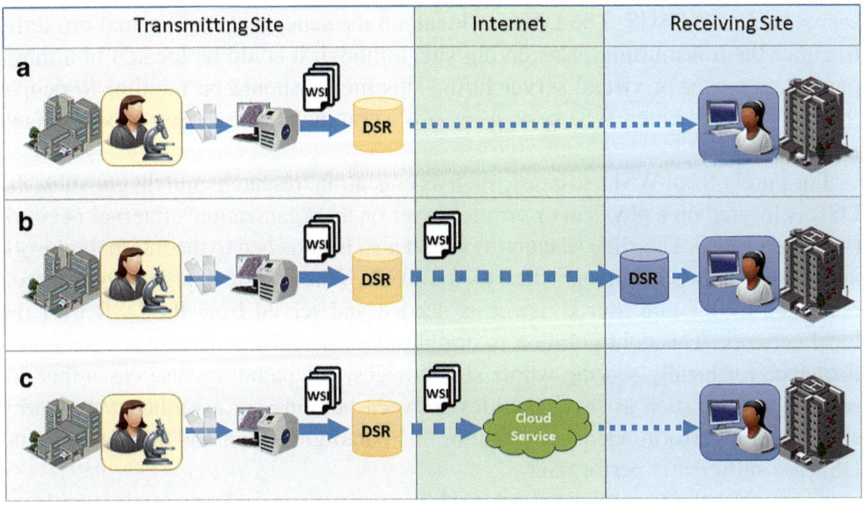

Fig. 3 Three methods of transmitting whole slide image data to remote receiving sites. This figure shows three strategies for transmitting whole slide image data from the transmitting site, depicted in the left lane, to the receiving site, depicted in the right lane. In this illustration, all data is transmitted between the sites via the Internet, depicted in the middle lane. (**a**) Glass slides are scanned to whole slide image files (WSI) and stored locally in a digital slide repository (DSR). WSI image data (i.e., image tiles) is sent directly to the client viewer at the receiving site via the Internet. (**b**) Again, glass slides are scanned to whole slide image files and stored locally in a digital slide repository (DSR). The entire whole slide image is sent via the Internet to a digital slide repository located at or near the receiving site. (**c**) Glass slides are scanned to whole slide image files. These files may be stored locally in a digital slide repository and then forwarded to a cloud service (as depicted) or may be sent directly to the cloud service. The pathologist at the receiving site then accesses the whole slide image data from the cloud service. The relative advantages and disadvantages of these three approaches are discussed in the text

replicating content to these distributed servers, and then delivering the content via the server closest to the end user. In this way, a CDN increases responsiveness but remains essentially transparent to the end user. CDNs are not, however, a free or automatic service, and entities requiring a CDN must contract with a CDN provider or implement their own solution. In addition to intentional use of CDNs, there is also a significant amount of caching of content at various levels that helps reduce bandwidth and latency for commonly retrieved content.

CDNs and caching make the consumer Internet experience much more enjoyable, but they raise expectations for the performance of telepathology systems. While off-the-shelf CDNs will likely not solve latency issues over long haul telepathology routes, there are approaches to transmitting WSI that address the latency issues by implementing a bespoke CDN-like solution.

Traditional Client-Server Solutions

By far, the most commonly implemented WSI arrangement is the client-server model. In this model, the server is a "locally" hosted DSR or other type of WSI server such as a PACS. The DSR is "local" in the sense that it is located proximal to either the transmitting or receiving site, although it could be located in a third-party data center or virtual server farm. This model should be familiar to people that have implemented WSI systems as it is a common arrangement used by many institutions.

For purely local WSI use cases, such as education, research, and diagnostics, the DSR is located on a physical or virtual server on an organization's internal network ("*on-premises*"). The slide scanner(s) would also be attached to the internal network and send whole slide image files to the DSR. Whole slide image tiles are then requested by the end user's viewer as needed and served from the DSR over the local network. This configuration is straightforward and should have adequate performance for locally serving whole slide images. Telepathology use cases that are relatively local, such as serving slides between buildings or even between nearby sites, should perform adequately within this paradigm as long as the network and DSR are sufficiently performant.

Even when the transmitting and receiving sites are on independent networks or the distance between them increases, the above configuration may still be adequate. In this instance, the slides are scanned and the whole slide images are stored at a DSR local to the transmitting site (Fig. 3a). The pathologist at the receiving site connects directly to the transmitting site's DSR and image tiles are sent over the Internet. This is the simplest configuration for telepathology and requires no additional infrastructure components beyond what already exists at the transmitting site. An advantage of this arrangement is that the whole slide images are available for review by the remote pathologist immediately after they are scanned. The biggest issue with this configuration is that it is sensitive to network latency. As latency increases, tiles will load in slowly, and the pathologist at the receiving site will eventually have a sluggish, "pixelated" viewing experience.

To overcome network latency issues, an additional step can be added to the process (Fig. 3b). This approach is similar to the approach CDNs use. As before, the slides are scanned and the whole slide images are stored in the transmitting site's local DSR. The whole slide image files are then transferred over the Internet to another DSR located at the receiving site. The pathologist at the receiving site then connects to the local DSR, and his/her viewing experience should be equivalent to any local WSI use case. The primary disadvantage to this approach is that it consumes far more bandwidth sending the entire whole slide image rather than just the image tiles that are needed. Even in the best circumstances, transferring the files will take considerable time, and they will not be immediately available for review by the remote pathologist. While the process is wasteful and slow, it may be the only way to implement a client-server model over high latency connections. This approach also has some additional advantages. For one, the DSR at the receiving site needs to be compatible with the whole slide image file format used, but it does not need to be the same as the DSR at the transmitting site. This allows the receiving site to better integrate the whole slide images into their existing digital pathology system and workflow. It also creates a local copy of the whole slide image, consuming storage but giving the receiving site direct control over digital slide retention policy. Finally, in instances where there are significant time zone differences, this model may allow decreased latency without affecting clinical workflows as the slides scanned in one time zone could be transferred in their entirety and still be made available at the beginning of the work day in the later time zone. Some international consultation services have made good use of time zone differences to effectively transfer whole slide images "after hours."

Cloud-Based Solutions

Cloud-based digital pathology platforms have emerged as an alternative to traditional locally hosted client-server models (Fig. 3c). Cloud-based digital pathology platforms reside on remote servers operated by third-party vendors and are typically built on top of commercial cloud services such as Microsoft Azure or Amazon Web Services. Cloud-based digital pathology platforms are a natural fit for telepathology and can address many issues, including efficient content delivery.

In this approach, the slides are scanned and the whole slide images are stored in the transmitting site's local DSR (alternatively, they could be sent directly to the cloud, bypassing a local DSR). The whole slide images are then transferred over the Internet to a cloud-based digital pathology platform. If necessary, the platform can then move or replicate the whole slide image files to cloud storage servers closer to the receiving site. The pathologist at the receiving site then connects to the cloud platform and reviews the slides using a web-based viewer.

Cloud-based digital pathology platforms have a number of inherent advantages. Since the slides are served from the cloud, they are not subject to the same constraints as WSI systems on locally hosted servers. Furthermore, because cloud-based platforms use standard web protocols, all network traffic occurs on ports 80 and 443, the default ports for HTTP and HTTPS. Since these ports are used for serving the world wide web, they are almost universally passed through firewalls. Cloud platforms also facilitate the sharing of slides and remote collaboration via telepathology. On the flip side of the argument, healthcare organizations and academic institutions remain wary of moving protected health information (PHI) to the cloud, and use of these services may require de-identification of any PHI (which comes with its own issues) and/or the use of HIPAA-compliant business associate agreements.

Telepathology and Cybersecurity

Over the past decade, cybersecurity has emerged as an important issue in health care, driving hospitals and physicians to address it in their work on a daily basis. From the use of two-factor authentication to the creation of large-scale cybersecurity teams, healthcare institutions have had to adjust to a new world order where cybercrime, cyberterrorism, and healthcare breaches are the norm. For example, in 2015 alone, it was estimated that one-in-three Americans were victims of a healthcare data breach [50].

WSI-based telepathology, being an inherently digital product, introduces new cybersecurity risks for pathology groups. One such concern is the use of public networks (the Internet) for data transfer and the need for the receiving site pathologists to access sensitive and potentially identified health information remotely. Given the requirement for positive patient identification in clinical use cases such as primary diagnosis and formal telepathology secondary consultation, telepathology solutions will have to migrate from what has traditionally been a pathology laboratory-focused to a more central IT-based implementation. These solutions will require rigorous IT security testing and should minimally include: (1) an architectural review of systems by the central IT cybersecurity team, (2) third party penetration testing with contract based remediation of identified vulnerabilities, and (3) regularly scheduled annual risk assessments.

Finally, given that cloud-hosted services are becoming more prevalent in digital pathology systems, there have been some organizations who are opting to fully de-identify slides and cases in public-facing and/or fully cloud-based WSI systems. While this reduces the likelihood of an accidental protected health information disclosure or breach, it also removes the two-identifier standard from whole slide images and weakens a pathologist's ability to positively confirm the patient context. No matter how one decides to implement a WSI system, cybersecurity will play a major role in its implementation and use in the future.

Telepathology Network Topology

The constituent parts (histology labs, slide scanners, pathologists) form a telepathology network, and the arrangement of these parts (the topology) can vary considerably depending on the goals of a particular organization. Three general topology models are discussed below while the connections between the nodes (sites) in the network could be implemented using the approaches previously described (Fig. 3).

Hub and Spoke Model

The hub and spoke model (Fig. 4a) is one approach to providing pathology services in a large, distributed health system or private practice. In its purest form, the hub and spoke model has all pathologists colocated in a central laboratory. The pathologists would have immediate access to the glass (or potentially digital) slides produced at the central lab. The satellite sites are all equipped with digital slide scanners, allowing any frozen section and/or any permanent slides to be digitized as needed for review at the central laboratory.

Reverse Hub and Spoke Model

The reverse hub and spoke model (Fig. 4b) is another approach to solving this issue. As the name implies, this is the inverse of the hub and spoke model. In its purest form, the reverse hub and spoke model places the pathologists at satellite sites and distributes slides digitally from a central laboratory. With this arrangement, all sites are staffed by pathologists who can address on-site responsibilities like tumor boards and frozen section coverage while remotely reviewing cases digitized at the central lab.

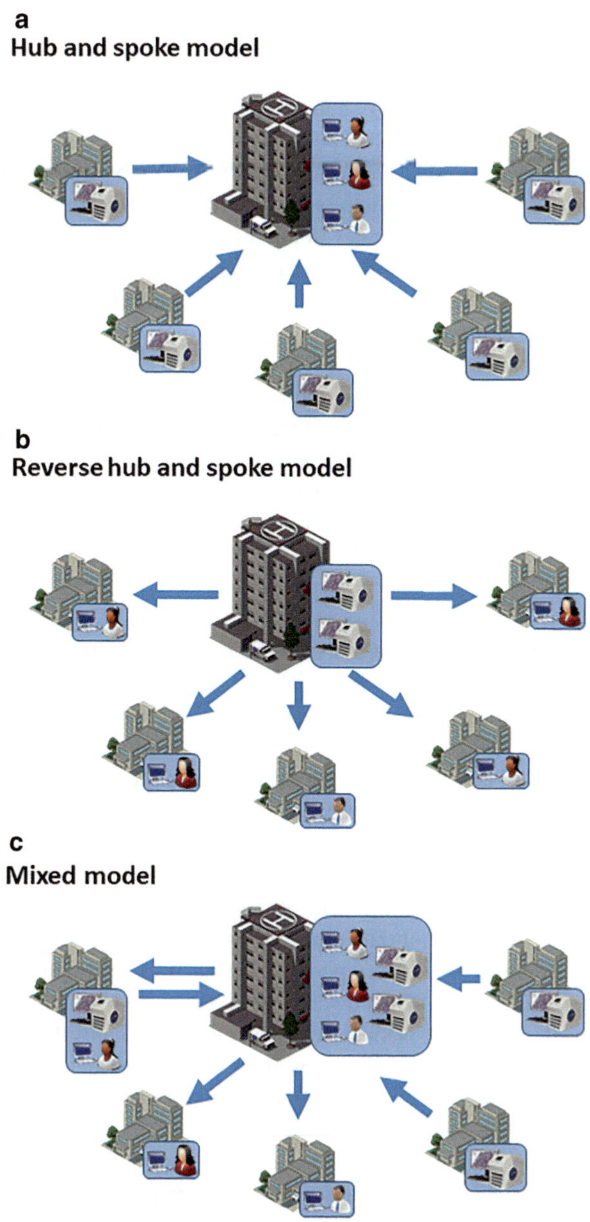

Fig. 4 Examples of telepathology network topologies. Within a telepathology network, there are a number of ways to deploy pathologists and scanning equipment. Depicted here are three approaches to using WSI for telepathology in a health system composed of a large central laboratory and several smaller satellite sites. (**a**) In a pure "hub and spoke" configuration, scanners are located at each satellite site and all the pathologists are located at the main laboratory. Slides from the satellite hospital are scanned and reviewed centrally. (**b**) The opposite configuration is a "reverse hub and spoke" configuration, where the pathologists are located at the satellite site and remotely read slides scanned at the central laboratory. (**c**) The "mixed model" combines the features of A and B, placing pathologist and scanners at locations that best suit the needs of the health system

Mixed Model

While pure versions of the hub and spoke or reverse hub and spoke models may work for symmetrically arranged health systems, the reality of today's large health systems is that they are increasingly heterogeneous and complex. For these reasons, a mixed model (Fig. 4c) is typically a better fit. In this model, pathologists and scanners are located at the central lab but are also provisioned to satellite sites as needed. For example, a hospital that requires only very infrequent frozen section coverage may be equipped with a slide scanner in lieu of an on-site pathologist. The wet tissue, blocks, and/or slides from that site may then be couriered to the central lab or processed locally, scanned, and signed out remotely at the central lab. In other cases, the hospital might be very distant or have other compelling reasons that demand full-time staffing of a local pathologist. This remote hospital could then scan excess caseload or subspecialty cases to be signed out at the central lab. Another remote hospital might have abundant on-site responsibilities, but few total cases. The hospital could be staffed locally by a pathologist with additional work or subspecialty cases sent from the central lab to be signed out remotely. There are endless possible permutations in the mixed model depending on the particular needs and size of a practice.

Regulatory and Legal Aspects of WSI Telepathology

While the practice of telepathology is subject to the same regulatory and legal requirements of clinical laboratory testing, there are some telepathology-specific concerns that must be taken into account prior to its clinical implementation. These separate regulatory and legal requirements are based largely on the fact that telepathology splits the diagnostic process between two distinct laboratory locations, the transmitting and receiving sites. In fact, from a strict regulatory perspective, the imaging modality used to perform telepathology (e.g., static, dynamic, or whole slide imaging) is less important than the actual declared clinical use case (e.g., FNA adequacy assessment, formal intraoperative/frozen section diagnosis, formal second opinion reporting, etc.). When discussing WSI-driven telepathology in particular, it is important to note that WSI devices, when used clinically, have been declared medical devices for specific intended uses and therefore subject to in vitro diagnostic (IVD) device regulation [51] in addition to laboratory-based regulatory measures.

Telepathology and In Vitro Device Regulation

In vitro diagnostic devices (IVDs) can be defined generally as medical devices intended for use in the in vitro examination of specimens derived from the human body, with the principal purpose of providing information about a physiological or pathological state or to monitor therapeutic measures [52]. IVDs are regulated by separate national agencies, such as the Food and Drug Administration (FDA) in the United States, Health Canada, the Pharmaceuticals and Medical Devices Agency

(PMDA) in Japan, the Member State Notified Bodies in the European Union, the Therapeutic Goods Administration (TGA) in Australia, etc., each governed by its own definitions, rules, and legislation. The FDA, for example, is charged with regulating the behavior and marketing practices of IVD manufacturers and vendors, but does not regulate the practice of medicine [53], whereas Health Canada is responsible for both device and health system regulation [54].

It is out of scope here to fully discuss the different ways and classes through which medical devices are regulated, including how WSI is regulated as a medical device in multiple countries. However, it is useful to briefly discuss the state of WSI device regulation in the United States as an example of the complexity involved with determining how to assess one's regulatory burden when implementing WSI-based telepathology.

Whole Slide Imaging, the FDA, and CLIA

After a long, and at times bumpy, journey, the first whole slide imaging system was De Novo granted by the FDA in the United States on April 12, 2017 to be marketed for primary diagnosis on formalin-fixed-paraffin-embedded (FFPE) tissue [11]. The details of this De Novo pathway submission, the rationale behind the FDA classification for WSI systems, and the vendor-performed non-inferiority pivotal study have all been previously described [55–57]. Briefly, this first system was cleared only for in vitro diagnostic use "as an aid to the pathologist to review and interpret digital images of surgical pathology slides prepared from formalin-fixed paraffin embedded (FFPE) tissue" [11, 12]. Notably, the system was cleared as a closed system, with the image acquisition (slide scanner) and workstation environment (image review software and display) subsystems only able to be marketed and sold as a combined system. Together, these subsystems must be validated in toto in order to preserve the pixel data pathway, which is defined as being the pixel data transmitted from the glass side, light source, and scanner through to the viewing software/workstation, monitor, and pathologist.

In the context of telepathology, this initial clearance of a WSI system by the FDA was important in that it gave pathology practices a way in which to perform primary diagnosis remotely without having to go through the CLIA-defined laboratory developed test (LDT) process [58]. While validation of a WSI system for a specific intended use (e.g., primary diagnosis) is necessary per CLIA guidelines regardless of whether the system has received FDA clearance, self-validation of WSI for a specific intended use would meet the criteria of an LDT and thus place the full risk and responsibility of the testing on the laboratory instead of being shared with the vendor. However, given the limited scope of the current FDA authorized intended uses for WSI (for primary diagnosis of FFPE tissue only; does not include frozen section, cytology, or non-FFPE hematopathology specimens), most practices performing telepathology for clinical purposes will most likely use a combination of FDA authorized and CLIA self-validated workflows. One could argue that, given this initial narrow intended use, if the LDT pathway is necessary for the most common telepathology applications, then FDA authorization is of secondary importance when considering WSI systems for telepathology.

Telepathology using WSI is further complicated by the closed system approach the FDA took with the initial De Novo process approach. As mentioned above, the pixel data pathway includes the display a pathologist must use to view WSI for primary diagnosis (Fig. 5). While sounding benign and reasonable, this actually introduces significant rigidity when implementing primary diagnosis telepathology. Given that the initial monitor cleared by the FDA had a retail price of over $5000 USD and was 3–4-year-old technology at the time of FDA authorization, practicing primary diagnosis telepathology using an FDA authorized WSI system adds financial and technical taxes to the process. With the clearance of additional WSI systems and further studies demonstrating the non-inferiority of additional displays, perhaps cleared independently as Digital Pathology Displays (IVD class PZZ), this rigidity should lessen and more flexible options will present themselves in the coming years [59].

At the time of this writing, there have been two additional significant FDA clearances for digital pathology. The first is the clearance of a second WSI system on May 20, 2019 through the FDA Class II 510(k) process [60]. This system was deemed substantially equivalent to the initial, de novo process system and thus is subjected to the same intended use (FFPE tissue only) and closed pixel pathway limitations [61]. The second clearance is for a software-only digital pathology module for a PACS system, the first approval of a device as Digital Pathology Image Viewing and Management Software (IVD class QKQ) [62].

In summary, one should fully evaluate one's use cases and needs in relation to primary diagnosis, secondary diagnosis, and current FDA authorizations and intended use criteria before initiating any clinical telepathology applications. Further, one should always review all regional, state, and local regulations, in addition to one's institutional policies and procedures, prior to starting a formal telepathology program.

Laboratory Accreditation and Telepathology

While the role of the FDA in telepathology is somewhat murky, the roles of CLIA (Clinical Laboratory Improvement Act/Amendments) and CMS (Center for Medicare and Medicaid Services) are better defined. This is exemplified by laboratory accreditation agencies, such as the College of American Pathologists (CAP), which has included telepathology within its Laboratory Accreditation Program (LAP) since 2007 [63]. There is merit discussing specific laboratory accreditation standards and their related checklist items in regards to telepathology as they can directly influence one's practice.

Telepathology Accreditation Standards

Telepathology services are covered under "Telepathology and Remote Data Assessment" in the Laboratory Computer Services section of the Laboratory General Checklist [7]. Importantly, this section has a robust set of instructions defining (1) the imaging modalities applicable to telepathology, (2) the applicable

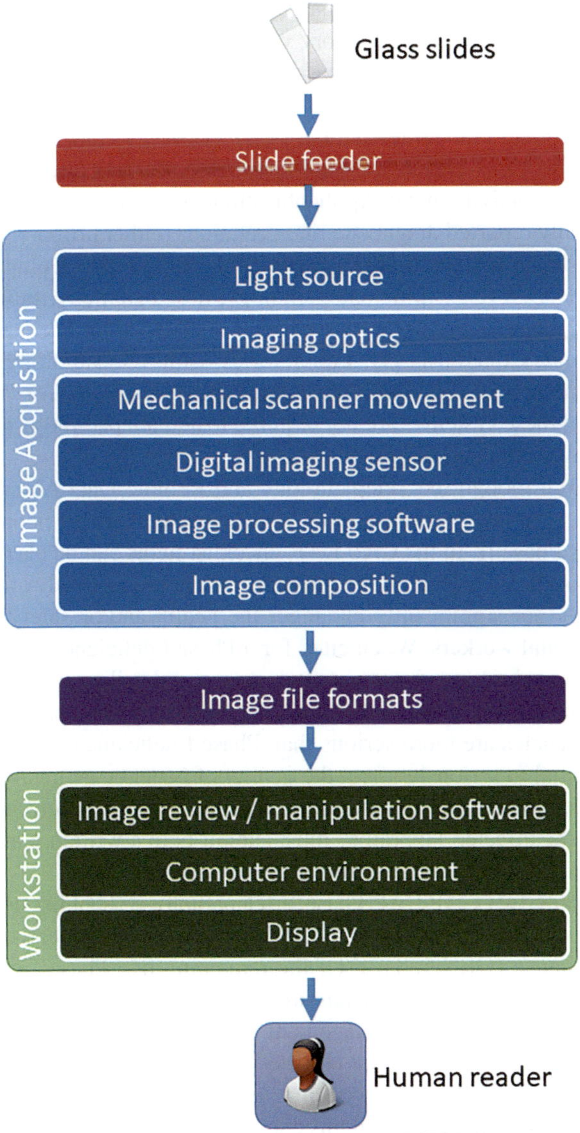

Fig. 5 The WSI "pixel pathway" as defined by the FDA. The FDA lists these as the typical components of WSI systems. The pathway can be divided into two major functional units. The image acquisition function is typically embodied by the WSI scanner. It takes in slides and outputs whole slide image files. The workstation is typically embodied by the computer, display, and image review software used by the receiving pathologist. Standardizing all aspects of this latter portion of the pixel pathway can be challenging in telepathology environments. (Adapted from the FDA [86])

clinical use cases for regulatory oversight of telepathology services, and (3) those clinical use cases for which regulatory oversight are not required. Overall, these instructions give pathology practices a clear idea of how to plan their approach to telepathology vis-à-vis accreditation.

Before beginning clinical telepathology services, laboratories must first assess their clinical use cases and, if they are applicable, declare telepathology on their formal laboratory activity menu. Applicable clinical use cases include telepathology used for formally reported diagnostic interpretations (either primary, frozen section, or secondary diagnoses), pathologist participation in ancillary techniques requiring image interpretation (e.g., in hematopathology, flow cytometry, molecular pathology, etc.), and the real time evaluation of FNA specimens for adequacy assessment and/or preliminary diagnosis [7]. Laboratories using telepathology for "informal reviews without formal reporting" (e.g., a virtual curbside) and/or "educational or research use of these systems" are not required to add telepathology to their activity menus, nor follow the checklist items [7].

Notably, even though the Telepathology and Remote Data Assessment section has been present for over 10 years, of the seven current checklist items, only two are categorized as Phase II. In the CAP LAP, checklist items can be classified as either Phase I or Phase II. Phase I items are those deemed not to seriously affect the quality of patient care, nor significantly endanger the health and/or safety of patients or laboratory/hospital workers. When cited for a Phase I deficiency, the affected laboratory is only required to submit a written response detailing a solution; however, documentation that the corrective action has been implemented is not required. Phase II deficiencies are more serious than Phase I deficiencies and are deemed to have the potential to seriously affect the quality of patient care and/or endanger the health and safety of patients or laboratory/hospital workers. When cited for a Phase II deficiency, the affected laboratory must submit both a written plan of corrective action and evidence of its implementation [64].

There are only two CAP LAP Phase II telepathology checklist items [7]. These concern positive patient identification (GEN.50057) and patient confidentiality/HIPAA compliance (GEN.52842). Of the remaining five Phase I checklist items, the most noteworthy include the requirement to (1) include one's telepathology services within the lab's quality management program (GEN.52860), (2) ensure the receiving site has access to relevant clinical information for the case (GEN.50614), and (3) validate telepathology systems used for clinical diagnostic purposes (GEN.50630). Given that Phase I items can be converted to Phase II status as laboratory practices evolve, telepathology practices should develop comprehensive policies and procedures to ensure all items in the checklist are followed.

Laboratory Validation of Telepathology Systems

The validation requirement for telepathology systems is significant for clinical laboratories given that the validation: (1) should closely emulate real-world clinical environments, (2) involve specimen preparation types and clinical settings relevant to the intended use(s) of the system, and (3) be carried out by one or more pathologists adequately trained to use the system. Notably, these criteria are distinct from the validation of whole slide imaging systems themselves, for which there is a separate checklist item in the WSI section in the Laboratory General CAP LAP checklist [7]. In short, this means that in most situations, one must perform two laboratory validations for WSI-based telepathology—one for the whole slide imaging system itself, followed by another for the intended use of telepathology.

In reviewing the above validation criteria, it becomes clear that defining the clinically relevant intended use(s) for the system is of extreme importance. For example, if the "real-world clinical environment" for which the technology will be used is for emulating frozen section diagnosis, then the validation cannot be subsequently applied to telepathology-based primary diagnosis of biopsies or formal secondary consult diagnosis. Further, each officially defined clinical intended use will also define where the telepathology will be deployed, including both expected imaging endpoints (transmitting and receiving sites). To emulate real-world circumstances, the actual endpoints should be validated.

When the potential for using ad hoc receiving sites (e.g., homes, hotels, conference sites, or any other site where pathologists may be asked to provide telepathology services) is present, validation of these sites may not be possible or feasible. In these cases, the clinical laboratory should consider limiting the use of ad hoc sites per policy or validating standard specific hardware for which telepathology services could be used. Further, when non-CLIA licensed sites are to be used, the laboratory might consider applying for a multiple site exception for their primary CLIA-certified laboratory [65]. However, the appropriateness of using a multiple site exception for telepathology services is not entirely clear, given that the most recent version of form CMS-116 (updated 09/2017) does not address telepathology directly. The authors recommend checking with the clinical laboratory's local CLIA office for interpretation of the multiple site exception.

Laboratory Validation of Whole Slide Imaging Systems

Finally, while virtual slides/whole slide imaging is listed as an imaging modality for the CAP LAP Telepathology and Remote Data Access section, there are currently no WSI-specific checklist items included within this section. Instead, as mentioned above, "whole slide imaging" is its own section and is only applicable to laboratories using WSI for diagnostic purposes (primary or secondary diagnosis, regardless of the use of telepathology) [7]. Similar to above, if one's lab is using WSI-based telepathology, WSI should be added to the laboratory's formal activity menu.

The WSI CAP LAP section currently consists of only two Phase I checklist items, one requiring WSI system validation/verification and one for proper system training prior to clinical implementation [7]. While WSI system validation is covered elsewhere in detail, it is worth mentioning that the CAP LAP only gives recommendations for WSI system validation, and the specifics of validation remain at the discretion of the CLIA-designated laboratory director. Two potential resources for WSI system validation include: (1) the CAP guidelines for validating WSI for diagnostic purposes and (2) the Clinical Guidelines for Telepathology issued by the American Telepathology Association [66, 67].

Overall, given the paucity of CLIA standards for WSI and related checklist items in the WSI section of the CAP LAP circa late 2021, the best recommendation for using WSI in any clinical application is to consult local regulatory agencies and the most recent literature before implementation. One would expect this section to expand as WSI is more widely adopted and becomes a more an integral part of the laboratory.

Image Retention and Telepathology

A notable gray area of telepathology regulation is the image retention requirement for whole slide images used in telepathology diagnosis. In 2016, the CAP LAP added whole slide images to its list of record retention requirements in the Anatomic Pathology Checklist [ANP.12500], with the stipulation that digital images used for primary diagnosis be retained for at least 10 years only if the original glass slides are "not available" [68]. However, the act of digitizing a glass slide does not directly change the CLIA/CAP requirement that glass slides be retained for a minimum of 10 years, that is, the requirement is not an "either/or" type of scenario.

To complicate matters further, neither CAP nor CLIA has provided requirements or guidance for retention of static images, dynamic imaging (live-video), or whole slide images for telepathology-based secondary diagnosis. With some WSI telepathology configurations (Fig. 3a, c), only a portion of the image tiles are transferred between sites, and the original whole slide image remains with the transmitting site or cloud service. This leaves the consulting pathologist without a record of the original scan, which could present a legal issue under certain circumstances. For example, if the transmitting site scanned a glass slide, but failed to include all the relevant diagnostic tissue, this may lead the consultant at the receiving site to make a misdiagnosis for reasons beyond his/her control.

Given the ambiguity surrounding image retention for telepathology, it is the authors' recommendation that, at the very least, CLIA-certified laboratories performing telepathology have a written policy indicating their position on the retention of whole slide images and other media used for telepathology. Additionally, since one can easily argue that medical images are a part of a patient's medical record, care should be made to research whether any institutional, local, state, and/or federal regulations for medical record retention are applicable to their practice of telepathology.

Medical Licensure

All forms of formal telediagnosis are subject to medical licensure requirements in the originating/transmitting site. Rules governing the intrastate, interstate/interprovincial, and international provision of medical services vary significantly from country to country and between countries [69]. An exhaustive discussion is beyond the scope of this chapter, which will instead focus on the situation in the United States.

In the United States, medical licensure is governed at the state level and lacks federal coordination. This system has produced 71 distinct medical licensing boards within the states and territories [70]. For the most part, the licensing requirements in the United States for WSI telepathology mirror those for glass slides. In the case of primary diagnosis, a pathologist should have a valid medical license for both the transmitting and receiving sites. Formal intraoperative diagnosis should be considered a form of primary diagnosis for the purpose of medical licensure [28].

Licensure requirements for interstate secondary diagnosis are less straightforward. The CAP has addressed this issue explicitly in its policy, "Licensure Requirements for Interstate Diagnosis, Including Interstate Telemedicine Practice" [71]. This CAP policy makes a clear distinction between the interstate practice of pathology and "intra-specialty consultation" performed by an out-of-state pathologist. The policy states that interstate practice of pathology requires a license in the state where the specimen is obtained. However, CAP makes an explicit exception for interstate consultation at the request of an in-state pathologist or when a primary diagnostic report has already been issued and the telepathologist is being asked to render a second opinion. The CAP policy, while it is informative and has been cited in legal precedent, does not overrule individual state medical statutes [71].

Hiemenz et al. attempted to directly address this issue of medical licensing for interstate practice of pathology in a study published in 2014 [72]. The authors describe their methodology:

> For all 50 states and the District of Columbia, we examined state medical practice acts, state medical board websites, and contacted each medical board for information regarding specific legislation or guidelines related to the interstate pathology practice [72].

Surveys were sent to the medical boards and were returned by all except Illinois. This study revealed three broad categories of licensure permissiveness for medical consultation. The most permissive group of states explicitly permitted either the limited practice of medicine (consultative or otherwise) without an in-state license ($n = 3$) or consultative practice by physicians located out-of-state without in-state medical licenses ($n = 33$). For the most part, these states align with the CAP policy on interstate consultation discussed above, although some states do place upper limits on the frequency of out-of-state consultation. The second most permissive group of states ($n = 9$) allow consultation without an in-state medical license, but only for physicians located in-state, which could be potentially problematic for telepathology services. The final group of states ($n = 5$) explicitly requires a medical license in their state for any physician performing a consultation. This study is worth reading, but the findings remain controversial, with many of the responses from states directly conflicting with the real-world experience of practices providing interstate expert opinion using glass slides.

Interstate Medical Licensure Compact

A number of states have tried to address the issue of interstate practice by creating the Interstate Medical Licensure Compact (IMLC), which provides an expedited pathway for obtaining licensure in multiple states [73]. The IMLC was created in 2014 and represents a voluntary agreement between the states and their Medical and

Osteopathic Boards. Member states join the IMLC by passing state legislation affirming participation in the compact. While the IMLC has the potential to significantly simplify obtaining a medical license in multiple states, it is important to note what the IMLC does not do. It does not replace state medical boards or individual state licenses, and it does not automatically confer licensure in all member states. Furthermore, it is not free. In addition to the IMLC's $700 fee, the applicant is still responsible for applicable state medical board license fees.

Physicians that want to apply to the IMLC must have an unrestricted medical license in a Compact Member State and must designate a state of principal licensure (SPL) that complies with IMLC requirements. The SPL is responsible for reviewing a physician's application and performing a federal criminal background check. The SPL then issues a Letter of Qualification that entitles the physician to obtain a license in any number of the IMLC member states. Twenty-nine states plus the District of Columbia and the Territory of Guam currently participate in the IMLC. The Compact began issuing Letters of Qualification in April 2017. Average turnaround time for licensure is currently about two weeks [73].

Privileging and Credentialing

Privileging is the process of authorizing physicians to provide specific services within a healthcare organization, while credentialing is the process of regularly confirming the validity of a physician's credentials to practice medicine. Hospitals must have privileging and credentialing processes in place that conform with CMS standards. Telepathology (and telemedicine in general) obviously complicates matters as various responsibilities in the process may now be split between the transmitting and receiving sites. In the best case, this might result in duplication of effort; however, in the worst case, it could result in each site having an incomplete view of relevant incidents occurring at the other site. This is especially pertinent in ongoing evaluation of the pathologist's remote practice.

To address these issues, CMS established rules in 2011 that govern credentialing and privileging for telemedicine services [74]. These rules specify that:

1. A written agreement is required when telemedicine services are provided remotely to a hospital.
2. The agreement must include provisions that the receiving entity uses a credentialing and privileging process that meets Medicare standards.
3. The individual physicians providing the telemedicine services must also hold privileges at the receiving site.
4. The transmitting site is required to convey any complaints about, or adverse events resulting from, telemedicine services to the receiving site.
5. The receiving site assumes the responsibility for conducting quality assurance reviews of the physicians providing services.

Similar to the above regulatory and licensing scenarios, pathologists should check with their healthcare organization's privileging and credentialing officials to ensure proper procedures are followed prior to initiating telepathology services.

Liability, Malpractice, and Malpractice Insurance

Proving a malpractice claim requires several criteria to be met: (1) a physician-patient relationship must have existed, (2) the physician must have been negligent in that relationship, (3) the negligence must have led to injury, and (4) the injury must have resulted in damage.

Of the above, the physician-patient relationship is sometimes debated in pathology practice since pathologists rarely interact directly with patients. Most people would agree that in the case of primary diagnosis, though, the primary pathologist has direct responsibility to the patient that is established by the presence of both a formal report and reimbursement for services. A physician-patient relationship becomes more tenuous with formal secondary diagnosis (with a formal report) and even more tenuous with informal consultation (without a report). As WSI telepathology might entail any of the above situations, pathology practices should ensure that they are properly complying with all potential FDA, CLIA, state, local, and institutional rules and regulations in order to minimize their potential liability.

Unfortunately, at the time of this writing, there is little legal precedent for telemedicine, and, for telepathology, there is none. For this reason, an overabundance of caution is warranted, including careful validation of one's telepathology practice. Finally, it is important to confirm that the medical malpractice insurance for you and your practice will cover telemedicine services prior to initiating clinical telepathology services. Coverage needs to specifically address the type of telepathology services you intend to provide as well as specific relationships between the transmitting and receiving sites, including intrastate versus interstate versus international practice.

Reimbursement

In the current practice, WSI telepathology services are generally considered to be equivalent to their local pathology equivalents. At present, this means that pathology services provided via digital pathology and/or telepathology are reimbursed at the same rate as services rendered using glass slides. As one can imagine, given the increased capital and operational costs associated with starting up either digital pathology and/or telepathology practices, equivalent reimbursement poses a significant impediment to implementing WSI-based services. In fact, a common question when discussing WSI and telepathology implementations is whether there will be increased payments to cover the increased cost of digital pathology in the future, perhaps as an increased technical component for the transmitting site.

CMS does have specific HCPCS/CPT codes related to telehealth [9]. Almost all of these codes are restricted to specific services and originating locations (either outside of a Metropolitan Statistical Area or is a rural Health Professional Shortage Area as defined by CMS). However, CMS has made no provision for pathology telehealth services. The current HCPCS/CPT codes cover telehealth equivalents of traditional face-to-face encounters between providers and medicare recipients. In fact, with only one exception, CMS specifically excludes using telehealth HCPCS/CPT codes for asynchronous "store and forward" technologies. This single exception is a newly-proposed HCPCS code, G2010, that covers "remote evaluation of recorded video and/or images submitted by an established patient (e.g., store and forward)" [67]. This code is not subject to any restrictions in location but is intended for use in patient evaluation and management services and would therefore not apply to telepathology. At this point, it is very unlikely that new medicare billing codes will emerge specifically for WSI telepathology.

Currently, the best strategy for reimbursement remains billing telepathology services as equivalent to traditional, local glass-based diagnostic services. Combined with potential drivers of telepathology, such as making more efficient use of one's existing workforce, expanding one's service area and test volume, and providing higher quality patient care, a surcharge may not be necessary or warranted. As digital pathology and WSI-based telepathology become more commonplace, the issue of reimbursement may eventually be directly addressed.

COVID-19 and Telepathology

In December of 2019, an outbreak of pneumonia developed in and around a seafood wholesale market in Wuhan, Hubei province, China [75]. The outbreak was due to a novel coronavirus (initially called 2019-nCoV and later SARS-CoV-2) resulting in a respiratory disease dubbed Coronavirus Disease 2019 (COVID-19) by the WHO. By early 2020, SARS-CoV-2 had spread rapidly and widely, resulting in the global COVID-19 pandemic. The first case in the United States was identified on January 19, 2020, and by January 31, 2020, the Department of Health and Human Services declared a public health emergency related to COVID-19 [76]. Growth of cases was initially slow in the United States, but as evidence for the pandemic mounted, the White House declared a national emergency on March 13, 2020 [77]. Shortly after that, states began issuing mandatory stay-at-home orders, beginning with California on March 19 [78]. Stay-at-home orders made exceptions for essential healthcare workers, but many healthcare organizations and employers also recognized that older adults were at increased risk from COVID-19. Indeed, the CDC reported that 8 out of 10 COVID-related deaths in the United States occurred in adults 65 years old and older [79, 80]. The pathology workforce is unique in health care in that it typically lacks direct patient contact and trends older than most medical specialties. The pathologist workforce has been shrinking for years, and is aging, with 32% of pathologists over the age of 55 and 12% over the age of 65 [81, 82]. Recognizing that telepathology could enable anatomic pathology services while supporting social distancing and stay-at-home orders, several pathology organizations, including the Alliance for Digital Pathology, the Association for Pathology Informatics (API), the Digital Pathology Association (DPA), and the CAP, lobbied the FDA and CMS to make regulatory exceptions for the use of telepathology during the crisis [83].

CMS responded by issuing the "Clinical Laboratory Improvement Amendments (CLIA) Laboratory Guidance During COVID-19 Public Health Emergency" memorandum on March 26, 2020 [84]. This memorandum outlined CMS's response to COVID-19, including their intention to exercise "enforcement discretion to adopt a temporary policy of relaxed enforcement [of CLIA] in connection with laboratories located at temporary testing sites…" and that "laboratories that choose to utilize temporary testing sites (e.g., for remote review and reporting of slides/images), may do so…" [84]. With respect to telepathology, relaxation of enforcement allows slides to be reviewed at temporary testing sites (including "the pathologist's home") provided that the work is done in association with a CLIA-licensed laboratory. While the memo allows temporary testing sites to be utilized without modifying one's CLIA license, it does not lift other CLIA requirements for telepathology, such as the need for proper verification or validation of a digital pathology system. Furthermore, the CMS memorandum is only in effect for the duration of the COVID-19 public health emergency although to date that has extended into late 2021.

About one month later, the FDA issued its guidance document, "Enforcement Policy for Remote Digital Pathology Devices During the Coronavirus Disease 2019 (COVID-19) Public Health Emergency" on April 24, 2020 [85]. Like the CMS, the FDA elected to exercise enforcement discretion with regards to the marketing of digital pathology systems suitable for telepathology, the intention of which was "to help expand the availability of devices for remote reviewing and reporting of scanned digital images of pathology slides… during this pandemic" [85]. The FDA guidance pertains to four types of digital pathology-related IVDs and makes it clear that the FDA does not intend to object to either (1) modifications to FDA-cleared indications, functionality, hardware, and/or software for use in a remote setting or (2) the marketing of new, digital pathology devices for use in remote settings that are not currently 510(k) cleared. As with the CMS, the FDA guidance is intended only for the duration of the declared HHS emergency.

The effects of the COVID-19 pandemic, social distancing, and the CMS and FDA relaxation of enforcement criteria for remote viewing of digital pathology slides will not be fully known for years. For those, the public emergency has highlighted a more urgent need to implement a digital pathology solution for disaster preparedness in addition to regular practice. For those with digital pathology systems in place, the issue of proper validation for remote use, either for telepathology or for remote diagnosis, has come to the forefront. As "working from home" practices evolve and establish themselves into mainstream healthcare business culture, WSI telepathology use will normalize and rise accordingly. Ultimately, one can hope the lessons learned during this time will help to inform future policy and further the practice of whole slide imaging and telepathology.

Summary

Whole slide imaging is a versatile technology particularly suited for telepathology—it provides a digital platform that can be interfaced with laboratory information systems, support primary, secondary, and intraoperative diagnosis, and is inherently able to overcome distance and other barriers. When implementing WSI telepathology, one must clearly identify the practice's intended use case(s), as this will inform one's technical configurations, hardware and networking requirements, regulatory, legal, licensing, and potential reimbursement/cost strategies.

References

1. Jordan DS. The principles of sciosophy. Science. 1900;11(281):763–72.
2. Weinstein RS. Prospects for telepathology. Hum Pathol. 1986;17(5):433–4.
3. Lancet. Teaching by television. Lancet. 1951;258(6678):335–6.
4. Allan R. Medical electronics: coming: the era of telemedicine: interactive audio/video telediagnosis is proven viable in both government- and privately-funded experiments. IEEE Spectr. 1976;13(12):31–6.
5. Freehe CL. Video microscopy with closed circuit television at the University of Washington Health Sciences Division. J Biol Photogr Assoc. 1960;28:15–20.
6. Murphy RL, Bird KT. Telediagnosis: a new community health resource. Observations on the feasibility of telediagnosis based on 1000 patient transactions. Am J Public Health. 1974;64(2):113–9.
7. College of American Pathologists. Laboratory General Checklist. CAP Accreditation Program. College of American Pathologists; 2018.
8. Lin O, Rudomina D, Feratovic R, Sirintrapun SJ. Rapid on-site evaluation using telecytology: a major cancer center experience. Diagn Cytopathol. 2019;47(1):15–9.
9. Centers for Medicare and Medicaid. Telehealth services [Internet]. Centers for Medicare and Medicaid. 2019 [cited 2019 Apr 4]. Available from: https://www.cms.gov/Outreach-and-Education/Medicare-Learning-Network-MLN/MLNProducts/Downloads/Telehealth-Services-Text-Only.pdf.
10. Centers for Medicare and Medicaid. Medicare carriers manual: section 15516, medicare payment for telehealth services [Internet]. 2003 [cited 2019 Jun 4]. Available from: https://www.cms.gov/Regulations-and-Guidance/Guidance/Transmittals/downloads/R1798B3.pdf.
11. FDA, Office of the Commissioner. FDA allows marketing of first whole slide imaging system for digital pathology [Internet]. FDA. 2017 [cited 2019 Jun 4]. Available from: http://www.fda.gov/news-events/press-announcements/fda-allows-marketing-first-whole-slide-imaging-system-digital-pathology.
12. Food and Drug Administration. 510(k) substantial equivalence determination decision summary: K172174 [Internet]. Food and Drug Administration. 2017 [cited 2019 Jun 4]. Available from: https://www.accessdata.fda.gov/cdrh_docs/reviews/K172174.pdf.
13. Flory LE. The television microscope. Cold Spring Harb Symp Quant Biol. 1951;16:505–9.
14. Light FW, Krigman MR. Microscopic telecommunication by closed-circuit television. Mil Med. 1967;132(1):28–33.
15. Weaver JM, Frost JK, Nieburgs HE. Television microscopy in cytopathology [Internet]. Washington: U. S. Public Health Service, Division of Chronic Diseases, Cancer Control Program; 1965 [cited 2019 Jun 4]. 6 p. Available from: https://catalog.hathitrust.org/Record/009370018.
16. Weinstein RS. Telemedicine: Back to the future - a 50 year perspective [Internet]. Northwest Regional Telehealth Resouce Center (NRTRC); 2015 Mar 30 [cited 2019 Jun 4]; Seattle,

WA. Available from: https://www.nrtrc.org/content/presentation-files/Telemedicine%20Back%20to%20the%20Future%20-%20a%2050%20Year%20Perspective.pdf.
17. Bashshur R. Technology serves the people: the story of a cooperative telemedicine project by NASA, the Indian Health Service and the Papago People. Indian Health Service, Staff Office of Planning, Evaluation and Research; 1979.
18. Freiburger G, Holcomb M, Piper D. The STARPAHC collection: part of an archive of the history of telemedicine. J Telemed Telecare. 2007;13(5):221–3.
19. Riley FE. STARPAHC. Part 1: final summary report [Internet]. 1974 Jun [cited 2019 Jun 4]. Available from: https://ntrs.nasa.gov/search.jsp?R=19750007223.
20. Viggiano LA. Diagnosis by satellite. Army Commun. 1986;11(1):54.
21. Weinstein R, Holcomb M, Krupinski E. Invention and early history of telepathology (1985–2000). J Pathol Inform. 2019;10(1):1.
22. Weinstein RS. Telepathology diagnostic network [Internet]. US5216596A, 1993 [cited 2019 Jun 4]. Available from: https://patents.google.com/patent/US5216596A/en?q=weinstein&q=telepathology&oq=weinstein+telepathology.
23. Nordrum I, Engum B, Rinde E, Finseth A, Ericsson H, Kearney M, et al. Remote frozen section service: a telepathology project in northern Norway. Hum Pathol. 1991;22(6):514–8.
24. Ghosh A, Brown GT, Fontelo P. Telepathology at the Armed Forces Institute of Pathology: a retrospective review of consultations from 1996 to 1997. Arch Pathol Lab Med. 2018;142(2):248–52.
25. Dunn BE, Choi H, Recla DL, Kerr SE, Wagenman BL. Robotic surgical telepathology between the Iron Mountain and Milwaukee Department of Veterans Affairs Medical Centers: a 12-year experience. Hum Pathol. 2009;40(8):1092–9.
26. Kaplan KJ, Burgess JR, Sandberg GD, Myers CP, Bigott TR, Greenspan RB. Use of robotic telepathology for frozen-section diagnosis: a retrospective trial of a telepathology system for intraoperative consultation. Mod Pathol. 2002;15(11):1197.
27. Evans AJ, Chetty R, Clarke BA, Croul S, Ghazarian DM, Kiehl T-R, et al. Primary frozen section diagnosis by robotic microscopy and virtual slide telepathology: the University Health Network experience. Hum Pathol. 2009;40(8):1070–81.
28. Pantanowitz L, Parwani A, Wiley C, Ahmed I, Cable W, Contis L, et al. Experience with multimodality telepathology at the University of Pittsburgh Medical Center. J Pathol Inform. 2012;3(1):45.
29. Bacus JW. jamesbacus.com BLISS system [Internet]. [cited 2019 Jun 4]. Available from: http://www.jamesbacus.com/page10.html.
30. Bacus JV, Bacus JW. Method and apparatus for creating a virtual microscope slide [Internet]. US6272235B1, 2001 [cited 2019 May 17]. Available from: https://patents.google.com/patent/US6272235B1/en.
31. Bacus JV, Bacus JW. Method and apparatus for acquiring and reconstructing magnified specimen images from a computer-controlled microscope [Internet]. US6101265A, 2000 [cited 2019 Jun 4]. Available from: https://patents.google.com/patent/US6101265A/en.
32. Ferreira R, Moon B, Humphries J, Sussman A, Saltz J, Miller R, et al. The virtual microscope. Proc AMIA Annu Fall Symp. 1997:449–53.
33. Kayser K, Beyer M, Blum S, Kayser G. Recent developments and present status of telepathology. Anal Cell Pathol J Eur Soc Anal Cell Pathol. 2000;21(3–4):101–6.
34. Wells CA, Sowter C. Telepathology: a diagnostic tool for the millennium? J Pathol. 2000;191(1):1–7.
35. Jukić DM, Bifulco CB. Telepathology and pathology at distance: an overview. Croat Med J. 1999;40(3):421–4.
36. Farahani N, Pantanowitz L. Overview of telepathology. Clin Lab Med. 2016;36(1):101–12.
37. Bashshur RL, Krupinski EA, Weinstein RS, Dunn MR, Bashshur N. The empirical foundations of telepathology: evidence of feasibility and intermediate effects. Telemed E-Health. 2017;23(3):155–91.
38. Bauer TW, Slaw RJ. Validating whole-slide imaging for consultation diagnoses in surgical pathology. Arch Pathol Lab Med. 2014;138(11):1459–65.

39. Bauer TW, Schoenfield L, Slaw RJ, Yerian L, Sun Z, Henricks WH. Validation of whole slide imaging for primary diagnosis in surgical pathology. Arch Pathol Lab Med. 2013;137(4):518–24.
40. Jones NC, Nazarian RM, Duncan LM, Kamionek M, Lauwers GY, Tambouret RH, et al. Interinstitutional whole slide imaging teleconsultation service development: assessment using internal training and clinical consultation cases. Arch Pathol Lab Med. 2015;139(5):627–35.
41. Zhao C, Wu T, Ding X, Parwani A, Chen H, McHugh J, et al. International telepathology consultation: three years of experience between the University of Pittsburgh Medical Center and KingMed Diagnostics in China. J Pathol Inform. 2015;6(1):63.
42. World Internet Users Statistics and 2019 World Population Stats [Internet]. [cited 2019 Jun 4]. Available from: https://www.internetworldstats.com/stats.htm.
43. Farris AB, Cohen C, Rogers TE, Smith GH. Whole slide imaging for analytical anatomic pathology and telepathology: practical applications today, promises, and perils. Arch Pathol Lab Med. 2017;141(4):542–50.
44. Fontelo P, Liu F, Yagi Y. Evaluation of a smartphone for telepathology: lessons learned. J Pathol Inform. 2015;6(1):35.
45. Monaco SE, Koah AE, Xing J, Ahmed I, Cuda J, Cunningham J, et al. Telecytology implementation: deployment of telecytology for rapid on-site evaluations at an Academic Medical Center. Diagn Cytopathol. 2019;47(3):206–13.
46. Michel R. Pathologists in China, U.S. linked by digital pathology [Internet]. The Dark Intelligence Group. 2012 [cited 2019 Jun 4]. Available from: https://www.darkintelligencegroup.com/the-dark-report/digital-pathology/pathologists-in-china-u-s-linked-by-digital-pathology/.
47. UCLA Health International Telepathology Brochure [Internet]. UCLA Health. 2016 [cited 2019 Jun 4]. Available from: http://pathology.ucla.edu/workfiles/Clinical%20Services/Telepathology/EnglishBrochure11-23.pdf.
48. Chlipala E, Elin J, Eichhorn O, Krishnamurti M, Long RE, Sabata B. Archival and retrieval in digital pathology systems [Internet]. Digital Pathology Association. 2011 [cited 2019 Jul 10]. Available from: https://digitalpathologyassociation.org/_data/files/Archival_and_Retrieval_in_Digital_Pathology_Systems.pdf.
49. Miller K. Calculating optical fiber latency [Internet]. [cited 2019 Jun 4]. Available from: http://www.m2optics.com/blog/bid/70587/Calculating-Optical-Fiber-Latency.
50. Frumento E. Cybersecurity and the evolutions of healthcare: challenges and threats behind its evolution [Internet]. springerprofessional.de. [cited 2019 Jul 10]. Available from: https://www.springerprofessional.de/en/cybersecurity-and-the-evolutions-of-healthcare-challenges-and-th/16506760.
51. FDA Product Classification, Whole slide imaging system [Internet]. [cited 2019 Jun 11]. Available from: https://www.accessdata.fda.gov/scripts/cdrh/cfdocs/cfpcd/classification.cfm?id=5048.
52. Administration AGD of HTG. IVD medical devices: Definitions & links [Internet]. Therapeutic Goods Administration (TGA). 2010 [cited 2019 Jun 9]. Available from: https://www.tga.gov.au/ivd-medical-devices-definitions-links.
53. Buckman Company v. Plaintiffs' Legal Committee - Amicus (Merits) [Internet]. 2014 [cited 2019 Jun 11]. Available from: https://www.justice.gov/osg/brief/buckman-company-v-plaintiffs-legal-committee-amicus-merits.
54. Canada H. Health Canada [Internet]. aem. 2019 [cited 2019 Jun 9]. Available from: https://www.canada.ca/en/health-canada.html.
55. Abels E, Pantanowitz L. Current state of the regulatory trajectory for whole slide imaging devices in the USA. J Pathol Inform [Internet]. 2017 May 15 [cited 2019 Jun 9];8. Available from: https://www.ncbi.nlm.nih.gov/pmc/articles/PMC5450449/.
56. Mukhopadhyay S, Feldman MD, Abels E, Ashfaq R, Beltaifa S, Cacciabeve NG, et al. Whole slide imaging versus microscopy for primary diagnosis in surgical pathology. Am J Surg Pathol. 2018;42(1):39–52.

57. Borowsky AD, Glassy EF, Wallace WD, Kallichanda NS, Behling CA, Miller DV, et al. Digital whole slide imaging compared with light microscopy for primary diagnosis in surgical pathology: a multicenter, double-blinded, randomized study of 2045 cases. Arch Pathol Lab Med. 2020;arpa.2019-0569-OA.
58. College of American Pathologists. All common checklist. CAP Accreditation Program. College of American Pathologists; 2018.
59. Food and Drug Administration. Product classification: Digital Pathology Display (PZZ) [Internet]. [cited 2020 Apr 27]. Available from: https://www.accessdata.fda.gov/scripts/cdrh/cfdocs/cfpcd/classification.cfm?id=5105.
60. Leica Biosystems Receives FDA 510(k) clearance to market a digital pathology system for primary diagnosis [Internet]. Leica Biosystems. [cited 2019 Jun 9]. Available from: https://www.leicabiosystems.com/news-events/news-details/article/leica-biosystems-receives-fda-510k-clearance-to-market-a-digital-pathology-system-for-primary-diag/News/detail/.
61. Food and Drug Administration. 510(k) substantial equivalence determination decision summary: K190332 [Internet]. Food and Drug Administration. 2019 [cited 2019 Jun 4]. Available from: https://www.accessdata.fda.gov/cdrh_docs/reviews/K190332.pdf.
62. Food and Drug Administration. 510(k) substantial equivalence determination decision summary: K193054 [Internet]. Food and Drug Administration. 2020 [cited 2020 Apr 27]. Available from: https://www.accessdata.fda.gov/cdrh_docs/reviews/K193054.pdf.
63. College of American Pathologists. Laboratory General Checklist. CAP Accreditation Program. College of American Pathologists; 2007.
64. Carlson DA. Laboratory inspections: the view from CAP. Lab Med. 2003;34(5):373–80.
65. Clinical Laboratory Improvement Amendments (CLIA) Application For Certification. Form CMS-116. [Internet]. Centers for medicare and medicaid services. 2017 [cited 2019 Jul 5]. Available from: https://www.cms.gov/Medicare/CMS-Forms/CMS-Forms/downloads/cms116.pdf.
66. College of American Pathologists. Validating Whole Slide Imaging for Diagnostic Purposes in Pathology. [cited 2021 Sep 21]. Available from: https://www.cap.org/protocols-and-guidelines/cap-guidelines/current-cap-guidelines/validating-whole-slide-imaging-for-diagnostic-purposes-in-pathology.
67. Pantanowitz L, Hassell L, Henricks W, Lennerz J, Lowe A, Parwani A, et al. American telemedicine association clinical guidelines for telepathology. J Pathol Inform. 2014;5(1):39.
68. College of American Pathologists. Anatomic pathology checklist. CAP Accreditation Program. College of American Pathologists; 2021.
69. Cornish TC, McClintock DS. Medicolegal and regulatory aspects of whole slide imaging-based telepathology. Diagn Histopathol. 2014;20(12):475–81.
70. FSMB | Contact a State Medical Board [Internet]. [cited 2019 Jun 13]. Available from: https://www.fsmb.org/contact-a-state-medical-board/.
71. Biereg J. Mr. Smith goes to Washington [Internet]. CAP Today Online. 2011 [cited 2019 Jun 13]. Available from: http://www.captodayonline.com/Archives/0311/0311d_mr_smith.html.
72. Hiemenz MC, Leung ST, Park JY. Crossing boundaries: a comprehensive survey of medical licensing laws and guidelines regulating the interstate practice of pathology. Am J Surg Pathol. 2014;38(3):e1–5.
73. Interstate Medical Licensure Compact | A faster pathway to medical licensure [Internet]. [cited 2019 Jun 4]. Available from: https://imlcc.org/.
74. Hamilton TE. Telemedicine services in hospitals and critical access hospitals (CAHs) [Internet]. Centers for Medicare and Medicaid. 2011 [cited 2018 Oct 6]. Available from: https://www.cms.gov/Medicare/Provider-Enrollment-and-Certification/SurveyCertificationGenInfo/downloads/SCLetter11_32.pdf.
75. Wu Y-C, Chen C-S, Chan Y-J. The outbreak of COVID-19: an overview. J Chin Med Assoc. 2020;83(3):217–20.

76. Azar AM. Determination that a public health emergency exists [Internet]. Depertment of Health and Human Services. 2020 [cited 2020 May 9]. Available from: https://www.phe.gov/emergency/news/healthactions/phe/Pages/2019-nCoV.aspx.
77. Trump DJ. Proclamation on declaring a national emergency concerning the novel coronavirus disease (COVID-19) outbreak [Internet]. 2020 [cited 2020 May 9]. Available from: https://www.whitehouse.gov/presidential-actions/proclamation-declaring-national-emergency-concerning-novel-coronavirus-disease-covid-19-outbreak/.
78. Kates J, Michaud J, Tolbert J. Stay-At-Home Orders to Fight COVID-19 in the United States: The risks of a scattershot approach | The Henry J. Kaiser Family Foundation [Internet]. 2020 [cited 2020 May 9]. Available from: https://www.kff.org/coronavirus-policy-watch/stay-at-home-orders-to-fight-covid19/.
79. CDC. Coronavirus Disease 2019 (COVID-19): Older adults [Internet]. Centers for Disease Control and Prevention. 2020 [cited 2020 May 9]. Available from: https://www.cdc.gov/coronavirus/2019-ncov/need-extra-precautions/older-adults.html.
80. Ehrlich H, McKenney M, Elkbuli A. Protecting our healthcare workers during the COVID-19 pandemic. Am J Emerg Med. 2020;S0735675720302527.
81. Robboy SJ, Weintraub S, Horvath AE, Jensen BW, Alexander CB, Fody EP, et al. Pathologist workforce in the United States: I. development of a predictive model to examine factors influencing supply. Arch Pathol Lab Med. 2013;137(12):1723–32.
82. Metter DM, Colgan TJ, Leung ST, Timmons CF, Park JY. Trends in the US and Canadian pathologist workforces from 2007 to 2017. JAMA Netw Open. 2019;2(5):e194337.
83. Alliance for Digital Pathology. CMS/CLIA allowing temporary remote signout [Internet]. [cited 2020 May 9]. Available from: https://digitalpathologyalliance.org/remote-signout.
84. Centers for Medicare & Medicaid Services. Clinical Laboratory Improvement Amendments (CLIA) laboratory guidance during COVID-19 public health emergency; Memo No. QSO-20-21-CLIA [Internet]. 2020 [cited 2020 May 5]. Available from: https://www.cms.gov/files/document/qso-20-21-clia.pdf-0.
85. Food and Drug Administration. Enforcement policy for remote digital pathology devices during the coronavirus disease 2019 (COVID-19) public health emergency - guidance for Industry, Clinical Laboratories, Healthcare Facilities, Pathologists, and Food and Drug Administration Staff [Internet]. 2020 [cited 2020 May 5]. Available from: https://www.fda.gov/media/137307/download.
86. Technical performance assessment of digital pathology whole slide imaging devices - guidance for Industry and Food and Drug Administration Staff [Internet]. April 2016 [cited 2019 Jun 13]. Available from: https://www.fda.gov/media/90791/download.

Whole Slide Imaging: Remote Consultations/Second Opinions

Giovanni Lujan, Anil V. Parwani, and Marilyn M. Bui

Introduction

Whole slides image (WSI) is a digital replica of a histopathology glass slide created by a whole slide image scanner which can be viewed via a computer monitor instead of the light microscope [1]. Remote consultation for second opinion is one of the most important utilities of whole slide image-based digital pathology [2]. This requires the participating pathology laboratories having the infrastructure of producing quality whole slides images, exchanging these images along with clinical and radiological information, and supporting case discussion and reporting in compliance with the regulatory as well as patient privacy policies and guides [3]. This allows consultation between pathologists in a central location and the affiliated locations and access to expert pathologists within the institution or outside the institution, region, or country. Guidelines for telepathology have been published by the American Telemedicine Association [4].

Anatomic pathology is an important branch of pathology which is a diverse and broad medial specialty. Anatomic pathologists make diagnosis, prognosis, and prediction of therapy based on the gross, microscopic, biochemical, immunohistochemical, genomic, and molecular study of organs, tissues, and cells of patients. In most pathology departments, pathologists practice as generalists, while in more resource-rich departments, they practice as subspecialists with expertise in defined

G. Lujan (✉)
College of Medicine, The Ohio State University Wexner Medical Center, Department of Pathology, Columbus, OH, USA
e-mail: Giovanni.Lujan@osumc.edu

A. V. Parwani
Department of Pathology, College of Medicine, The Ohio State University Wexner Medical School, Columbus, OH, USA

M. M. Bui
Moffitt Cancer Center, Department of Pathology, Tampa, FL, USA

A. V. Parwani (ed.), *Whole Slide Imaging*,
https://doi.org/10.1007/978-3-030-83332-9_8

organ systems (such as gastrointestinal, breast, etc.) or by credential (surgical pathology, cytopathology, hematopathology, molecular pathology, etc.). With the rapid and massive advance of knowledge in anatomic pathology in the era of precision medicine, it has become more and more challenging for practicing pathologists to keep up with the demands of ever-increasing workload while maintaining the proficiency and knowledge in every aspect of pathology. However, providing timely and accurate diagnostic, prognostic, and predictive information holds the key to effective management of patients. Due to the critical value of a pathology diagnosis, it is a standard practice in pathology to conduct consultation for second opinion for quality assurance. This includes intradepartmental, external, and international consultation.

Importance of Consultation for Second Opinions

There have been a number of publications in the last few decades highlighting the importance of consultation for second opinion and consultations in surgical pathology, especially those provided by an expert in the field; this can be paramount when the diagnosis carries a big impact in treatment and prognosis [5]. Cancer diagnosis is an area which is susceptible to misdiagnosis, discordance, and misclassifications since those can significantly alter treatment decisions for the patient [6]. Also, the implications in the cost have been analyzed many times, and the conclusions have been along the lines that big savings are directly related to an accurate and precise diagnosis before treatment is implemented [5, 7–9].

Second opinions and consultations play a key role in pathology. It is partly related to the workflow by which the diagnosis in surgical pathology is rendered. Anatomical pathology in particular is based on pattern recognitions, observations, and interpretation. The pathologist, depending on their knowledge and experience, will make comparisons with known or learned images [1]. The process of comparisons, recognition, and knowledge will then lead to fine-tuning of the diagnosis. There are several pre-analytical factors such as slide preparation, fixation, embedding, and staining which will also impact the diagnostic process. Ultimately, with all the factors in place and a review, the case is signed out or released into the medical records.

Many studies through the years have analyzed this variability and have come up with mechanisms to reduce the potential of severe misleading interpretation [10, 11].

One common solution on how to address this variability is to search for a second independent reading [7, 12], either as a second opinion from a peer in the same institution, consensus opinion if many pathologist of similar expertise are available to be consulted simultaneously, or individually or in what could be a more formal level of second opinion by requesting the opinion of an expert in such organ or system. Some large hospitals and institutions have a mandatory review of any image rendered diagnosis before implementing any significant treatment. [10, 13].

The most effective way by which this variability can be reduced is when the interpretation is left to so-called experts on the area in question. These 'experts' however, developed usually from an initial formal training, which lays the foundation, usually under supervision of a mentor who is already an expert on the subject; this initial period is followed by a lifetime of experience devoted to mostly or largely interpreting images on that particular subject and then becoming aware of the many nuances of the interpretation process of those diagnosis that are difficult to reproduce. Many areas of specialized pathology have published their own studies highlighting the facts of utilizing experts in certain type of diagnosis to address variability, impact on patient's treatment, and cost. Some important studies have been in areas like thyroid pathology [14], dermatopathology [15], uropathology [16–18], breast pathology [19, 20], head and neck pathology [10, 21, 22], liver pathology [23], gastrointestinal pathology [24], and others.

These "experts", however, are not readily available, and in many instances, they are completely out of reach. Telepathology has been envisioned as the solution in order to make expert consultants available to provide that sought-after expertise in difficult to interpret cases [25–27].

Shortage of Pathologists in General Around the World

In developing countries and even in most industrialized nations, there is a shortage of pathologists in general, and most countries completely lack expert pathologists in all. In The United States, the number of active pathologists decreased between 2007 and 2017 by about 17.5% (JAMA Network Open) [28].The number of active pathologists dropped from 15,568 to 12,839 between 2007 and 2017, and in relative terms, that translates to a decline from 5.16 professionals per 100,000 in the population to 3.94 per 100,000 in 2017. In comparison, the number of pathologists in Canada increased by 20.45% (rising from 1467 to 1767), and the number of pathologists per 100,000 in the population increased from 4.46 to 4.81. While the number of pathologists has declined, workload demands have been on the rise. The number of new cancer cases managed by pathologists rose by 41.73% in the United States between 2007 and 2017 versus 7.06% in Canada, the researchers noted. In contrast with physician specialties where the workload is limited by the number of patients who can be seen and treated, pathologists working in laboratories must manage all clinical specimens and materials from clinical colleagues within a specified period of time [28].

To make the situation worse, In the United States, the number of graduating medical students applying for pathology positions dropped by 27.5% between 2008 and 2017; thus pathology is also experiencing a pipeline issue [29].

In The United Kingdom, The Royal College of Pathologists (RCP) published a report that found nationwide histopathology staff shortage; only 3% of histopathology departments that responded to the RCP's workforce census reported enough staff to meet the work load; shortage of pathologist contributes to record-long waiting periods in starting cancer treatment in England [30].

The pathologist number in the world is predicted to decrease according to scientificpathology. weebly.com, which more severely impacts in developing countries [31] (Fig. 1).

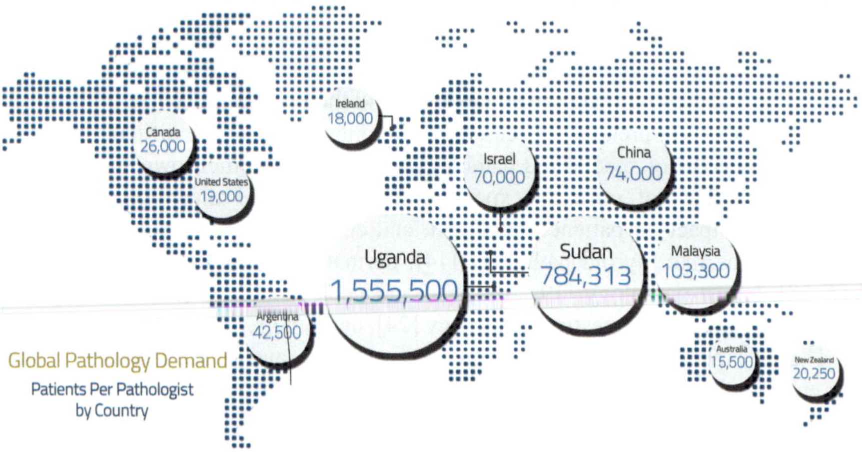

Fig. 1 Pathology demand map. Efforts by countries or groups of countries launching large-scale initiatives for consultations. (Image courtesy of David West, with permission [31])

Whole slide imaging and telepathology have the capabilities to revolutionize consultations and second opinions.

Telepathology technologies including whole slide imaging have the potential to provide easier access to pathology subspecialists around the United States and other countries where there is lack of expert pathologists or lack of pathologists in general. Experts from academic institutions can share in a matter of minutes their expertise across the hall with their colleagues or across the world. Basically, telepathology bypasses the barriers of distance and time [32]. Consensus conferences among groups of pathologists will be as easy as clicking into a software, opening the case, and sharing in real time or in a more passive fashion by sending a link that can be opened and studied by the consultant at his own leisure. Consultations from satellites hospitals with solo practice or small number of pathologists have immediate access to expert consultation at their fingertips. Interaction will be possible from everyone to everyone. Diagnosis of known low reproducibility and high stakes could be brought to a consensus diagnosis between experts either from the same institutions or interinstitutional [33, 34].

In China, for example, telepathology may play an important role in pathology consultation and quality control for cancer diagnosis, as the country has the largest population of cancer patients worldwide. The results of 2 years implementation indicated that telepathology could solve the problem of uneven distribution of pathology resources and become an invaluable tool to improve the quality of pathology diagnosis [35].

Worldwide Initiatives

One initiative within large geographic participation has proposed the creation of a program of Worldwide Excellence in Breast Pathology. This will have the objective of improving medical care services, particularly to medically underserved women and those living in countries with limited resources. This initiative emphasizes effectively the talent and expertise of pathologists around the globe to provide a cost-effective way to diagnose breast cancer, particularly at advanced stages. For example, pathologists can sample lesions by fine-needle aspiration biopsy (FNAB), stain the resulting smears, and provide an immediate bedside diagnosis. This is a valid contribution; however, this exercise requires the availability of a pathologist with experience in breast cytopathology. Alternatively, the pathologist may seek consultations from more experienced pathologists. Developing strategies to better recognize the importance of high-quality breast pathology services and to train qualified and innovative breast pathologists is an ambitious task [36].

In Europe, there is an active project to create the European Centre for Pathology which could function as a stimulating pathological consultation center and office of the European Society of Pathology. The creation of such institution, that perhaps would have been a counterpart of the now disappeared Armed Forces Institute of Pathology, will undoubtedly be a powerful breakthrough in European pathology [37].

In Asia, there is a plan to create the Asiatic Center of Pathology as a basis of progress of Asiatic pathology in the future. This could function as a "brain" center and, at the same time, be an office of the Asian continent's pathologists [38].

In Japan there has been a recent economic evaluation of telemedicine; the results have been to undertake specific policy measures to promote telemedicine further including telepathology and teleradiology [39].

In Canada, the Eastern Québec Telepathology Network was created to provide uniform diagnostic telepathology services in a huge territory with a low population density. This has maintained a high-quality pathology services and rapid turnaround time to more than 20 sites disseminated on a huge territory. A second phase is now underway to expand telepathology to other regions across the province [40, 41].

Developing countries usually lack the manpower, expertise, infrastructure, and monetary resources to initiate their own programs. In places where there is one pathologist per million of habitants, the odds are strongly against to have any pathologist (let alone an expert pathologist) review someone's biopsy or anatomo-pathological specimen. These odds may eventually change when the advent of telepathology and the nascent large networks of expert consultation are being created in wealthy areas, some of whom have already expressed an interest and are actively developing a path to assist those less fortunate countries [36, 42, 43].

Some Examples of a Work Already in Progress

Among the different subspecialties, dermatopathology appears to be making strides in creating consultation networks, acknowledging the importance of second opinions, and taking full advantage of internet-based communications and WSI technologies to decrease barriers and facilitate and open access to the best expertise; in order to accomplish that, software has been developed to frame and streamline the consultation process to secure a fast turnaround time [44]. These online consultation services use WSI envisions to compensate for the shortage of dermatopathologists and other subspecialties that deal with cases that tend to be difficult or controversial, like gastrointestinal pathology, uropathology, and gynecologic pathology [45]. A review article titled "Practice of Teledermatopathology: A Systematic Review," published in 2018, concluded, after extensive review of available literature dating from 2012 to the time the article was written, that telepathology increases access to specialists, reduces interpretive errors and healthcare expenditures, improves the efficiency of workflow, and optimizes patient outcomes. Also listed as conclusion was that teledermatopathology facilitates international collaboration by widening global access to dermatopathology services and providing educational resources in underserved areas. The study highlighted at the time that regulations and quality of digital images in teledermatopathology needed to be improved [46].

In California, UCLA has published a detailed account of the implementation of a regional digital pathology subspecialty consultation network in a hub and spoke consultation system, which included UCLA Medical Center as the main hub and six spoke sites UC San Diego, UC Irvine, UC Davis, Northridge Hospital Medical Center, Olive View Medical Center, and Children's Hospital Los Angeles. Their experience at the time of the publication in 2019 included a total of 165 consultations between May 2017 and July 2018, noting an improved TAT over conventional carrier mail; it was specially advantageous for preliminary kidney biopsy diagnosis where the average TAT was only 0.7 day. Other benefits for the spoke sites in addition to shortened consultation TAT included financial savings over hiring faculty with expertise to support a potentially low-volume service. For the hub site, the value includes exposure to educationally valuable cases, additional caseload volume to support specialized services, and improved communication with referring facilities over traditional carrier mail [47].

At an international level, one of the best documented examples is a retrospective study that summarizes the telepathology experience and diagnostic consultation results between the University of Pittsburgh Medical Center in the United States and KingMed Diagnostics, the largest independent pathology medical laboratory in China. During a period of 3 years from January 2012 to December 2014, they documented 1561 telepathology consultation cases; they noted that from all those cases, 61.4% were referred by pathologists, 36.9% by clinicians, and 1.7% by patients. Hematopathology received the largest number of consultations (23.7%) followed by bone and soft tissue (21%) and gynecologic/breast (20.2%) subspecialties. Average turnaround time (TAT) per case was 5.4 days, which decreased from 6.8 days during 2012 to 5 days in 2014. In 855 cases (54.7%), a primary diagnosis or impression was provided by the referring institution in China; from those cases the final diagnosis rendered by UPMC pathologist was identical in 25.6% of cases and significantly modified (alterations in the treatment plan) in 50.8% of cases. These results, concluded by the authors of the review study from both institutions, indicate that international telepathology consultation can significantly improve patient care by facilitating access to pathology expertise. They also concluded that the overall experience was encouraging for the practice of international second opinions via telepathology. They attribute the success of the enterprise to a strong commitment and support from leadership, information technology expertise, and dedicated pathologists who understood the language and culture on both sides. They cited lack of clinical information, missing gross pathology descriptions, and insufficient tissue sections submitted for evaluation were the main reasons for indefinite final diagnosis [3].

Digital Pathology as a Window into Computational Pathology

Once the images have been scanned, they become part of the digital realm, and as such they are also amenable to be analyzed by software; currently there is a rapid development of algorithms that aid to classify, count, measure, and identify cellular and tissue components within those images; this serves as the base for computational pathology which will produce more sophisticated layers of analysis and evaluation. As the level of sophistication increases, perhaps more consultations might be necessary as the tools of analysis, at least initially may not be available to small practices and hospitals. The scope of all of these avenues is increasing manyfold in rapid succession [48]. The ultimate goal is to utilize artificial intelligence to help analyze the image from the pixel's perspective and provide more wholesome, reproducible diagnosis with new information that will be incorporated in the initial diagnosis and then used as an aid to select therapy, later in follow-up after treatment to assess the result of the chosen therapy, and finally in evaluating the patient for possible recurrence or residual disease [49–51].

Telepathology and COVID-19 Pandemic

The COVID-19 pandemic impacted the workflow of anatomic pathology laboratories by decreasing staff due to social distancing, especially affecting the senior pathologists, which is reported that 12% pathologists being 65 years of age or older [52, 53].

This shortage of pathologists disproportionally affects subspecialty areas, particularly in rare disease subspecialty or subspecialty with high numbers of older pathologists. In addition, the hospitals with more large number of COVID-19 cases must balance the COVID-19 testing itself and associated demands of COVID-19 patient care in addition to the medical needs of routine patient cares, especially cancers. Due to the COVID-19 pandemic, the College of American Pathologists successfully advocated a temporary relaxing of remote sign out for pathologists including using telepathology from Centers for Medicare & Medicaid Services (CMS) and the Department of Health and Human Services (HHD) [54].

Conclusions

Whole slide imaging for telepathology/secondary opinion/consultation has proven to be a powerful tool for pathologists to access peer review in a timely manner to improve the quality care of their patients. There are established guidelines and numerous good practice examples to follow in the United States as well as around the world. The digital health environment and the new challenges of the COVID-19 pandemic provide new opportunities to accelerate the adoption of telepathology.

References

1. Zarella MD, Bowman D, Aeffner F, et al. A practical guide to whole slide imaging: a white paper from the digital pathology association. Arch Pathol Lab Med. 2019;143(2):222–34.
2. Ghosh A, Brown GT, Fontelo P. Telepathology at the armed forces Institute of Pathology: a retrospective review of consultations from 1996 to 1997. Arch Pathol Lab Med. 2018;142(2):248–52.
3. Zhao C, Wu T, Ding X, et al. International telepathology consultation: three years of experience between the University of Pittsburgh Medical Center and KingMed Diagnostics in China. J Pathol Inform. 2015;6:63.
4. Pantanowitz L, Dickinson K, Evans AJ, et al. American telemedicine association clinical guidelines for telepathology. J Pathol Inform. 2014;5(1):39.
5. Middleton LP, Feeley TW, Albright HW, Walters R, Hamilton SH. Second-opinion pathologic review is a patient safety mechanism that helps reduce error and decrease waste. J Oncol Pract. 2014;10(4):275–80.
6. Cook IS, McCormick D, Poller DN. Referrals for second opinion in surgical pathology: implications for management of cancer patients in the UK. Eur J Surg Oncol. 2001;27(6):589–94.
7. Peck M, Moffat D, Latham B, Badrick T. Review of diagnostic error in anatomical pathology and the role and value of second opinions in error prevention. J Clin Pathol. 2018;71(11):995–1000.
8. Renshaw AA, Gould EW. Measuring the value of review of pathology material by a second pathologist. Am J Clin Pathol. 2006;125(5):737–9.
9. Frable WJ. Surgical pathology–second reviews, institutional reviews, audits, and correlations: what's out there? Error or diagnostic variation? Arch Pathol Lab Med. 2006;130(5):620–5.
10. Kronz JD, Westra WH, Epstein JI. Mandatory second opinion surgical pathology at a large referral hospital. Cancer. 1999;86(11):2426–35.
11. Liu YJ, Kessler M, Zander DS, Karamchandani DM. Trends in extramural consultation: comparison between subspecialized and general surgical pathology service models. Ann Diagn Pathol. 2016;24:20–4.
12. Sohani AR, Sohani MA. Static digital telepathology: a model for diagnostic and educational support to pathologists in the developing world. Anal Cell Pathol (Amst). 2012;35(1):25–30.
13. Strosberg C, Gibbs J, Braswell D, et al. Second opinion reviews for cancer diagnoses in anatomic pathology: a Comprehensive Cancer Center's experience. Anticancer Res. 2018;38(5):2989–94.

14. Hamady ZZ, Mather N, Lansdown MR, Davidson L, Maclennan KA. Surgical pathological second opinion in thyroid malignancy: impact on patients' management and prognosis. Eur J Surg Oncol. 2005;31(1):74–7.
15. Gaudi S, Zarandona JM, Raab SS, English JC 3rd, Jukic DM. Discrepancies in dermatopathology diagnoses: the role of second review policies and dermatopathology fellowship training. J Am Acad Dermatol. 2013;68(1):119–28.
16. Gordetsky J, Collingwood R, Lai WS, Del Carmen Rodriquez Pena M, Rais-Bahrami S. Second opinion expert pathology review in bladder cancer: implications for patient care. Int J Surg Pathol. 2018;26(1):12–7.
17. Ramsey SD, Zeliadt SB, Fedorenko CR, et al. Patient preferences and urologist recommendations among local-stage prostate cancer patients who present for initial consultation and second opinions. World J Urol. 2011;29(1):3–9.
18. Chan TY, Epstein JI. Patient and urologist driven second opinion of prostate needle biopsies. J Urol. 2005;174(4 Pt 1):1390–4; discussion 1394; author reply 1394
19. Elmore JG, Longton GM, Carney PA, et al. Diagnostic concordance among pathologists interpreting breast biopsy specimens. JAMA. 2015;313(11):1122–32.
20. Tosteson ANA, Yang Q, Nelson HD, et al. Second opinion strategies in breast pathology: a decision analysis addressing over-treatment, under-treatment, and care costs. Breast Cancer Res Treat. 2018;167(1):195–203.
21. Kronz JD, Westra WH. The role of second opinion pathology in the management of lesions of the head and neck. Curr Opin Otolaryngol Head Neck Surg. 2005;13(2):81–4.
22. Westra WH, Kronz JD, Eisele DW. The impact of second opinion surgical pathology on the practice of head and neck surgery: a decade experience at a large referral hospital. Head Neck. 2002;24(7):684–93.
23. Torbenson MS, Arnold CA, Graham RP, et al. Identification of key challenges in liver pathology: data from a multicenter study of extramural consults. Hum Pathol. 2019;87:75–82.
24. Villanacci V, Salemme M, Stroppa I, Balassone V, Bassotti G. The importance of a second opinion in the diagnosis of Barrett's esophagus: a "real life" study. Rev Esp Enferm Dig. 2017;109(3):185–9.
25. Wilbur DC, Madi K, Colvin RB, et al. Whole-slide imaging digital pathology as a platform for teleconsultation: a pilot study using paired subspecialist correlations. Arch Pathol Lab Med. 2009;133(12):1949–53.
26. Cornish TC, Swapp RE, Kaplan KJ. Whole-slide imaging: routine pathologic diagnosis. Adv Anat Pathol. 2012;19(3):152–9.
27. Wells CA, Sowter C. Telepathology: a diagnostic tool for the millennium? J Pathol. 2000;191(1):1–7.
28. Metter DM, Colgan TJ, Leung ST, Timmons CF, Park JY. Trends in the US and Canadian pathologist workforces from 2007 to 2017. JAMA Netw Open. 2019;2(5):e194337.
29. Jajosky RP, Jajosky AN, Kleven DT, Singh G. Fewer seniors from United States allopathic medical schools are filling pathology residency positions in the Main Residency Match, 2008-2017. Hum Pathol. 2018;73:26–32.
30. Communications Team TRCoP. College Report Finds UK wide histopathology staff shortages. 2018.
31. West D. Taking Pathology to The Cloud. 2015. Proscia Inc. Accessed at https://s3.amazonaws.com/proscia-viewer/Taking+Pathology+to+the+Cloud.pdf on June 23, 2020.
32. Aeffner F, Blanchard TW, Keel MK, Williams BH. Whole-slide imaging: the future is here. Vet Pathol. 2018;55(4):488–9.
33. Cross SS, Dennis T, Start RD. Telepathology: current status and future prospects in diagnostic histopathology. Histopathology. 2002;41(2):91–109.
34. Weinstein RS, Graham AR, Lian F, et al. Reconciliation of diverse telepathology system designs. Historic issues and implications for emerging markets and new applications. APMIS. 2012;120(4):256–75.

35. Chen J, Jiao Y, Lu C, Zhou J, Zhang Z, Zhou C. A nationwide telepathology consultation and quality control program in China: implementation and result analysis. Diagn Pathol. 2014;9 Suppl 1(Suppl 1):S2.
36. Masood S. The expanding role of pathologists in the diagnosis and management of breast cancer: worldwide excellence in breast pathology program. Breast J. 2003;9(Suppl 2):S94–7.
37. Zubritsky AN. European Centre of Pathology as a basis of progress of European pathology in the future. Pathol Res Pract. 1996;192(11):1079–80; discussion 1081
38. Zubritsky AN. Asiatic Center of Pathology as a basis of progress of Asiatic pathology in the future. Pathol Int. 1999;49(3):270–1.
39. Miyahara S, Tsuji M, Iizuka C, Hasegawa T, Taoka F, Teshima M. An economic evaluation of Japanese telemedicine, focusing on teleradiology and telepathology. J Telemed Telecare. 2006;12(Suppl 1):29–31
40. Perron E, Louahlia S, Nadeau L, et al. Telepathology for intraoperative consultations and expert opinions: the experience of the Eastern Québec Telepathology Network. Arch Pathol Lab Med. 2014;138(9):1223–8.
41. Têtu B, Perron É, Louahlia S, Paré G, Trudel MC, Meyer J. The Eastern Québec Telepathology Network: a three-year experience of clinical diagnostic services. Diagn Pathol. 2014;9 Suppl 1(Suppl 1):S1.
42. Ahmed Z, Yaqoob N, Muzaffar S, Kayani N, Pervez S, Hasan SH. Diagnostic surgical pathology: the importance of second opinion in a developing country. J Pak Med Assoc. 2004;54(6):306–11.
43. Vargas HI, Anderson BO, Chopra R, et al. Diagnosis of breast cancer in countries with limited resources. Breast J. 2003;9(Suppl 2):S60–6.
44. Zembowicz A, Ahmad A, Lyle SR. A comprehensive analysis of a web-based dermatopathology second opinion consultation practice. Arch Pathol Lab Med. 2011;135(3):379–83.
45. Nakayama I, Matsumura T, Kamataki A, et al. Development of a teledermatopathology consultation system using virtual slides. Diagn Pathol. 2012;7:177.
46. Saleh J. Practice of teledermatopathology: a systematic review. Am J Dermatopathol. 2018;40(9):667–70.
47. Chong T, Palma-Diaz MF, Fisher C, et al. The California Telepathology service: UCLA's experience in deploying a regional digital pathology subspecialty consultation network. J Pathol Inform. 2019;10:31.
48. Abels E, Pantanowitz L, Aeffner F, et al. Computational pathology definitions, best practices, and recommendations for regulatory guidance: a white paper from the digital pathology association. J Pathol. 2019;249(3):286–94.
49. Sirintrapun SJ. Preparing for a computational pathology future through informaticians and a computational technologist workforce. Am J Clin Pathol. 2018;149(5):369–72.
50. Koelzer VH, Sirinukunwattana K, Rittscher J, Mertz KD. Precision immunoprofiling by image analysis and artificial intelligence. Virchows Arch. 2019;474(4):511–22.
51. Ramamurthy B, Coffman FD, Cohen S. A perspective on digital and computational pathology. J Pathol Inform. 2015;6:29.
52. Robboy SJ, Gupta S, Crawford JM, et al. The pathologist workforce in the United States: II. An interactive modeling tool for analyzing future qualitative and quantitative staffing demands for services. Arch Pathol Lab Med. 2015;139(11):1413–30.
53. Robboy SJ, Weintraub S, Horvath AE, et al. Pathologist workforce in the United States: I. Development of a predictive model to examine factors influencing supply. Arch Pathol Lab Med. 2013;137(12):1723–32.
54. Pathologists CoA. COVID-19 remote sign-out guidance. College of American Pathologists: Chicago; 2020.

Quality Assurance and Quality Improvement Enabled by Whole Slide Imaging

Philipp W. Raess and S. Joseph Sirintrapun

Introduction

Whole slide imaging (WSI) underpins a technological revolution which is transforming the practice of pathology. The microscope has been the primary method of histopathologic interpretation for hundreds of years, is the primary modality with which essentially all pathologists have received their training, and still is the primary diagnostic methodology for the vast majority of surgical pathology cases. However, WSI has matured technologically and can now be used for primary diagnosis in surgical pathology in many countries [1–4]. Since this modality is accepted for use in clinical practice and is being integrated into clinical workflows, robust quality assurance (QA) and quality improvement (QI) programs are necessary to ensure excellent clinical care. The defining feature of WSI is that digitization of glass slides obviates interpreting physical glass slides for pathologic evaluation. The "virtual" nature of a WSI workflow alleviates physical constraints and creates unique QA opportunities such as enabling the remote viewing of slides, enabling slide sorting functionalities, and creating disruptive approaches to objective analysis and computational approaches to quality efforts. The QA opportunities afforded by these unique characteristics of WSI are detailed below in the context of the three phases of testing.

P. W. Raess (✉)
Oregon Health & Science University, Department of Pathology, Portland, OR, USA

S. J. Sirintrapun
Memorial Sloan Kettering Cancer Center, Department of Pathology, New York, NY, USA

A. V. Parwani (ed.), *Whole Slide Imaging*,
https://doi.org/10.1007/978-3-030-83332-9_9

WSI in the Pre-analytical Phase of Testing

WSI and Patient/Specimen Identification

Patient and specimen misidentification in anatomic pathology is a significant source of error, affecting up to 1% of specimens in some settings [5]. Tight integration of WSI image management platforms with laboratory information systems (LISs) is necessary to ensure synchronization for case, specimen, and slide accountability with proper identification. This synchronization must stay robust even through system enhancements and changes to interface design [4]. Ideally, scanned images from the multitude of scanner vendors would be supported by and integrated within the LISs as a common standard. Unfortunately, this is not the case, and integration of scanned images with LISs is currently limited to a select few scanner vendors. Tight integration starts with implementation of bar code slide asset tracking which becomes the necessary functionality for LISs to enable positive identification of slides and reduce specimen identification errors [6].

While use of bar code slide asset tracking alleviates slide mix-up between and within cases, several caveats apply. A bar code system will not necessarily prevent "wrong tissue on glass" errors created at the microtome, and lack of human oversight in organizing cases removes an opportunity for quality control via comparison of similarity in tissue between levels of the same block. Bar codes etched onto a slide remove the possibility of the wrong label being manually placed on a slide (as opposed to a bar-coded label being manually affixed to a slide). More experience or systematic investigation is needed to ensure etched bar codes do not have increased read failure rates compared to bar codes manually printed and affixed to a slide. Furthermore, bar code read errors create the possibility of having slides grouped with the wrong case or not grouped with a case at all. While pathologist attention to case identifiers during sign out will catch the first two of these errors, a bar code read error resulting in failure to identify a slide will create additional work for a laboratory technician to identify the slide and re-scan it or manually group it with the correct case. Bar code asset tracking is also predicated on interchangeability of bar coding systems within an institution. It is possible to coordinate bar code tracking systems within a single AP laboratory (e.g., histology and immunohistochemistry), but this harmonization may require considerable effort and expense depending on the legacy systems in place at the time of WSI implementation.

Extramural consultation cases pose an additional challenge due to bar code non-interchangeability or, worse, interchangeability but with different encoded data leading to specimen or patient misidentification. All institutions which intend to scan and archive extramural consultation cases must then create and utilize additional workflows and resources to relabel physical slides for scanning with internally recognized barcode labels. This additional layer of physical handling introduces additional opportunities for mislabeling of extramural consultation glass slides with internally recognized bar codes. Furthermore, the majority of scanner vendors utilize low-resolution bar code reading cameras positioned only to read the slide label region. This creates inflexibility and does not allow placement of the internally recognized bar code on empty areas of the glass slide outside the slide label region. In resolving this constraint, the original outside label must be covered by the internally recognized bar code; removing or covering the label for extramural clients is a common source of tension, however. For future development, image pattern recognition of bar codes should be performed on the initial low resolution scan of the physical slide rather than relying on installation of a bar code reading camera. This development would alleviate the necessity of overlaying extramural labels and provide the flexibility to programmatically recognize internally generated bar codes affixed outside the slide label region.

Case Assignment and Distribution

Assigning a reasonable daily workload for diagnosticians (pathologists and cytotechnologists) is an important part of a quality assurance program. Limits on the number of slides screened by cytotechnologists are required by CLIA '88 and are intended to prevent diagnostic fatigue and inattention during case review. A digital workflow can also enable real-time equitable case distribution to pathologists. By combining specimen type and complexity information from the LIS with digital slide delivery, flexible workflow models could be created that divert a subset of cases to subspecialists or balance work based on assigned complexity metrics [7, 8]. Workloads that are equitably distributed based on case complexity by a digital workflow are a very disruptive concept. Unfortunately, translating academic models of case complexity into existing antiquated LISs is a significant barrier. For many institutions, only WSI viewers are integrated into LISs, limiting the promises of a digital workflow. For the few institutions which have chosen to use WSI image management platforms like a PACS to drive digital sign out workflows, capturing and translating case complexity shift the burden away from the LISs and towards the PACS. However, metrics required for capture of case complexity currently reside within LISs, further emphasizing the need for tight integration between WSI image management platforms (rather than just WSI viewers) and LISs.

Physical glass slide delivery that is traditionally performed in batch mode after case organization can shift towards a digital delivery model, with increased efficiency for laboratory technicians and clerical staff. With a WSI-supported digital workflow, slides are "delivered" to pathologists' electronic sign out queues after image quality has been confirmed in real time. This "just-in-time" workflow has been shown to benefit turnaround time, a key quality indicator [9]. In addition, significant time and cost savings have also been shown to result from a digital workflow. In the experience of one intermediate-sized pathology laboratory, 19 person-hours of time were saved per day, primarily in routine case organization, distribution, and filing [10].

A fully digital workflow realizes additional benefits through obviating the need for retention of glass slides in physical proximity to pathologists. Slide loss or damage that occurs during manual handling, transportation, or archival processes is minimized with a WSI archival workflow. Retrospective WSI of key archived slides has been used during frozen section analysis, resulting in decreased requests for physical glass slides, faster turnaround times for large resection cases (for which the outside consultation biopsy was digitally archived), and even decreased ordering of immunohistochemical stains because of the immediate retrieval of prior cases enabled by WSI archiving [11].

Quality Assurance of Physical Glass Slides with Histology and Immunohistochemistry

In the past, an AP quality assurance program relied on subjective, highly manual pathologist assessment of histochemical and immunohistochemical staining quality to identify slides with suboptimal or non-diagnostic staining. Subsequent improvements in QA programs have relied on time- or volume-based triggers to replace reagents (reagent expiration date, changing solutions at specified slide, or time intervals).

Technical standardization, of both routine stains and digital images, represents an untapped area in which WSI can contribute to quality assurance in anatomic pathology. Variability in H&E staining characteristics is a well-known phenomenon in routine clinical surgical pathology practice and is due to a variety of pre-analytical (ischemic time, duration, and type of tissue fixation and processing) and analytical (specific staining reagents used, staining protocol, tissue thickness) factors. WSI allows objective assessment of staining parameters and can be used for staining quality control and quality assurance. Investigations into the use of WSI for quality assurance and quality control demonstrate that there is significant variability between laboratories in H&E color characteristics but also between both stainers and whole slide scanners within a laboratory [12]. When combined with an automated and objective assessment of digital images, WSI has the ability to routinely perform quality control on stained sections and serve as the measure of a staining quality assurance program. Color calibration slides have been developed which aid the reproducibility of image display [13, 14]. The FDA has recommended the use of a target slide for color quality control in digital pathology [2016 guidance statement], underlining the importance of this component of WSI. In addition to standardization of glass slide staining and image acquisition, standardization of image display is an important component of quality assurance in digital pathology [15–17].

Robust quality assurance measures are also critical for interpretation of immunohistochemical stains, particularly those for which semi-quantitative or quantitative analysis has direct impact on patient care such as Her2/neu. Although more work has been focused on digital evaluation of the quality of H&E-stained slides, similar principles clearly apply to immunohistochemical stains. Recent work has focused on developing color normalization and image standardization protocols to minimize interbatch variability of staining intensity [18–20]. Clinical application of these techniques would allow prospective measurement of staining intensity of known positive control tissue and automated quality control, rather than relying on pathologists' interpretations of control staining. These technologies could also underpin further efforts to objectively quantitative stain intensity of frequency of positivity using automated image analysis algorithms [21].

With WSI, automated prospective tools for QA and quality control can be integrated into the digital workflow. In an ideal scenario, a slide with suboptimal staining characteristics or one that does not meet pre-specified quality thresholds would be flagged by the LIS upon digitization (before slide delivery to the pathologist), and creation of a replacement slide could be expedited. Monitoring of quality control metrics (e.g., number of H&E slides failing to meet quality standards) can be performed in a prospective and objective manner with WSI, directly contributing to increases in quality in the pre-analytical phase. Moreover, computational pathology tools are intended for automated evaluation and standardization of staining, color intensity, scan quality, and other parameters in development. Such computational tools are likely incorporated more easily into a flexible PACS environment rather than a digital LIS environment, since LISs are highly dependent on proprietary and often restrictive WSI viewers.

Quality Assurance of Digital Images

Standardization of image quality has long been recognized as a critical component to successful utilization of WSI [22, 23]. The most common source of image quality problems with WSI was failed autofocusing by WSI scanners resulting from either imprecise tissue detection or erroneous focus depth, as reported by one of the largest PACS-driven digital pathology laboratories (2). Failed autofocusing is especially problematic with cytological and hematopathology smears or slides with faint immunohistochemical staining intensity.

For WSI scanners, the most widely used autofocusing mechanism determines optimal focus for a number of automatically selected focus points and then extrapolates by triangulation to the entire slide area. This is used because the alternative through selection of optimal focus for each capture unit (image tile or line, depending on the scanning mode) is prohibitively time-consuming. Scanners have since improved, leveraging autofocusing techniques to determine optimal focus in parallel with image acquisition, thus saving valuable time and enabling larger number of focus points to be used [24]. However, commercially available WSI scanner autofocusing mechanisms still do not provide robust performance in all clinical use cases, such as cytology and hematopathology smears.

Early attempts at developing standards for acceptable image quality involved relying on subjective assessments of image quality by pathologists which were quantitated and applied to subsequently digitized images [25]. Objective analysis is preferred, however, due to efficiencies gained in terms of pathologist time as well as reproducibility and interinstitutional applicability. Referenceless methods of image quality evaluation are preferred as it is not feasible to obtain a reference image with WSI. Objective methods that evaluate for blur, noise, and focus errors have been developed [26, 27]. More recently, this work has been extended to use machine learning to prevent artifacts such as tissue folds or air bubbles from spuriously decreasing image quality measurements [28]. Other groups have also used statistical learning methods to evaluate image quality and automatically identify regions of interest that require additional focus points [29]. Integrating automated image quality evaluation into a WSI workflow obviates the need for subjective, time-consuming slide quality evaluation by a pathologist or technician and acts as a critical complement to quality assurance measures in glass slide production.

WSI in the Analytical Phase of Testing

Intramural and Extramural Consultation

The benefits of WSI are most readily apparent when considering robust consultative practices at geographically disparate sites within a distributed health system. One of the key QA benefits of WSI is the increased availability of pathologists with subspecialty expertise to review challenging cases, and not be constrained by physical location with flexibility to work remotely. At the University of Arizona, a QA program was instituted to provide same-day re-review of new malignancies and challenging cases encountered at a satellite location staffed by a single part-time pathologist. WSI-enabled same-day consensus re-review of these cases at the flagship hospital resulted in greater than 90% complete concordance with less than 2% major discrepancies [30]. Importantly, less than 2% of cases were deferred for examination of the glass slides at the flagship institution. In-depth analysis of breast biopsies performed at the satellite location showed similar complete concordance, discrepancy, and deferral rates [31]. Same-day re-review resulted in important quality gains in cases of diagnostic discrepancies. Additionally, subspecialty pathologists without special training in breast pathology who were stationed at the satellite location reported subjective increases in job satisfaction, presumably due to increased diagnostic confidence following subspecialist review.

Extramural consultative practices can also benefit from adoption of WSI. WSI can be integrated into the workflow in one of two ways in this scenario: scanning is performed either at the referring institution or performed at the consulting institution following physical receipt of glass slides. WSI performed at the referring institution has the benefit of theoretically faster case delivery to the consulting institution (and therefore improved overall turnaround time). In addition, WSI performed at the referring institution minimizes bias introduced by selection and submission of static images limited to areas of interest by the referring pathologist, with the possible exclusion of important diagnostic findings in non-submitted material.

For WSI to be utilized by both referring and receiving institutions, the digitized images must be compatible at least with the receiving institution's LIS and/or WSI image management system. A large barrier is the lack of widely accepted consensus file format standards for image capture, storage, and exchange, although efforts in this area are underway [32]. Consensus for standardization through DICOM is far less developed in pathology than in radiology. Increasing this complexity in WSI are the plethora of WSI vendors, each with their own pathology slide image capture and file formats containing image and image metadata; some of these vendors use proprietary formats that are unlockable by other WSI systems. This complexity in the variety of histology laboratories and scanning platforms hampers harmonization of image exchange between referring and receiving institutions. When limitations in receiving WSI files are encountered at institutions with extramural consultative practices, the workflow reverts to reliance on physical slide receipt, effectively defeating the purpose of a WSI workflow for extramural consultation.

Several successful instances of extramural consultation services with WSI have been recently described [33–38]. The most successful instances have involved "trusted" partnerships where the referring and receiving institutions have established relationships and a steady pipeline of referral cases. This effectively lowers the potential for security breaches and decreases the complexity for reimbursement because both parties are familiar and accountable to each other. In one such example, the authors showed non-inferiority of a WSI-based subspecialty extramural consultative service [34]. Key factors in the performance of this service included technologist quality control of WSI images prior to pathologist review and pathologist familiarity with the WSI interface following a training period. WSI review of extramural consultative cases within select subspecialties showed a major discrepancy rate with WSI of less than 3%, including a subset of errors made due to inadvertent lack of review of diagnostic WSI images.

More "open" extramural consultation services, though promising, have fared less well for a multitude of reasons. "Open" extramural consultation can disrupt pathology practices through an additional stream of case volume and revenue. This model can capture the attention of institutional leadership and identify pathology departments as a driver for patient capture and revenue growth. However, for the parties involved (particularly referring institutions), the "open" model raises the level of constraints for patient data governance, security, and exchange in comparison to "trusted" partnerships because parties are less familiar and accountable to each other. In addition, "open" extramural consultation services require continual marketing services, catering to clients, and reputation building to expand the service, whereas "trusted" partnerships are usually based on established relationships and initial agreements to a steady case volume.

Transitioning from the traditional analog workflow with microscopes to one of WSI incorporation will involve a considerable shift in mindset for pathologists. The vast majority of pathologists are trained and sign out using traditional analog workflows. Earning their trust for WSI adoption therefore takes time. As WSI becomes more commonplace, future generations of pathologists should become accustomed with WSI workflows, particularly with the incorporation of sign out workflow enhancements like seamless digital consultation and integrated computational-assisted diagnostics. Remote case sign out with WSI is arguably the most disruptive change in the pathology workforce in the foreseeable future. Interestingly, regulatory stakeholders and not the technology will prove the most critical factor in making remote sign out possible in the USA [39–41]. The transformation of radiology from film to digital created a disruptive shift in the radiology workforce in allowing for remote work. Regulatory stakeholders such as state medical boards raised the barriers to performing remote primary reads of radiologic studies across state lines. State medical boards also affect WSI consultation portals, where some states may demand any deliverance of care to require a license with the state corresponding to the patients needing a consultation as it relates to primary diagnosis [42]. Furthermore, reimbursement issues are currently problematic in radiology when insurance companies may refuse to reimburse charges if interpretation is performed in another state [43].

Another regulatory stakeholder that factors into WSI intramural and extramural consultation in pathology is CLIA'88. CLIA'88 has never applied to radiology, and thus radiologists are able to sign out from home. This is not true in pathology, where any physical location in which a pathologist performs the interpretation requires a separate CLIA'88 license. Because CLIA became law prior to the digital era, it is difficult to extrapolate these regulations to contemporary practice involving WSI. It may be debatable whether non-primary diagnosis tasks such as frozen section interpretation, WSI-enabled telepathology consultation, or QA procedures are subject to CLIA'88 regulations [1].

Intradepartmental Quality Assurance Programs

Intradepartmental case re-review constitutes a key component of an anatomic pathology QA system. There are several advantages of WSI over re-review of glass slides. AP LISs currently have the capability to prospectively flag a specified percentage of cases for re-review prior to finalization, a practice currently used to meet standards for cytotechnologist quality assurance. At Memorial Sloan Kettering Cancer Center, manually selected representative slides are scanned for every surgical pathology case, including extramural cases that require re-review for patient care referrals. The WSIs of these cases are available for instant retrieval in the LIS through integration with a WSI viewer. Once WSI of these cases was made available, physical glass slide requests (mainly used for comparison to frozen sections and for comparison of resection specimens with prior biopsies) decreased to essentially zero. The immediacy of WSI of previously reviewed consultation cases had several additional benefits. The number of immunohistochemical stains that were ordered decreased because prior tumor biopsies were available for comparison. Turnaround times for resections specimens were cut by 1/3 because review of prior biopsies was no longer delayed by physical retrieval. Pathologist satisfaction, familiarity with WSI, and cultural trust all increased as this "on-demand" model of WSI case re-review via was accepted in clinical workflows.

There is utility in going further than this "on-demand" model of case re-review in implementing a systemized prospective or second review of cases prior to report finalization. Retrospective re-review of cases may not identify errors in a sufficiently timely manner to prevent harm to the patient or performance of an unnecessary procedure. WSI allows simultaneous independent review of cases by multiple pathologists, therefore enabling prospective QA review and helping to identify and correct errors before they reach the patient. In addition, prospective or concurrent re-review of cases can be configured to hide the prior diagnosis. This configuration is beneficial in order to minimize bias known to be introduced by knowledge of the prior diagnosis [44]. In addition, the original or concurrent pathologist can also be anonymized to eliminate another source of potential bias. Many practices also require a second pathologist to review cases with newly diagnosed malignancies or cases known to be diagnostically challenging or especially litiginous as part of their QA plan. The use of WSI allows pathologists to manually identify these critical cases for re-review within the LIS and deliver them instantly to the sign out queue of a colleague, obviating the need for manual transfer of glass slides between pathologists. Turnaround time would be expected to improve while maintaining QA standards.

The practice of prospective re-review for even physical glass slides is not as widespread in anatomic pathology due to several reasons. Most importantly, pre-finalization re-review of pathologist cases is not mandated by accrediting agencies (in contrast to cytotechnologist cases with significant findings) and also the logistical considerations of transferring physical glass slides to a second pathologist. Prospective scanning of cases prior to sign out requires a major shift in operations and significant resources. For institutions that have LIS-driven digital pathology workflows, functionalities in LISs have not yet been built that enable prospective re-review of cases prior to report finalization. Even retrospective scanning of physical glass slides for WSI case QA re-review requires significant resources in terms of capital equipment, operational costs, and personnel.

Increased quality achieved with a digital workflow optimized for consultation and case re-review can not only increase diagnostic accuracy but also normalize diagnostic standards. This theoretical advantage will be most beneficial among pathology groups that do not routinely review cases together, whether due to lack of physical proximity or other barriers. When WSI is combined with other readily available technologies (screen sharing, conference calling), a "virtual consensus conference" could take place within a physically disparate group of pathologists. One can envision this occurring within a large health system or even to standardize diagnostic practice across institutions [45]. In large health systems where there are sites separated by physical distance and access to expert consultation, the potential benefits of diagnostic standardization become readily apparent.

Increased Diagnostic Efficiency

WSI enhances quality through higher diagnostic efficiency of primary diagnosis and intramural and extramural consultation. As discussed prior, large-scale retrospective case archival of representative slides through WSI implementation improves turnaround times and reduces immunohistochemical ordering [11]. Instantaneous access to prior cases through WSI creates improvements in the diagnostic process. Clerical and administrative time searching for old cases during routine sign out can be minimized by linking historical scanned cases to the current case within the AP LIS. The utility of this capability is readily apparent when considering extramural cases that are reviewed when a patient transfers their care or undergoes a complex surgery therapy. WSI enable the digital retention of glass slides that are returned to the referring institution, allowing comparison of the original biopsy specimen with the current case to confirm diagnosis, to compare a possible metastatic lesion to a previously reviewed primary lesion, and to assess the effect of neoadjuvant therapy more precisely. WSI-enabled digital storage of historical intramural cases also allows rapid comparison with current cases. It is anticipated that comparison with prior digitized cases would decrease immunohistochemical stain ordering and improve turnaround time. Additionally, challenging intraoperative (frozen section) specimens may be more confidently evaluated following consultation with WSI of prior specimens.

Digital workflows driven by WSI image management systems like a PACS are more optimized to increase diagnostic efficiency than digital pathology workflows driven by LISs. Functionalities of PACS include easily accessible annotation, allowing regions of interest to be recorded. This function can improve efficiency when cases are shared between pathologists for intramural consultation on challenging cases, at digital consensus conferences, and multidisciplinary tumor board. In addition, routine histological sections can be displayed simultaneously with immunohistochemical stains. This functionality could be further optimized by co-registration of the immunohistochemical and histochemical WSI in order to allow efficient high-magnification comparison of regions of interest across all images.

WSI in the Post-analytical Phase of Testing

Although many of the more readily conceived QA functions of WSI occur in the pre-analytical and analytical test phases, WSI also has value in the post-analytical phase of testing. Review of prior cases for tissue triage, at multidisciplinary tumor boards, for correlation between cytology and surgical pathology specimens, and clearer diagnostic audit trails are several examples of QA improvements with a digital workflow.

At Memorial Sloan Kettering Cancer Center, WSI is used to triage specimens for next-generation sequencing (NGS) through selection and digitization of select tissue blocks. These WSI are available for triage by molecular pathologists, and specimens with insufficient tumor quantity are stopped from proceeding down the NGS pipeline in order to save resources.

WSI de-identification for research and educational purposes possesses several advantages over recutting or manually de-identifying glass slides. Digital de-identification removes constraints placed by limited histology resources, increasing the number of cases for research and education. With nearly all scanner vendor systems, however, de-identification is currently a manual process, leaving many institutions to resort to physically de-identifying glass slides before re-scanning, essentially duplicating effort. Ideally, future iterations of scanning software will possess digital de-identification capabilities.

Cytologic/histologic correlation is a critical component of a QA plan and is required by regulatory standards and accrediting agencies [46]. This process functions to identify areas for quality improvement at the institutional and individual level by identifying discrepant cytologic and histologic findings in paired specimens. This QA correlation is generally performed by comparing prior concurrent cytology and histology cases and is retrospective in nature. Digitization in cytology through streaming telecytology has clear benefits in service efficiency and quality despite the notable restrictions in proper selection of regions of interest, particularly where assessments are rendered [47, 48]. Digitization through WSI for cytologic specimens currently faces inherent technical challenges like vendor flexibility for z-stacking and other issues as discussed previously [2, 24]. Thus WSI is less widely adopted than WSI of histology slides to date [48, 49]. Nonetheless, use of digitized histologic slides is expected to result in efficiencies gained in cytologic/histologic correlation in terms of time spent retrieving and organizing archived histologic slides.

An additional QA benefit of a WSI-enabled digital workflow is greater ease in performing diagnostic audits. While systematic retrospective audits have been described in the preceding section to facilitate comparison with prospective QA review, sentinel event and root cause analysis can also benefit from a digital workflow. Certain specialized WSI viewers integrated with LISs and advanced integrated PACS systems are configurable to audit when cases were accessed digitally, for how long, and whether every slide in a case has been viewed. This digital trace of pathologist activity within the WSI environment may be quite helpful in differentiating interpretive errors from errors of omission [34].

WSI and Quality Assurance: Future Considerations with Computational Pathology

Many significant advances have been made in WSI and digital pathology over the last several years, with much more to continually arrive. Many believe the field of pathology is at an inflection point, with WSI underpinning significant changes in pathologists' daily workflow. Quality assurance will always be a critical contribution to the healthcare team by pathologists, and many new technologies to improve QA lie just over the horizon. Efforts to explore and enhance pathologists' interfaces with digital images are underway through emerging computational pathology tools.

As previously discussed, computational pathology tools enhance quality in the pre-analytic phase of testing through tools for ensuring proper image focus [27, 50, 51]. Visual interpretation of WSI is of increasing interest in computational pathology. At the most basic QA level, WSI viewers can be configured to ensure that the pathologist visualizes all areas of tissue with WSI, thus performing a vital QC function to help alleviate diagnostic errors of omission. Tracking pathologists gaze when evaluating WSI is more accessible than with a conventional microscope, and gaze patterns have been shown to correlate with diagnostic expertise and case difficulty [52–55]. Studying gaze patterns and visual strategies of expert pathologists provides data to develop tools to help improve diagnostic accuracy using WSI. Gaze patterns, alone or in combination with histopathological image classification, may inform future computational methods which can predict areas most likely to have diagnostic regions of interest; early iterations of these algorithms have been described [56, 57]. Successful prediction algorithms have the possibility of reducing computational load, improving diagnostic accuracy, and acting as quality control decision support tools for pathologists.

WSI has only recently enabled financial opportunities through grant-funded academic research for digital pathology commons like in the Cancer Genome Atlas (https://cancergenome.nih.gov/), partnerships with pharmaceutical companies (for biomarker discovery, companion diagnostics, and immune-oncology), and collaborations with artificial intelligence companies in development and validation of AI applications. Traditional business use cases for digital pathology with logistical advances (including cost reductions due to fewer staff requirements and better turnaround time) have further substantiated this trend [58].

AI companies and digital pathology vendors are now entering the computational pathology space through the realization of revenue opportunities to make data-driven decisions, make faster decisions, and achieve better financial results. Paige. AI, started in 2018 with $25 million in venture capital funding, is one example of a company focused on using AI for clinical cancer diagnosis and treatment (https://paige.ai/). IBEX is another example that deployed the first AI-based digital pathology cancer diagnosis system in a clinical setting (https://ibex-ai.com/). IBEX has developed an algorithm to evaluate prostate needle core biopsies; the algorithm essentially functions as a second read system for quality control. The trend of AI incorporation into pathology is expected to continue as more AI companies compete in the computational pathology arena.

WSI has opened many challenges and opportunities for pathology. The most critical of these is fostering pathologist trust through quality diagnostic effectiveness and well-developed integration into digital pathology workflows. Dynamic QA programs are a key step to gain this trust and to demonstrate the clinical value of WSI. Additional challenges include leading regulatory agencies through the AI transformation. The future of pathology is exciting, and digital applications integrated into pathology workflows hold the promise to pre-screen, optimize, perform quality control functions, and enable decision support for pathologists to continue to deliver high-quality diagnostic patient care. The incorporation of WSI and AI into pathology will define the coming disruptive shift and will have profound, positive impacts for continual quality assurance and improvement.

References

1. Evans AJ, et al. US food and drug administration approval of whole slide imaging for primary diagnosis: a key milestone is reached and new questions are raised. Arch Pathol Lab Med. 2018;142(11):1383–7.
2. Stathonikos N, et al. Going fully digital: perspective of a Dutch academic pathology lab. J Pathol Inform. 2013;4:15.

3. Thorstenson S, Molin J, Lundstrom C. Implementation of large-scale routine diagnostics using whole slide imaging in Sweden: digital pathology experiences 2006-2013. J Pathol Inform. 2014;5(1):14.
4. Cheng CL, et al. Enabling digital pathology in the diagnostic setting: navigating through the implementation journey in an academic medical centre. J Clin Pathol. 2016;69(9):784–92.
5. Valenstein PN, Sirota RL. Identification errors in pathology and laboratory medicine. Clin Lab Med. 2004;24(4):979–96, vii
6. Heher YK, et al. Achieving high reliability in histology: an improvement series to reduce errors. Am J Clin Pathol. 2016;146(5):554–60.
7. Cloetingh D, Schmidt RA, Kong CS. Comparison of three methods for measuring workload in surgical pathology and cytopathology. Am J Clin Pathol. 2017;148(1):16–22.
8. Ducatman BS, Parslow T. Benchmarking academic anatomic pathologists: the Association of Pathology Chairs Survey. Acad Pathol. 2016;3:2374289516666832.
9. Fraggetta F, et al. Routine digital pathology workflow: the Catania experience. J Pathol Inform. 2017;8:51.
10. Baidoshvili A, et al. Evaluating the benefits of digital pathology implementation: time savings in laboratory logistics. Histopathology. 2018;73(5):784–94.
11. Hanna MG, et al. Implementation of digital pathology offers clinical and operational increase in efficiency and cost savings. Arch Pathol Lab Med. 2019;143(12):1545–55.
12. Gray A, et al. Quantification of histochemical stains using whole slide imaging: development of a method and demonstration of its usefulness in laboratory quality control. J Clin Pathol. 2015;68(3):192–9.
13. Bautista PA, Hashimoto N, Yagi Y. Color standardization in whole slide imaging using a color calibration slide. J Pathol Inform. 2014;5(1):4.
14. Clarke EL, Treanor D. Colour in digital pathology: a review. Histopathology. 2017;70(2):153–63.
15. Krupinski EA, et al. Observer performance using virtual pathology slides: impact of LCD color reproduction accuracy. J Digit Imaging. 2012;25(6):738–43.
16. Hirschorn DS, Krupinski EA, Flynn MJ. PACS displays: how to select the right display technology. J Am Coll Radiol. 2014;11(12 Pt B):1270–6.
17. Peck D, Flynn M. TU-E-217A-01: informatics 1: DICOM and the QMP, assessment of color displays. Med Phys. 2012;39(6Part24):3916.
18. Van Eycke YR, et al. Image processing in digital pathology: an opportunity to solve inter-batch variability of immunohistochemical staining. Sci Rep. 2017;7:42964.
19. Khan AM, et al. A nonlinear mapping approach to stain normalization in digital histopathology images using image-specific color deconvolution. IEEE Trans Biomed Eng. 2014;61(6):1729–38.
20. Xu J, et al. Sparse non-negative matrix factorization (SNMF) based color unmixing for breast histopathological image analysis. Comput Med Imaging Graph. 2015;46(Pt 1):20–9.
21. Van Eycke YR, et al. Segmentation of glandular epithelium in colorectal tumours to automatically compartmentalise IHC biomarker quantification: a deep learning approach. Med Image Anal. 2018;49:35–45.
22. Yagi Y, Gilbertson JR. Digital imaging in pathology: the case for standardization. J Telemed Telecare. 2005;11(3):109–16.
23. Kayser K, et al. Image standards in tissue-based diagnosis (diagnostic surgical pathology). Diagn Pathol. 2008;3:17.
24. Montalto MC, McKay RR, Filkins RJ. Autofocus methods of whole slide imaging systems and the introduction of a second-generation independent dual sensor scanning method. J Pathol Inform. 2011;2:44.
25. Shrestha P, et al. A quantitative approach to evaluate image quality of whole slide imaging scanners. J Pathol Inform. 2016;7:56.
26. Hashimoto N, et al. Referenceless image quality evaluation for whole slide imaging. J Pathol Inform. 2012;3:9.

27. Campanella G, et al. Towards machine learned quality control: a benchmark for sharpness quantification in digital pathology. Comput Med Imaging Graph. 2018;65:142–51.
28. MS Hossain., et al., Practical image quality evaluation for whole slide imaging scanner. Proceedings Biomedical Imaging and Sensing Conference. 2018. Vol. 10711.
29. Moles Lopez X, et al. An automated blur detection method for histological whole slide imaging. PLoS One. 2013;8(12):e82710.
30. Graham AR, et al. Virtual slide telepathology for an academic teaching hospital surgical pathology quality assurance program. Hum Pathol. 2009;40(8):1129–36.
31. Lopez AM, et al. Virtual slide telepathology enables an innovative telehealth rapid breast care clinic. Hum Pathol. 2009;40(8):1082–91.
32. Clunie D, et al. Digital imaging and communications in medicine whole slide imaging connectathon at digital pathology association pathology visions 2017. J Pathol Inform. 2018;9:6.
33. Wilbur DC, et al. Whole-slide imaging digital pathology as a platform for teleconsultation: a pilot study using paired subspecialist correlations. Arch Pathol Lab Med. 2009;133(12):1949–53.
34. Jones NC, et al. Interinstitutional whole slide imaging teleconsultation service development: assessment using internal training and clinical consultation cases. Arch Pathol Lab Med. 2015;139(5):627–35.
35. Baidoshvili, A., et al. Validation of a whole-slide image-based teleconsultation network. Histopathology, 2018.
36. Zhao C, et al. International telepathology consultation: three years of experience between the University of Pittsburgh Medical Center and KingMed Diagnostics in China. J Pathol Inform. 2015;6:63.
37. Chen J, et al. A nationwide telepathology consultation and quality control program in China: implementation and result analysis. Diagn Pathol. 2014;9(Suppl 1):S2.
38. Nahal A, et al. Setting up an ePathology Service at Cleveland Clinic Abu Dhabi: Joint Collaboration With Cleveland Clinic, United States. Arch Pathol Lab Med. 2018;142(10):1216–22.
39. Abels E, Pantanowitz L. Current state of the regulatory trajectory for whole slide imaging devices in the USA. J Pathol Inform. 2017;8:23.
40. Leung, S. and T. Allen, Legal/Regulatory. 2016. in Digital pathology, K.J. Kaplan, L.K.F. Rao (eds.): p. 79–86.
41. Cornish TC, McClintock DS. Medicolegal and regulatory aspects of whole slide imaging-based telepathology. Diagn Histopathol. 2014;21(12):475–81.
42. Hiemenz MC, Leung ST, Park JY. Crossing boundaries: a comprehensive survey of medical licensing laws and guidelines regulating the interstate practice of pathology. Am J Surg Pathol. 2014;38(3):e1–5.
43. Li KC, et al. Digitization of medicine: how radiology can take advantage of the digital revolution. Acad Radiol. 2013;20(12):1479–94.
44. Renshaw AA, Lezon KM, Wilbur DC. The human false-negative rate of rescreening pap tests. Measured in a two-arm prospective clinical trial. Cancer. 2001;93(2):106–10.
45. Ho J, et al. Use of whole slide imaging in surgical pathology quality assurance: design and pilot validation studies. Hum Pathol. 2006;37(3):322–31.
46. Crothers BA. Cytologic-histologic correlation: where are we now, and where are we going? Cancer Cytopathol. 2018;126(5):301–8.
47. Sirintrapun SJ, et al. Successful secure high-definition streaming telecytology for remote cytologic evaluation. J Pathol Inform. 2017;8:33.
48. Sirintrapun SJ, et al. Robotic telecytology for remote cytologic evaluation without an on-site cytotechnologist or cytopathologist: an active quality assessment and experience of over 400 cases. J Pathol Inform. 2017;8:35.
49. Van Es SL, et al. Constant quest for quality: digital cytopathology. J Pathol Inform. 2018;9:13.
50. Janowczyk A, Basavanhally A, Madabhushi A. Stain normalization using sparse AutoEncoders (StaNoSA): application to digital pathology. Comput Med Imaging Graph. 2017;57:50–61.
51. Kather JN, et al. New colors for histology: optimized bivariate color maps increase perceptual contrast in histological images. PLoS One. 2015;10(12):e0145572.

52. Shin D, et al. PathEdEx - uncovering high-explanatory visual diagnostics heuristics using digital pathology and multiscale gaze data. J Pathol Inform. 2017;8:29.
53. Brunye TT, et al. Eye movements as an index of pathologist visual expertise: a pilot study. PLoS One. 2014;9(8):e103447.
54. Brunye TT, et al. Accuracy is in the eyes of the pathologist: the visual interpretive process and diagnostic accuracy with digital whole slide images. J Biomed Inform. 2017;66:171–9.
55. Schaumberg AJ, et al. DeepScope: nonintrusive whole slide saliency annotation and prediction from pathologists at the microscope. Comput Intell Methods Bioinform Biostat (2016). 2017;10477:42–58.
56. Mercan E, et al. Localization of diagnostically relevant regions of interest in whole slide images: a comparative study. J Digit Imaging. 2016;29(4):496–506.
57. Zheng Y, et al. Histopathological whole slide image analysis using context-based CBIR. IEEE Trans Med Imaging. 2018;37(7):1641–52.
58. L., P., Turning research repository images into gold: winning strategies for funding WSI research infrastructure & programs. Pathology Informatics Summit 2018. 2018.

Whole Slide Imaging in Cytopathology

Zaibo Li and Liron Pantanowitz

Introduction

Whole slide imaging (WSI) success in surgical pathology is exemplified by FDA approval for primary diagnosis, development of guidelines for standardizing clinical validation and telepathology, etc. [1]. However, WSI in cytopathology has not been as pervasive [2–4]. Validation studies have proven that WSI is not inferior to the conventional microscope in diagnosing surgical pathology cases [5, 6], but comparative studies have demonstrated that glass slides were more accurate and faster than WSI in diagnosing cytopathology cases [7, 8]. Several unique barriers in cytopathology have limited the application of WSI technology including image acquisition challenges (focus, resolution) and complex cytology workflow (multiple slide preparations, screening). This chapter addresses these challenges and discusses current and future applications of using WSI in cytopathology practice.

Challenges of WSI in Cytopathology

Focus

Surgical pathology slides with 4–5 micron thick tissue sections have little variation topologically; therefore, scanning these slides with one Z-focus level to generate a two-dimensional (2D) WSI is generally sufficient to have almost everything in focus, except for occasional tissue folds. In contrast, cytology slides often include

Z. Li (✉)
Department of Pathology, The Ohio State University Wexner Medical Center, Columbus, OH, USA
e-mail: Zaibo.Li@osumc.edu

L. Pantanowitz
Department of Pathology, University of Michigan, Ann Arbor, MI, USA

A. V. Parwani (ed.), *Whole Slide Imaging*,
https://doi.org/10.1007/978-3-030-83332-9_10

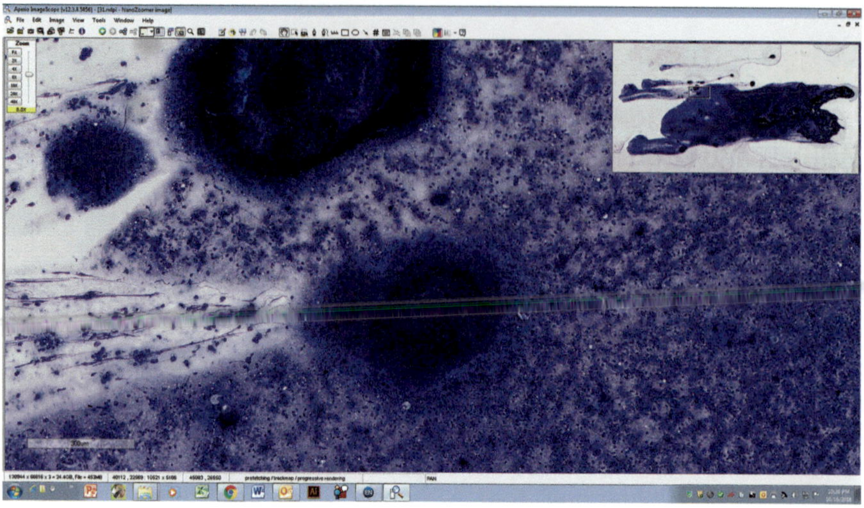

Fig. 1 A WSI of a Diff-Quik-stained smear from a lymph node FNA. The smear is hypercellular and thick in areas with abundant cellular material and 3D clusters of cells

thick smears and/or contain three-dimensional (3D) cell groups (Fig. 1), making it more difficult to have all cells/material in focus if acquiring an image with only one Z-plane. Although liquid-based cytology (LBC) slides usually have monolayers of cells, 3D cell clustering still occurs, especially when sample cellularity is high [9]. In addition, there may be further confounding factors that negatively impact focus such as obscuring material (blood, mucus, etc.), dotting pen marks, and cellular material extending beyond the coverslip on smeared slides.

Cytopathologists/cytotechnologists usually focus up and down the vertical or Z-axis to focus on 3D cell clusters or thick smears when using a conventional light microscope to interpret cytology slides. Therefore, it is important to be able to scan cytology slides in both horizontal (X and Y) and vertical (Z) axes in order to ensure that all cytology material is in focus [10, 11]. Z-stacking can overcome this problem by scanning glass slides at multiple focus levels (planes) and then generating a final composite file with images atop each other (Z-stack) (Fig. 2). WSIs scanned with Z-stacking make it possible for cytologists to digitally focus up and down the different acquired planes just like a conventional light microscope. Nowadays, many WSI scanners offer Z-stacking capability (Table 1).

However, Z-stacking comes with additional costs and challenges. The scan time for Z-stacking is much longer, and the generated WSI file size is much larger than a single Z-level scan. Z-stacking typically increases file size linearly by the number of levels scanned. It has been reported that it takes around 40 minutes to scan a SurePath Pap slide with Z-stacking of seven planes and that such a scan will produce a WSI file size of 11 GB [12]. Such large WSI files may cause high demand on storage needs, and limited network bandwidth may result in pixilation and freezing when viewing images.

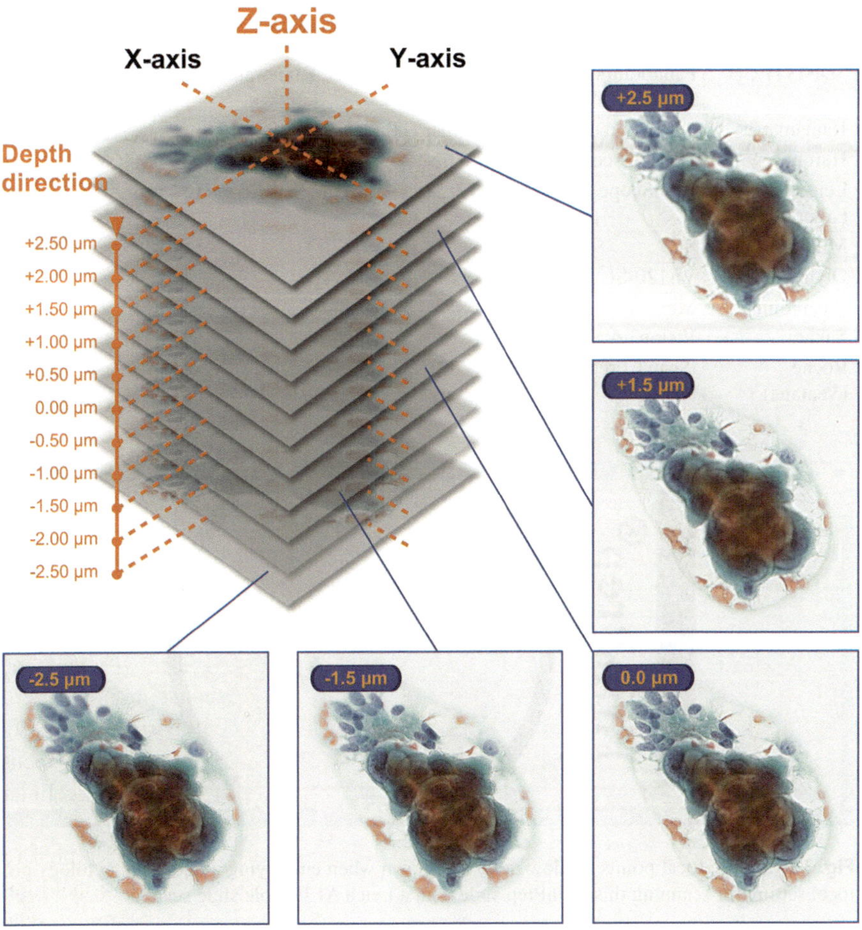

Fig. 2 Z-stacking images are acquired at multiple planes along the Z-axis above and below the "optimal" focal plane, which in turn are used to create a 3D image. (Reproduced with permission from Hamamatsu Inc. (http://www.hamamatsu.com/jp/en/C9600.html))

The optimal number of Z-focal planes required when digitizing cytology slides has been investigated by several groups, but this parameter has not yet been standardized. One study found that WSIs with 21 Z-focal planes (at 1.5 micron intervals) showed better quality than WSIs with 5 Z-focal planes (at 1 micron intervals) for LBC Pap slides [8]. Another study found that WSIs with three Z-focal planes (at 1 micron intervals) were adequate for LBC Pap test slides [11]. The discrepancy may be related to different scanners used in these studies. However, even the same scanner may not always produce the exact same WSI each time when the same slide is scanned, likely because scanning may not always occur at the exact same Z-focal plane [13]. Some scanners (e.g., Leica AT2) have a dedicated cytology scan

Table 1 Some WSI scanners with Z-stacking capability

Vendor	Scanner model
3DHISTECH	Pannoramic Desk II, Pannoramic MIDI II, Pannoramic SCAN II, Pannoramic 250 Flash II, Pannoramic 1000
Hamamatsu	Nanozoomer RS, Nanozoomer HT, Nanozoomer XR
Huron	TISSUEscope 4000, TISSUEscope 4000XT, TISSUEscope TM4000XT
Leica (Aperio)	ScanScope AT, Aperio AT2, ScanScope CS, ScanScope FL, versa
Mikroscan	SL5
Olympus	VS120-SL
PreciPoint	M8
Sakura	VisionTek, VisionTek M6
Roche (Ventana)	iScan Coreo, iScan HT

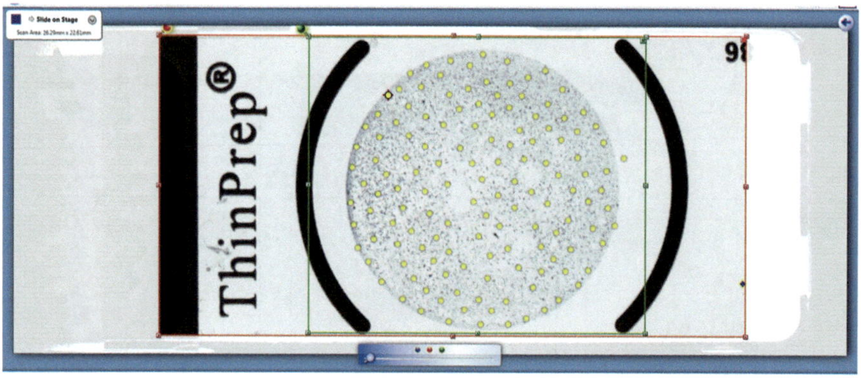

Fig. 3 Multiple focal points (yellow dots) are shown when employing a dedicated cytology protocol setting for scanning this ThinPrep slide with a Leica AT2 whole slide scanner

protocol that drops abundant focal points on the slide which greatly improves the final focus of scanned slides even with one Z-plane (Fig. 3).

The Panoptiq digital slide imaging system (ViewsIQ, Canada) provides an alternative solution to Z-stacking (Fig. 4). The Panoptiq system can digitize glass slides in real time while examining them on traditional light microscope at any objective (2× to 100×) by stitching together multiple fields of view into a single panoramic image. This requires a digital camera to be attached via a C-mount to any existing conventional light microscope. Furthermore, the Panoptiq setup uses high frame rate videos to capture Z-stacks for selected regions and integrates them into the digitized panoramic image. However, the scanning process needs to be performed manually including selecting regions of interest for Z-stacked videos. Hence, image acquisition requires experienced personnel with cytology expertise in order to capture representative images [14–17].

Although Z-stacking is preferred for cytology slides with 3D cell clusters (e.g., Pap tests with hyperchromatic crowded groups), some cytology slides with

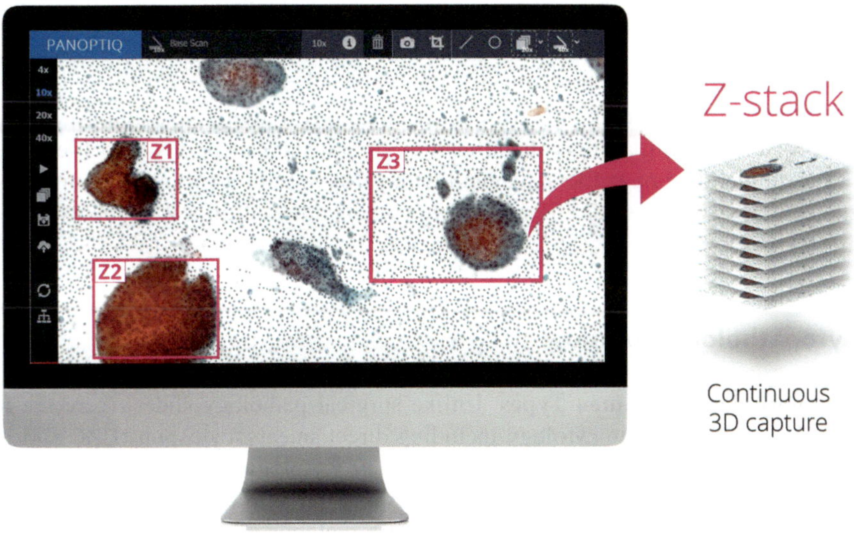

Fig. 4 The Panoptiq digital slide imaging system uses high frame rate video to capture Z-stacks for selected regions of interest and integrates them into digitally mapped panoramic slides. (Image courtesy of ViewsIQ Inc. and adapted from "Whole-slide imaging: widening the scope of cytopathology" El-Gabry et al. [67])

abundant cellular material may not require Z-stacking in order to make a diagnosis (e.g., hypercellular fine-needle aspiration smear with adenocarcinoma) as long as sufficient cellular material is in focus. Indeed, one study has shown that Z-stacking may have negligible return on diagnostic yield [5]. Our unpublished experience with scanning cytology slides without Z-stacking supports this notion. Of interest, a workaround solution proposed in one study was to scan only cell block sections for cervical cytology specimens as a replacement for processing and scanning LBC Pap test slides [18].

Magnification and Resolution

WSI with scanning at a 20x magnification usually suffices for digitizing surgical pathology slides. However, scanning at 40x magnification is often necessary to obtain higher optical resolution in order to examine cytology slides at the cellular level. Higher optical resolution can be further obtained by using objectives with greater numerical aperture (NA). In addition, image quality can be further enhanced by increasing digital resolution, which depends on the scanner's digital camera sensor and display monitor [19]. WSI size is dependent on the following parameters: the scanner's objective lens magnification (including NA), size/number of individual pixels of the digital camera sensor, number of Z-stacks, and image compression. It has been reported that higher diagnostic accuracy and lower interpretation time were obtained from reviewing WSIs scanned at 40x with 0.75 NA and 0.23 micron/pixel resolution when compared to reviewing WSIs scanned at 20x with 0.5 NA and 0.46 micron/pixel resolution (8). Therefore, it is necessary to assess both objective magnification and digital camera sensor resolution when evaluating a WSI scanner intended for digitizing cytology slides. Of course, scanning at high magnification significantly increases WSI file size. For example, the image file associated with a 20x scan of a 15 mm × 15 mm tissue can be as large as 2.7 GB while a 40× scan can result in a WSI file as large as 10 GB.

Cytopathology Workflow

Cytopathology Specimen Types Unlike surgical pathology slides, there are a variety of slide types in cytology including direct smears, cytospins, LBC slides (ThinPrep or SurePath), and cell block sections. Cytology slides can also contain very scant single cells or abundant cellular material with crowded 3D cell clusters. Moreover, there are typically more stain methods encountered in cytology including Diff-Quik stain, Papanicolaou stain, and H&E stain, among others. Hence, managing all of the slides from one fine-needle aspiration case (e.g., Diff-Quik-stained smears, Pap-stained smears, H&E-stained cell block sections, and immunostained slides) can become a very complex process, making routine high-volume digitization very challenging. In addition, in most cytology laboratories, many slides (e.g., smears) may not be barcoded, prohibiting their routine automated scanning.

Screening, Navigation, and Annotation Unlike surgical pathology cases, key target cells that need to be detected (e.g., carcinoma cells) in cytology specimens are often hidden among abundant normal cells or buried within background material. This is why each cytology slide needs to be carefully and entirely screened, and these targeted cells annotated (e.g., dotted). The screening process is usually performed by a cytotechnologist. However, screening digital slides using a computer mouse is tedious and time-consuming [20]. Keyboard-controlled navigation together with displaying a thumbnail image to confirm complete slide coverage has been reported to facilitate the screening process [21]. In addition, built-in tracking tools can be used to reassure screeners that they have screened all areas of a WSI. Several other methods such as trackballs, touch pads, gaming controls, and touchscreens have proven to facilitate navigating surgical pathology slides, but they have not been fully explored using digital cytology slides [22]. Many WSI viewers offer the ability to annotate images using different shapes and colors that can be leveraged similar to screener's dotting cells of interest on glass slides [21]. With WSI, additional functions can be added to annotation such as incorporating text (e.g., with specific morphologic features and interpretation). Also, one can opt to use hidden annotations that can be revealed later for education and proficiency test purposes.

Clinical Applications

Primary Diagnosis

WSI for primary diagnosis of surgical pathology has been adopted by several pathology labs [23–25]. The US Food and Drug Administration (FDA) also approved of the Philips IntelliSite Pathology Solution (PIPS) for primary diagnosis of "tissue slides" in 2017 [26]. However, making routine primary diagnoses for cytology cases using WSI has not been reported yet. Nevertheless, multiple studies have suggested that a WSI is indeed sufficient for cytologists to make reliable diagnostic decisions [27–30].

Secondary Diagnosis

Cytology cases are amenable to telecytology for second opinion consultation. Recent improvements in telepathology diagnostic concordance (accuracy) are linked to advancements in technology, better user training, and familiarity with such systems. Globally, the remote interpretation of digital images has the potential to provide effective screening and clinical triage for individuals in underserved populations [3, 31]. Telecytology for non-gynecologic cases using only cell blocks has been shown to be feasible and sufficient to provide a meaningful second opinion interpretation in many cytology cases [32]. Cell block-only consultations solve focus issues typically plagued by cytology whole slide imaging. Cell blocks also provide a valuable source of material for performing immunohistochemistry and are thus highly recommended for second opinion teleconsultation.

Rapid on-Site Evaluation (ROSE)

There is increased utilization of cytopathology to provide rapid on-site evaluation (ROSE) of fine-needle aspiration (FNA) and touch preparations of small biopsies. A well-executed ROSE procedure can significantly impact the diagnostic quality and appropriate specimen triage of procured biopsy materials. Given the demand to offer this service, many institutions employ some form of telecytology to facilitate ROSE. There are four modes of telecytology that could be used: static image capture system, live video steaming system, live/real-time robotic microscope, and WSI system [27, 28, 33]. Each of these systems has its advantages and disadvantages.

For static image capture systems, static (still) images are captured by means of a digital camera or smartphone and transmitted to a remote individual/site via e-mail or other methods. The advantage of this system is low cost, simple implementation, and maintenance. The disadvantages include inability to review the entire slide (i.e., relying on only select images to render a diagnosis) and the need to have an experienced cytologist on-site, and focusing is problematic with static images.

Live video streaming systems require a light microscope, mounted digital camera and compatible software such as the NetCam (Olympus), iMedHD2 (Remote

Medical Technologies), and CytoXpress (Spot Imaging) systems. Video streaming using smartphones (e.g., FaceTime) with an adapter attached to a microscope is feasible. These systems rely on streaming a high-definition image [34, 35]. Their advantage includes relatively low cost (relative to WSI), ability to review the entire slide, and interaction with the sender/driver in real time who can focus on cells/materials. The disadvantages include dependency on network connection, inability of the remote cytopathologists to control examining the slide themselves, and a need to have an experienced cytologist onsite.

Examples of live/real-time robotic microscope and WSI hybrid devices include the VisionTek (Sakura), LV1 (Leica), M8 (PreciPoint), SL5 (Mikroscan), and Glissando (Objective Imaging). Advantages of these systems include their ability to allow users to review the entire slide while controlling the examination process, ability to focus on all cells/materials, and no need for on-site cytology expertise. The disadvantage includes higher cost [36, 37]. WSI systems without hybrid live viewing capability are advantageous for similar reasons. They allow the entire slide to be reviewed and archived without the need for having on-site cytology expertise. However, the disadvantage of employing a WSI scanner for telecytology is its high cost, the fact that images may not be immediately available for review, and relying on Z-stacking for focus.

Currently, the most frequently used platforms for ROSE are live video streaming systems [38]. By comparison, hybrid live robotic/WSI scanners can alleviate the shortcoming of such "webcam"-type solutions by negating the need for an on-site person to "drive" the slide. All that is required is for an individual on-site to prepare a slide and insert it into the scanner. These hybrid devices have proven to be acceptable for frozen section telepathology including brain smears at many institutions [39] and more recently have also been explored as a telecytology solution for ROSE [37]. To the best of our knowledge, no literature has reported the utilization of non-hybrid WSI systems as a telecytology solution for ROSE. Our unpublished data supports single Z-stacked WSI as a feasible solution for ROSE. Once scanned, the entire slide of a WSI is immediately available for the cytopathologist to review. However, the disadvantage with this method is the time required to scan a slide, which can take up to 10 minutes for a conventional smear slide and even longer with Z-stacking [40]. Moreover, WSI generates large file size, which may warrant large network bandwidths for transmission. Thus, for these reasons, Z-stacked scanning is impractical to apply for ROSE [12, 33]. Some studies have also shown that Z-stacked images may have a negligible return in diagnostic yield [12]. In the near future, it is anticipated that advances dedicated to digital cytology slide scanning technology will help overcome some of these challenges [41].

Non-clinical Applications

Education

WSI has successfully replaced traditional classrooms equipped with microscopes in medical education at many institutions, including allied healthcare schools such as cytotechnology schools [42–45]. WSI virtual teaching sets can be accessed both inside and outside the classroom, whenever it is convenient for the student to do so, and WSIs can be easily annotated to facilitate instruction. In education, WSIs offer significant advantages over traditional glass slides. Digital slides are easier to share simultaneously with multiple users [46]. Cytology glass slides, except for cell block section recuts, are impossible to replicate or replace [47]. Several online education programs now offer WSIs, such as the International Academy of Cytology (IAC) [27, 31, 48]. More customized virtual cytology rotations for trainees can be similarly created by digitizing cytology slides [47, 49–54].

Proficiency Testing

Proficiency testing (PT) is an important component of a cytology quality assurance program. The Clinical Laboratory Improvement Amendments Act of 1988 (CLIA '88) requires cytopathologists and cytotechnologist to participate and pass an annual national PT test for gynecologic cytology. Currently, these national PT programs need a large number of well-vetted cytology glass slides and complex logistics to handle the administration of the test to thousands of laboratories dispersed in a large geographic area and manage the data collected from thousands of participants. Gynecologic cytology PTs are available from the College of American Pathologists (CAP) or American Society for Clinical Pathology (ASCP) [55, 56]. Ideally, all PT participants should be examined with same materials akin to those slides they are likely to encounter in routine clinical practice in order to fairly assess their diagnostic skills. This is almost impossible to guarantee with certain cytology specimens (e.g., direct smears, liquid-based preparations) because each cytology slide is likely to contain distinct diagnostic material, even from the same case. However, employing WSI can provide a solution to this challenge because digital slides can be replicated and/or made accessible to an unlimited number of PT participants. WSIs have accordingly been recommended for use in PT programs [48, 57]. So far, several studies have demonstrated that image-based testing was equivalent to using glass slides and hence feasible for PT in cytology [56, 58].

Quality Assurance

Quality assurance (QA) is an important part of cytopathology practice. Cytology QA includes intra-, inter-, and/or extra-departmental second review of select cases [59, 60]. Studies have revealed that discrepancy rates based on second review within the same institution may underestimate actual error rates because of potential biases, such as the reviewer often knowing the original diagnosis and/or the identity of the sign out pathologist [48, 61–63]. Nevertheless, it is attempting to try to establish a uniform level of quality across an entire institution, especially for large, multiple facility healthcare systems. However, one of the major challenges for establishing such a multi-facility QA program is the expense and difficulty managing and transferring slides between facilities. WSI may provide a solution to this challenge [28, 31, 56, 59, 64, 65]. If necessary, WSIs can hide all identifiable information (e.g., case number, sign out pathologist, original diagnosis, etc.) in order to avoid any potential bias.

Cytology Slide Archiving

WSI can be used for permanently archiving slides. This is more important for cytology slides than it is for surgical pathology slides since most cytology slides cannot be easily replaced if lost or damaged. Archived slides can be readily accessed when cytologists need to compare/review a patient's previous case and or perform cytological-histological correlation. An ideal opportunity to scan slides is when they are requested and/or received for outside institution or medicolegal consultation, in order to maintain a permanent digital record. On occasion, it may be necessary to scrape off cytology material from a glass slide in order to perform molecular testing. Before such a glass slide gets sacrificed, it is advisable to have it scanned and archived [66]. There are currently no official guidelines on how long digitized cytology slides should be stored.

Conclusion

WSI success in pathology has largely been dedicated to surgical pathology. However, WSI has the potential to also broaden its scope to cytopathology. This technology has been implemented and validated in several areas of cytology including ROSE, teleconsultation, proficiency testing, QA and education. For the purpose of remotely performing ROSE, several medical centers have opted to employ hybrid live robotic WSI devices to aid with real-time focusing. For teleconsultation work the use of only cell block sections has been advocated as a feasible solution in order to address focus issues. Several WSI vendors now offer technical solutions such as Z-stacking and alternate scanning protocols to produce high quality cytology digital slides. However, cytopathologists/cytotechnologists still need to become more proficient at using WSI for routine practice (e.g. screening slides). When cytology laboratories commit to finally going fully digital they will begin to reap some of the benefits of digital pathology such as workflow efficiency, workload balancing, easy sharing of images, and computational cytology (e.g. computer-assisted diagnosis).

References

1. Pantanowitz L, Sinard JH, Henricks WH, Fatheree LA, Carter AB, Contis L, et al. Validating whole slide imaging for diagnostic purposes in pathology: guideline from the College of American Pathologists Pathology and Laboratory Quality Center. Arch Pathol Lab Med. 2013;137(12):1710–22.

2. El-Garby EAPA, Pantanowitz L. Whole slide imaging: widening the scope of cytopathology. Diagn Histopathol. 2014;20:456–61.
3. Zhao C, Wu T, Ding X, Parwani AV, Chen H, McHugh J, et al. International telepathology consultation: Three years of experience between the University of Pittsburgh Medical Center and KingMed Diagnostics in China. J Pathol Inform. 2015;6:63.
4. Amin MPA, Pantanowitz L. In: PA P, editor. Digital imaging. New York: Springer; 2014.
5. Bauer TW, Schoenfield L, Slaw RJ, Yerian L, Sun Z, Henricks WH. Validation of whole slide imaging for primary diagnosis in surgical pathology. Arch Pathol Lab Med. 2013;137(4):518–24.
6. Snead DR, Tsang YW, Meskiri A, Kimani PK, Crossman R, Rajpoot NM, et al. Validation of digital pathology imaging for primary histopathological diagnosis. Histopathology. 2016;68(7):1063–72.
7. House JC, Henderson-Jackson EB, Johnson JO, Lloyd MC, Dhillon J, Ahmad N, et al. Diagnostic digital cytopathology: are we ready yet? J Pathol Inform. 2013;4:28.
8. Evered A, Dudding N. Accuracy and perceptions of virtual microscopy compared with glass slide microscopy in cervical cytology. Cytopathology. 2011;22(2):82–7.
9. Fan Y, Bradley AP. A method for quantitative analysis of clump thickness in cervical cytology slides. Micron (Oxford, England : 1993). 2016;80:73–82.
10. Pantanowitz L, Parwani AV, Khalbuss WE. Digital imaging for cytopathology: are we there yet? Cytopathology. 2011;22(2):73–4.
11. Donnelly AD, Mukherjee MS, Lyden ER, Bridge JA, Lele SM, Wright N, et al. Optimal z-axis scanning parameters for gynecologic cytology specimens. J Pathol Inform. 2013;4:38.
12. Wright AM, Smith D, Dhurandhar B, Fairley T, Scheiber-Pacht M, Chakraborty S, et al. Digital slide imaging in cervicovaginal cytology: a pilot study. Arch Pathol Lab Med. 2013;137(5):618–24.
13. Donnelly A, Mukherjee M, Schneider J, Lyden E, Lele S, McGaughey M, et al. Z-Axis scanning parameters: an investigation of consistency. J Am Soc Cytopathol. 2014;3(5):S79.
14. Goswami R, Pi D, Pal J, Cheng K. Hudoba De Badyn M. performance evaluation of a dynamic telepathology system (Panoptiq) in the morphologic assessment of peripheral blood film abnormalities. Int J Lab Hematol. 2015;37(3):365–71.
15. Pradhan D, Monaco SE, Parwani AV, Ahmed I, Duboy J, Pantanowitz L. Evaluation of panoramic digital images using Panoptiq for frozen section diagnosis. J Pathol Inform. 2016;7:26.
16. Hanna MG, Monaco SE, Cuda J, Xing J, Ahmed I, Pantanowitz L. Comparison of glass slides and various digital-slide modalities for cytopathology screening and interpretation. Cancer Cytopathol. 2017;125(9):701–9.
17. Groen R, Abe K, Yoon HS, Li Z, Shen R, Yoshikawa A, et al. Application of microscope-based scanning software (Panoptiq) for the interpretation of cervicovaginal cytology specimens. Cancer Cytopathol. 2017;125(12):918–25.
18. Tawfik O, Davis M, Dillon S, Tawfik L, Diaz FJ, Amin K, et al. Whole-slide imaging of pap cellblock preparations is a potentially valid screening method. Acta Cytol. 2015;59(2):187–200.
19. Sellaro T, Filkins R, Hoffman C, Fine J, Ho J, Parwani A, et al. Relationship between magnification and resolution in digital pathology systems. J Pathol Inform. 2013;4(1):21.
20. Pantanowitz L, Nayar R, Auger M, Schmitt F, Wasserman P, Wilbur DC, et al. Evaluation of the international academy of cytology (IAC) virtual slide library. J Pathol Inform. 2012;3:46.
21. Khalbuss WE, Cuda J, Cucoranu IC. Screening and dotting virtual slides: a new challenge for cytotechnologists. Cyto J. 2013;10:22.
22. Yagi Y, Yoshioka S, Kyusojin H, Onozato M, Mizutani Y, Osato K, et al. An ultra-high speed whole slide image viewing system. Stud Health Technol Inform. 2012;179:239–49.
23. Cheng CL, Azhar R, Sng SH, Chua YQ, Hwang JS, Chin JP, et al. Enabling digital pathology in the diagnostic setting: navigating through the implementation journey in an academic medical Centre. J Clin Pathol. 2016;69(9):784–92.
24. Stathonikos N, Veta M, Huisman A, van Diest PJ. Going fully digital: perspective of a Dutch academic pathology lab. J Pathol Inform. 2013;4:15.

25. Thorstenson S, Molin J, Lundstrom C. Implementation of large-scale routine diagnostics using whole slide imaging in Sweden: digital pathology experiences 2006-2013. J Pathol Inform. 2014;5(1):14.
26. Evans AJ, Bauer TW, Bui MM, Cornish TC, Duncan H, Glassy EF, et al. US Food and Drug Administration approval of whole slide imaging for primary diagnosis: a key milestone is reached and new questions are raised. Arch Pathol Lab Med. 2018;142(11):1383–7.
27. Wilbur DC, Madi K, Colvin RB, Duncan LM, Faquin WC, Ferry JA, et al. Whole-slide imaging digital pathology as a platform for teleconsultation: a pilot study using paired subspecialist correlations. Arch Pathol Lab Med. 2009;133(12):1949–53.
28. Lee ES, Kim IS, Choi JS, Yeom BW, Kim HK, Han JH, et al. Accuracy and reproducibility of telecytology diagnosis of cervical smears. A tool for quality assurance programs. Am J Clin Pathol. 2003;119(3):356–60.
29. Galvez J, Howell L, Costa MJ, Davis R. Diagnostic concordance of telecytology and conventional cytology for evaluating breast aspirates. Acta Cytol. 1998;42(3):663–7.
30. Hedvat CV. Digital microscopy: past, present, and future. Arch Pathol Lab Med. 2010;134(11):1666–70.
31. Pantanowitz L. Digital images and the future of digital pathology. J Pathol Inform. 2010;1:PMC2941968.
32. Mosquera-Zamudio A, Hanna M, Monaco S, Xing J, Harper T, Zhao C, et al. International telecytology feasibility using digitally scanned cell block slides. J Am Soc Cytopathol. 2017;6(5):S53.
33. Lin O. Telecytology for rapid on-site evaluation: current status. J Am Soc Cytopathol. 2018;7(1):1–6.
34. Agarwal S, Zhao L, Zhang R, Hassell L. FaceTime validation study: low-cost streaming video for cytology adequacy assessment. Cancer Cytopathol. 2016;124(3):213–20.
35. Alsharif M, Carlo-Demovich J, Massey C, Madory JE, Lewin D, Medina AM, et al. Telecytopathology for immediate evaluation of fine-needle aspiration specimens. Cancer Cytopathol. 2010;118(3):119–26.
36. Cai G, Teot LA, Khalbuss WE, Yu J, Monaco SE, Jukic DM, et al. Cytologic evaluation of image-guided fine needle aspiration biopsies via robotic microscopy: a validation study. J Pathol Inform. 2010;1:4.
37. Sirintrapun SJ, Rudomina D, Mazzella A, Feratovic R, Alago W, Siegelbaum R, et al. Robotic Telecytology for remote Cytologic evaluation without an on-site cytotechnologist or Cytopathologist: a tale of implementation and review of constraints. J Pathol Inform. 2017;8:32.
38. Steinberg DM, Ali SZ. Application of virtual microscopy in clinical cytopathology. Diagn Cytopathol. 2001;25(6):389–96.
39. Bauer TW, Slaw RJ, McKenney JK, Patil DT. Validation of whole slide imaging for frozen section diagnosis in surgical pathology. J Pathol Inform. 2015;6:49.
40. Rojo MG, Garcia GB, Mateos CP, Garcia JG, Vicente MC. Critical comparison of 31 commercially available digital slide systems in pathology. Int J Surg Pathol. 2006;14(4):285–305.
41. McKay RR, Baxi VA, Montalto MC. The accuracy of dynamic predictive autofocusing for whole slide imaging. J Pathol Inform. 2011;2:38.
42. Zwonitzer R, Hofmann H, Roessner A, Kalinski T. Virtual 3D microscopy in pathology education. Hum Pathol. 2010;41(3):457–8.
43. Romer DJ, Suster S. Use of virtual microscopy for didactic live-audience presentation in anatomic pathology. Ann Diagn Pathol. 2003;7(1):67–72.
44. Stewart J, Bevans-Wilkins K, Bhattacharya A, Ye C, Miyazaki K, Kurtycz DFI. Virtual microscopy: an educator's tool for the enhancement of cytotechnology students' locator skills. Diagn Cytopathol. 2008;36(6):363–8.
45. Saco A, Bombi JA, Garcia A, Ramirez J, Ordi J. Current status of whole-slide imaging in education. Pathobiology. 2016;83(2–3):79–88.
46. Dee FR. Virtual microscopy in pathology education. Hum Pathol. 2009;40(8):1112–21.

47. Fonyad L, Gerely L, Cserneky M, Molnar B, Matolcsy A. Shifting gears higher--digital slides in graduate education--4 years experience at Semmelweis University. Diagn Pathol. 2010;5:73.
48. Pantanowitz L, Hornish M, Goulart R. The impact of digital imaging in the field of cytopathology. Cyto J. 2009;6(1):6.
49. Foster K. Medical education in the digital age: digital whole slide imaging as an e-learning tool. J Pathol Inform. 2010;1:14.
50. Heidger PM Jr, Dee F, Consoer D, Leaven T, Duncan J, Kreiter C. Integrated approach to teaching and testing in histology with real and virtual imaging. Anat Rec. 2002;269(2):107–12.
51. Kang HP, Hagenkord JM, Monzon FA, Parwani AV. Residency training in pathology informatics: a virtual rotation solution. Am J Clin Pathol. 2009;132(3):404–8.
52. Li L, Dangott BJ, Parwani AV. Development and use of a genitourinary pathology digital teaching set for trainee education. J Pathol Inform. 2010;1:2.
53. Weinstein RS, Graham AR, Richter LC, Barker GP, Krupinski EA, Lopez AM, et al. Overview of telepathology, virtual microscopy, and whole slide imaging: prospects for the future. Hum Pathol. 2009;40(8):1057–69.
54. Daniel C, Garcia Rojo M, Bourquard K, Henin D, Schrader T, Della Mea V, et al. Standards to support information systems integration in anatomic pathology. Arch Pathol Lab Med. 2009;133(11):1841–9.
55. Eversole GM, Moriarty AT, Schwartz MR, Clayton AC, Souers R, Fatheree LA, et al. Practices of participants in the College of American Pathologists interlaboratory comparison program in cervicovaginal cytology, 2006. Arch Pathol Lab Med. 2010;134(3):331–5.
56. Gagnon M, Inhorn S, Hancock J, Keller B, Carpenter D, Merlin T, et al. Comparison of cytology proficiency testing: glass slides vs. virtual slides. Acta Cytol. 2004;48(6):788–94.
57. Wilbur DC, Black-Schaffer WS, Luff RD, Abraham KP, Kemper C, Molina JT, et al. The Becton Dickinson focal point GS imaging system: clinical trials demonstrate significantly improved sensitivity for the detection of important cervical lesions. Am J Clin Pathol. 2009;132(5):767–75.
58. Marchevsky AM, Khurana R, Thomas P, Scharre K, Farias P, Bose S. The use of virtual microscopy for proficiency testing in gynecologic cytopathology: a feasibility study using ScanScope. Arch Pathol Lab Med. 2006;130(3):349–55.
59. Kalinski T, Sel S, Hofmann H, Zwönitzer R, Bernarding J, Roessner A. Digital workflow management for quality assessment in pathology. Pathol Res Pract. 2008;204(1):17–21.
60. Allen KA. Evaluation methods for assessing cytotechnology students' screening skills. Diagn Cytopathol. 2000;23(1):66–8.
61. Raab SS, Nakhleh RE, Ruby SC. Patient safety in anatomic pathology: measuring discrepancy frequencies and causes. Arch Pathol Lab Med. 2005;129(4):459–66.
62. Stewart Iii J, Miyazaki K, Bevans-Wilkins K, Ye C, Kurtycz DFI, Selvaggi SM. Virtual microscopy for cytology proficiency testing: are we there yet? Cancer. 2007;111(4):203–9.
63. Marsan C. Quality control in cytopathology applied to screening for cervical carcinoma. Pol J Pathol. 1995;46(4):245–8.
64. Archondakis S, Georgoulakis J, Stamataki M, Anninos D, Skagias L, Panayiotides I, et al. Telecytology: a tool for quality assessment and improvement in the evaluation of thyroid fine-needle aspiration specimens. Telemed e-Health. 2009;15(7):713–7.
65. Marchevsky AM, Wan Y, Thomas P, Krishnan L, Evans-Simon H, Haber H. Virtual microscopy as a tool for proficiency testing in cytopathology: a model using multiple digital images of Papanicolaou tests. Arch Pathol Lab Med. 2003;127(10):1320–4.
66. Pantanowitz L. Leveraging digital pathology for molecular testing. Cancer Cytopathol. 2018;12:965–6.
67. El-Gabry EA, Parwani AV, Pantanowitz L. Whole-slide imaging: widening the scope of cytopathology. Diag Histopathol. 2014;20(12):456–61.

Whole Slide Imaging and Research Applications

Bryan Dangott

While clinical use of whole slide imaging is governed by medical device regulations, non-clinical uses have fewer constraints, and there is far more flexibility in this domain. As a result the newest technology in whole slide imaging may become available to research laboratories and investigators well before it is available in the clinic. For many years in the United States, there were no digital pathology scanners available that had been approved or cleared by the FDA. During this time, scanners were primarily used for education and research. This chapter will focus on the some of the research applications of whole slide imaging including advanced imaging methods, algorithmic research, and clinical/preclinical research.

Analog vs Digital

Some of the most notable benefits of whole slide imaging in the domain of research stem from the creation of a digital version of an analog slide. Inherent weaknesses of working with glass slides include fragility, stain degradation, cover slip separation, singular availability, and limitations of analog/manual interpretation methods. In contrast a digital scan of an analog slide allows long-term preservation without degradation, easy reproduction and sharing, and access to computational image analysis. For researchers, the ability to copy and share the exact same image and to analyze those images with computational methods allows improved experimental reproducibility. In contrast, glass slides using manual interpretation may face challenges in trying to obtain consistent results several years later due to slide degradation, breakage, loss, or variability in manual interpretation. Both inter- and intra-observer variability can impact interpretation and scoring of both glass and digital histology and immunohistochemistry studies. To address these sources of

B. Dangott (✉)
Mayo Clinic – Jacksonville, Department of Laboratory Medicine and Pathology, Jacksonville, FL, USA

A. V. Parwani (ed.), *Whole Slide Imaging*,
https://doi.org/10.1007/978-3-030-83332-9_11

variability, some experiments may benefit from a hybrid design where digital slides are interpreted by a manual reader in combination with computational methods. This design may allow cohorts to be compared over time using both a manual interpretation which is the current standard of care and an algorithmic approach to provide a thread of consistency between cohorts. Use of computational methods allows the same algorithms to be applied to samples acquired at different time points. The algorithmic approach allows a somewhat objective and quantitative measure over long time frames which may be difficult with manual methods due to changes in personnel or due to variability inherent in manual methods.

Researchers new to digital pathology may wonder about the reliability of using digital slides to perform interpretations when glass slides have been the de facto standard for primary diagnosis for so long. It may help to know that some scanners have been approved for primary diagnosis in major regulatory environments including CE mark since 2012 [1] and the FDA since 2017 [2]. In addition, whole slide scanners have been used for manual reads of a digital slide for immunohistochemistry for several years prior to the primary diagnosis approvals. There are even IVD-approved quantitative algorithms for specific biomarkers which predate the primary diagnosis approvals. In general, whole slide scanners can be qualified for a particular study by performing a glass vs digital study to establish performance expectations. The validation studies submitted for primary diagnosis regulatory approvals in the United States compared the diagnosis between glass and whole slide images. Since there are many histologic features which contribute to a diagnosis, there are some studies which examine the comparability of the microscopic features between glass and digital. The FDA has conducted long-term research studies using a platform called eeDAP (evaluation environment for digital and analog pathology). In the eeDAP studies, regions of interest (ROIs) are evaluated by trained pathologists on both glass and whole slide images. The pathologists perform paired evaluations for predefined parameters of both digital and glass ROIs which may include morphologic features of individual cells. By using predefined parameters and well-defined ROIs, the study aims to eliminate variability by standardizing terminology and fields of view [3]. By performing correlations between digital and glass on features instead of diagnosis, this platform can provide a more granular comparison and may help identify subtle differences between digital and glass. This research may also help in defining the resolution requirements for whole slide images and may contribute to greater acceptance of digital pathology by regulatory agencies.

Manual Methods

Manual stain evaluation involves visual examination of various staining characteristics which may include intensity, specificity, cellular localization, population of interest, and spatial relationships. Intensity is a measure of the amount of chromogen bound to the cells. Using HER-2 as an example, the intensity has a range which includes scores of 0, 1+, 2+, and 3+. Specificity is a measure of how well the stain avoids precipitation on non-target tissue. Sensitivity is a measure of how well the stain detects expression of a target when it is present. Using the HER-2 example, high specificity would mean there is no staining in non-target tissue such as lymphocytes or stroma while high sensitivity would mean expression of HER-2 is detected in tissues which are known to have low levels of HER-2 expression. Cellular localization is a representation of where the marker of interest is demonstrated in the cell. This could be discretely nuclear, membranous, or cytoplasmic localization. Some biomarkers demonstrate staining in multiple compartments. Understanding the cellular localization is useful when studying therapeutic targets in that a membranous marker will have different physiologic and delivery considerations than a nuclear marker which may need intracellular transport. One issue to note here is that histology sections are comprised of slices of tissue and thus cells are cut leaving nuclei exposed and readily accessible for stains. This is in contrast to whole cells in vivo or whole cells in flow cytometry in which the nuclei are relatively protected from the outside environment and thus not as available for studying biologic markers without using special techniques. This distinction can account for differences in performance of the same biomarker in flow cytometry vs histology. For example, in flow cytometry, the cell must be permeabilized to study markers like TdT which are localized to the nucleus by IHC.

It is important to define the cells of interest when investigating a new biomarker and establishing new scoring criteria. A percentage positive score should define whether the percentage represents the subset of positive tumor cells or the subset of positive total cells which may include tumor, stroma, inflammatory cells, and normal epithelium. In oncology, the population of interest is most frequently confined to the tumor being studied. However, there are also applications in fields such as immuno-oncology where the non-tumor inflammatory infiltrate is also of interest. Some markers will only highlight tumor while others will only highlight a component of the inflammatory cells. There are also biomarkers such as PD-L1 which integrate both tumor and mononuclear inflammatory cells in the scoring paradigm. Spatial relationships between the tumor and inflammatory infiltrate may also be important in immuno-oncology. Assessing spatial relationships is a difficult if not impossible task using glass slides. Digital pathology can evaluate spatial relationship by using slide annotation and measurement tools. In addition, algorithms can be used to make assessments of positivity within a boundary, radius, or annotation. Algorithms become especially useful when quantifying a mix of biomarkers and spatial relationships. Techniques to study multiple populations and spatial relationships will be discussed below.

Clinical and Research Applications for Biomarkers

Researching complex biological interactions will often require multiple biomarkers. In the clinical setting, multiple biomarkers are often used diagnostically for characterizing tumors. For example, a Hodgkin lymphoma case may be evaluated by integrating the morphology with the pattern of staining using a mix of biomarkers such as CD20, CD15, CD30, and PAX5. The right panel of biomarkers can generate incredibly important and often required information to contribute to a diagnosis. Phenotypic patterns also have therapeutic implications in the right clinical context. For example, antibody analogs of CD20 may be used in the treatment of CD20-positive tumors such as mature B-cell lymphomas. In diagnostic evaluations, immunohistochemistry (IHC) studies are traditionally performed using a single section for each antibody. In the research setting, the simultaneous application of several antibodies may be of value to visualize and understand the complex interactions of tumor with adjacent inflammatory cells. This technique is known as multiplexing.

Multiplexing Techniques

Researchers may want to visualize the cellular expression profiles of tumor, normal epithelium, inflammatory cells, and stroma to characterize the infiltrating border of a tumor. While this can be done on individual slides, researchers may find greater utility in the information gained by running the biomarkers simultaneously. This can be helpful for understanding co-expression of some biomarkers and for identifying cell phenotypes in immuno-oncology. The research setting allows some flexibility in running biomarkers simultaneously which is important since there are very few multiplexing assays labeled for IVD clinical use. In addition, there may be experimental design considerations for multiplexing driven by limited tissue availability. It is important to understand both the drivers and expectations for data points from multiplexing assays before establishing the components of the multiplexed panel. A thorough understanding of the experimental design and the available techniques can help guide the experiment and deliver better results.

Techniques to study multiple biomarkers include serial sectioning, colorimetric multiplexing, fluorescence multiplexing, and sequential staining [4]. Serial sectioning is analogous to the diagnostic setting where individual biomarkers are applied individually to serial slides. The data from serial sections may be integrated manually or digitally. However, due to slight tissue variations between sections, the ability to assess co-expression can be limited. Additional artifacts such as tissue folds or tissue drop out may also be introduced in the production of serial sections. Colorimetric multiplexing includes using two or more biomarkers on the same slide. With immunohistochemistry this can be done by using different chromogens. While brown is traditionally used in singleplex studies, additional chromogens may include green, red, and blue. This technique is limited by the ability to visually separate colors in close proximity. It works best with a limited number of markers that are separated by cell type or cellular compartment. For example, tumor and stroma may have distinct biomarker expression profiles which helps geographically separate the biomarkers on the slide. This technique can add processing time and complexity to the assay. In some settings multiplexed IHC can be combined with multiplexed fluorescence to expand the number of markers that can be used [5]. An alternative way to achieve multiple biomarkers on the same slide is via sequential staining [6]. This technique involves repeated cycles of staining with an antibody, slide imaging, and biomarker removal. The resulting whole slide images comprise a library of biomarker signals from the same section of tissue.

Immunofluorescence

To address some of the limitations of multiplexing with immunohistochemistry, a fluorescence multiplexing approach may be used. Antibodies tied to different color fluorophores can be separated by using a combination of tuned light sources, fluorophores with distinct excitation and emission spectra, and filters [4]. The ability to separate signals allows cleaner attribution to a specific biomarker which can be challenging with colorimetric methods. Signal separation also allows better evaluation of biomarker co-expression. Fluorescence scopes equipped with photomultiplier tubes may also provide a quantitative measure of emitted light for each channel. All of these features contribute to a greater ability to perform more meaningful spatial analysis with fluorescence compared to colorimetric methods. A potential disadvantage of using fluorescence is that prolonged viewing can diminish the signal. This disadvantage can be mitigated with fluorescence whole slide scanning to create a digital archive.

Other Techniques

Other imaging techniques may allow sub-compartmentalization and focused analysis of tissue. There are several relevant applications of performing sub-compartment analysis which are highlighted in Table 1. If a research team is interested in

Table 1 Potential applications of sub-compartment analysis

Cell population profiling (Discrete cell molecular profiling applies to LCM)	Hodgkin lymphoma T-cell-rich large B-cell lymphoma Erythroid precursors Megakaryocytes Micrometastases Mitoses Plasma cells Angioimmunoblastic T-cell lymphoma Immune/inflammatory cell profiling
Architectural	Tumor profile mapping Central vs leading edge Necrotic vs viable Primary tumor vs metastatic Tumor bud analysis Tumor micro-environment Tumor vs normal Intratumoral vs peritumoral lymphocytes Angiogenesis Desmoplasia vs uninvolved stroma Dysplasia vs tumor Reactive/hyperplastic change vs neoplasia
Therapeutic monitoring	Treated vs untreated Time point studies

comparing the molecular profiles of tissue sub-compartments, one technique to consider includes laser capture microdissection (LCM). This technology allows the physical separation of tissue from a glass slide using a laser. A whole slide image of the slide can be obtained prior to LCM to maintain a record of the original histology. The regions for dissection can be manually annotated, and some techniques allow the DAB precipitate from immunohistochemistry to enhance the cell selection process through selective heating [7]. After the laser isolates the tissue of interest, the tissue can be removed from the slide and collected into a microtainer for further research. This process allows enrichment of the cells of interest, and even individual cells can be collected and sent for molecular profiling if so desired. Following LCM, the original slide can be re-scanned to show where the tissue was removed. By comparing the digital slides prior to LCM and after LCM, the histology of the tissue extracted from the slide can be isolated [7]. This is a powerful combination in that the histology that contributed to the molecular profile can be examined with machine learning techniques. Using these techniques, libraries of digital histology can be built which are correlated with molecular signatures. Machine learning techniques have been used to establish correlations between histologic features and survival outcomes. Features such as nuclear shape, texture, density of tumor infiltrating lymphocytes, stromal features, mitotic figures, glandular morphology, and epithelial features have been used in various studies to predict tumor behavior [8]. It should be noted that this machine learning correlation between histology and molecular profiles can be performed without microdissection. In addition, microdissection can be performed using manual dissection of glass slides. However, manual techniques are less precise, are more time-consuming, and may have more difficulty isolating the exact cells of interest.

Other techniques have been developed which expand on the concept of isolating tissue sub-compartments. One technology which allows multiple probes to be studied was developed by NanoString. The technique is called Digital Spatial Profiling and uses a platform called GeoMx™ [9]. The platform performs a scan of the tissue while also allowing the tissue to be investigated with multiple antibody or RNA probes. These probes are specially designed to be linked to a secondary oligonucleotide probe which acts as a unique identifier/bar code that can be quantified in subsequent steps. One of the keys to this technology is that the linker between the primary probe and the secondary oligonucleotide probe is sensitive to UV light. This allows the planned and controlled dissociation of the primary probe and the secondary oligonucleotide probe when exposed to UV light. This is roughly analogous to LCM in that regions of interest are determined via software which guides the UV light. There is an important difference in that GeoMx™ platform leaves the tissue intact and only separates the oligonucleotide bar codes from the slide. These oligos are then quantitatively processed on the NanoString nCounter® platform. One big advantage of this system is that the process is not destructive and leaves the tissue intact for further study. It also allows quantitative multiplexing of antibody and RNA probes. A potential disadvantage is that the NanoString system may not allow as much flexibility as LCM in ROI selection or number.

Tissue Microarrays (TMAs)

Acquiring appropriate tissue for study is one of the challenges with performing medical research. In some cases, tissue blocks can be acquired from commercial vendors for specific disease indications. Medical centers may also have tissue banks which may be able to supply tissues for academic and commercial research. It is important to identify tissues which represent the spectrum of clinical presentations which are seen in the disease state being investigated. Normal tissues and negative control tissues should also be included in study design. Additional questions for study design may be seen in Table 2. While TMAs are remarkably efficient for studying the staining characteristics of small regions of tissue, they are often difficult to navigate on glass. A tissue microarray is organized via a coordinate system generally using a grid of letters and numbers which contributes to glass navigation challenges. Other limitations encountered with glass TMAs may include fatigue due to the volume of sections on one slide and constraints on performing slide-to-slide comparisons.

In some studies it may be appropriate to consider using TMAs instead of, or in addition to, whole slide sections of tissue. In the clinical setting, whole sections are used to allow morphologic examination of tissue for pleomorphism, mitotic activity, calcification, lymphovascular invasion, neural invasion, necrosis, desmoplasia, margins, and architecture. In clinical practice, whole sections are essential for clinical diagnosis, grading, and classification. In the research setting, TMAs may be constructed to focus on specific tumor types or regions of tissue. One TMA block can be constructed to represent dozens or even hundreds of samples. In some cases, discrete TMA cores from different patients can be considered individual samples for validation studies. This property can contribute to efficiency in biomarker development and clinical trial studies. It is common for TMAs to contain multiple cores from each sample to help address heterogeneity, sampling error, and defects which occur during histologic sectioning. TMAs can be used for H&E, IHC, FISH, CISH, and RNA and DNA studies. This allows cost savings in that it is cheaper to acquire one TMA slide/block than dozens or hundreds of whole section slides/blocks. In addition, there is less labor involved in cutting one block, and the reagent expense for running biomarker investigations is reduced. There is also increased control and consistency in the protocol in that after TMA creation, each core on the TMA slide is exposed to the same temperature, pH, storage conditions, reagents, and protocols.

Table 2 Questions to explore during study design

What types of tissue should be included?
How many samples are needed?
What sample types are needed? Paraffin section, fresh, fine needle, core biopsy
What studies need to be performed? H&E, FISH, IHC, flow, molecular analysis, fluorescence, microdissection
How is performance determined? Specificity, sensitivity, accuracy, reproducibility
What methods are currently considered the reference standard?
What is the budget?
Are there plans to transfer the research to a clinical setting?
What regulatory pathways need to be navigated?

TMAs may not work as well if there is a lot of heterogeneity in the tissues being investigated or if the results are dependent on evaluation of large regions of tissue architecture. For these reasons, it is important to consider the advantages and disadvantages of TMAs during the experimental design.

TMA construction is traditionally a manual process using glass slides and paraffin blocks. As the glass slides of whole tissue sections are reviewed, a mark is made on the slide which allows the TMA technician to extract a core of tissue from the paraffin block roughly corresponding to the spot marked on the slide. This process is time-consuming, requires specialized tools and skills, and may be prone to imprecision in the tissue extracted from the block. The size of the TMA core can be adjusted slightly (roughly 0.6 mm^2 to 2.0 mm^2) based on the needs of the study. More recently digital pathology has been used in conjunction with automation of specialized TMA hardware for high-throughput TMA creation. The Institute of Pathology at the University of Bern has established a next-generation tissue microarray protocol (ngTMA) which integrates digital pathology images with the creation of TMAs [10]. Using this method the digital slides can be annotated with predefined tools which create circles of different colors which correspond to different tissue types for the TMA. An automated punch then uses the coordinates from the annotations to retrieve precise core samples from the original block to construct the TMA. This allows high-throughput TMA creation.

Digital pathology also excels for review of TMA histology, and there are many advantages over glass when using digital pathology for review of TMAs. Some of these advantages are highlighted in Table 3. In most cases, digital pathology is

Table 3 Comparison of glass TMAs vs WSI TMAs

Task	Conventional glass	Digital whole slide
Core location/ identification	Manual switching magnification, refocusing, and navigation on glass can be slow. Any disruption may require repositioning and confirmation of location which contributes to fatigue	Fast switching between low and high power without refocusing. Low-power thumbnail image confirms location even at full magnification
Interpretation	Glass has historically been the standard method of interpretation	Roughly equivalent to glass and adequate for most biomarker research
Antibody/stain comparison	Very difficult to perform direct comparison due to navigation constraints of glass. Only one glass slide can be viewed at time	Side-by-side comparison is possible which makes direct comparison possible
Throughput	Manual requires dedicated blocks of time to move through the TMA to maintain coordinates of the core of interest	Viewing two or more slides side by side allows the rapid parallel interpretation of all markers of interest for each core. Core coordinates are easily confirmed and synced across slides
Digital processing	Not available	Each TMA core can be automatically detected, digitally extracted, and organized into a library to correlate with other studies. Virtual TMAs may be constructed from serial sections to integrate cores from several slides into a single display [11]

preferable to glass when performing high-volume TMA review. In the optimal scenario, multiple digital slides from TMAs can be linked, navigated, and reviewed simultaneously. Possibilities may include simultaneous review of H&E, negative control, and several antibodies. Alternatively during protocol development, each protocol can be compared side by side to evaluate relative performance. This approach markedly increases throughput and allows relative interpretations of intensity and specificity across slides which is simply not practical with glass slide review.

TMAs may also be used to develop control slides. These TMAs can be used for proficiency testing and inter-lab comparability studies for IHC and other assays. One property of TMAs cores is that the tissue region in each core is very focused and thus the each section will closely approximate adjacent sections. This can be used in digital pathology to establish performance of assays across batches or across days. It may even be possible to deliver a digital TMA as part of proficiency testing to evaluate consistency of scoring across readers.

Summary

Research applications of whole slide imaging are plentiful, and this chapter highlights a few of the most common scenarios. The benefits of digital pathology in research are facilitated by the electronic nature of the medium and the relaxed regulatory environment compared to the diagnostic setting. Creative uses of whole slide imaging will continue to evolve, and this is one of the most interesting and exciting areas of pathology and medical research.

References

1. https://www.selectscience.net/product-news/aperio-scanscope-systems-ce-marked-as-a-primary-in-vitro-diagnostic-aid/?artID=25313. Accessed 09/07/2021.
2. https://www.fda.gov/news-events/press-announcements/fda-allows-marketing-first-whole-slide-imaging-system-digital-pathology. Accessed 09/07/2021.
3. Gallas B, Cheng W, Gavrielides M, Ivansky A, Keay T, Wunderlich A, Hipp J, Hewitt S. eeDAP: an evaluation environment for digital and analog pathology. Proceedings of SPIE, 9037, 903709-903709-12; 2014.
4. Himmel LE, Hackett TA, Moore JL, Adams WR, Thomas G, Novitskaya T, Caprioli RM, Zijlstra A, Mahadevan-Jansen A, Boyd KL. Beyond the H&E: advanced technologies for in situ tissue biomarker imaging. ILAR J. 2018;59(1):51–65.
5. Blom S, Paavolainen L, Bychkov D, et al. Systems pathology by multiplexed immunohistochemistry and whole-slide digital image analysis. Sci Rep. 2017;7(1):15580. Published 2017 Nov 14. https://doi.org/10.1038/s41598-017-15798-4.
6. Bolognesi MM, Manzoni M, Scalia CR, et al. Multiplex staining by sequential immunostaining and antibody removal on routine tissue sections. J Histochem Cytochem. 2017;65(8):431–44. https://doi.org/10.1369/0022155417719419.
7. Grafen M, Hofmann TR, Scheel AH, et al. Optimized expression-based microdissection of formalin-fixed lung cancer tissue. Lab Invest. 2017;97(7):863–72. https://doi.org/10.1038/labinvest.2017.31.

8. Bera K, Schalper KA, Rimm DL, Velcheti V, Madabhushi A. Artificial intelligence in digital pathology - new tools for diagnosis and precision oncology. Nat Rev Clin Oncol. 2019;16(11):703–15. https://doi.org/10.1038/s41571-019-0252-y.
9. Gupta S, Zugazagoitia J, Martinez-Morilla S, Fuhrman K, Rimm DL. Digital quantitative assessment of PD-L1 using digital spatial profiling. Lab Invest. 2020;100(10):1311–7. https://doi.org/10.1038/s41374-020-0424-5
10. Zlobec I, Suter G, Perren A, Lugli A. A next-generation tissue microarray (ngTMA) protocol for biomarker studies. J Vis Exp. 2014;(91):51893. Published 2014 Sep 23. https://doi.org/10.3791/51893.
11. Quintayo M, Starczynski J, Yan F, Wedad H, Nofech-Mozes S, Rakovitch E, Bartlett J. Virtual tissue microarrays: a novel and viable approach to optimizing tissue microarrays for biomarker research applied to ductal carcinoma in situ. Histopathology. 2014;65(1):2–8.

Whole Slide Image Analysis

Bryan Dangott

Whole slide imaging is a technology that has seen adoption in pathology education and research over the past few decades. Image analysis in these settings has allowed for development and exploratory uses for quantitative biomarker applications. The use of whole slide scanners and image analysis for diagnostic purposes has been limited until relatively recently for various reasons. One of the main barriers to using image analysis clinically is the adoption rate for fully digital workflows in pathology which has hinged on regulatory approvals. Primary diagnosis for digital pathology was first approved in Europe in June 2012 [1] with the first FDA approval of digital pathology in the United States in April of 2017 [2]. These approvals are essential for allowing companies to market these devices for clinical use and for allowing laboratories to use them diagnostically. As these technologies are more broadly implemented for primary diagnosis, workflow changes will facilitate greater use of image analysis. Currently most institutions in the United States are still using glass slides as their primary method of diagnosis. This means extra steps are required to scan a glass slide prior to running any image analysis algorithms. These steps take time, equipment, software, and personnel which combined may overshadow the interest and benefit in running algorithms. However, with fully digital workflows, these elements are already in place, and the barrier to using algorithms is much lower. In fact, some algorithms may even be performed automatically or routinely as part of the workflow while others are performed on demand.

Beginning in early 2020, the world experienced a pandemic of coronavirus disease (COVID-19) which challenged established paradigms in many industries. In response to the pandemic, companies, organizations, and governments enacted policies to reduce the transmission and spread of the virus. Many of these policies encouraged or required remote work where possible. For pathologists in the United States, a temporary CMS waiver was issued in March of 2020 which relaxed the

B. Dangott (✉)
Mayo Clinic – Jacksonville, Department of Laboratory Medicine and Pathology, Jacksonville, FL, USA

A. V. Parwani (ed.), *Whole Slide Imaging*,
https://doi.org/10.1007/978-3-030-83332-9_12

requirements for use of digital pathology hardware and for remote sign out [3]. Prior to this waiver, it was not possible in the United States to perform diagnostic sign out at home without a CLIA license for that address. While use of digital pathology in other parts of the world had already been established for several years, the conditions and policies developed in response to COVID-19 also created an environment where adoption and use of digital pathology were widely encouraged for diagnostic use. With many institutions delving into digital pathology in response to COVID-19, this represents the first large-scale clinical test of digital pathology in the United States. Hopefully, some of the lessons gained from this temporary waiver will lead to permanent and lasting improvements in how pathology is practiced and how digital pathology is used.

Regulatory

The regulatory approval of whole slide images for primary diagnosis will expand the use of digital pathology and also increase opportunities to use image analysis. However, there are separate regulatory requirements around using image analysis in a clinical setting. The College of American Pathologists (CAP) has several items in the 2018 Anatomic Pathology Checklist regarding use of image analysis [4]. Factors to consider include performance verification/validation, scanner calibration, control tissues/calibration, quality control reviews, selecting regions for analysis, and annotations. A big component of successful image analysis implementation is having very good quality control processes around the inputs. Table 1 highlights factors that may impact tissue staining. For pathology, image analysis input actually starts in the operating room when the specimen is removed from the body. Cold ischemia time, fixation time/quality, gross room processing, tissue processor programs, sectioning, histology processing, and staining all impact the quality of the slide. At best, the scanner can only yield output as good as the input slide. Usually there is some anticipated degradation of the image between glass and digital. The final digital image is dependent on illumination, the optical pathway, scan magnification, and file compression techniques. Table 2 summarizes some of the factors which may impact the digital image. Because of these factors, there is some variability inherent in digital images produced by different scanners. Figure 1 shows the same glass slide scanned across various different commercially available scanners. There are differences in color, detail, and sharpness which will impact some image analysis techniques.

There are a lot of variables inherent in tissue processing and slide scanning that make it challenging to produce an algorithm that performs reliably across many different labs. Even algorithms which have been cleared by the FDA need to be verified within the lab prior to implementation. Commercial algorithms that have been submitted to the FDA generally specify the antibody clone, staining hardware, and scanning hardware. In order to implement the algorithm according to the manufacturer label, the elements described in the package insert need to be preserved. In other words, the antibody clone, staining platform, scanner hardware, and algorithm

Table 1 Factors that may impact staining

Tissue factors which may impact staining
Biologic heterogeneity
Fixation quality
Necrosis
Blood or hemorrhage (nonspecific staining)
Inflammatory infiltrate (nonspecific staining)
Preparation type (cytology cell block, tissue section, core/fine needle biopsy)
Edge artifact
Crush artifact
Sampling bias
Slide preparation factors which may impact staining
Antigen retrieval
Antibody selection
Use of blocking agents
Chromagen selection, multi-chromagen protocols
Lot-to-lot or day-to-day variability in reagents
Microfluidics of stain platform (covertiles, tissue folds, large sections which interfere with the edge of the slide, viscosity)
Environmental factors (temperature, humidity, atmospheric pressure)
Floaters
Slide drying, tissue lifting, or deparaffinization variability
Personnel performing procedure
Hardware platform variability
Age of paraffin section (oxidation)
Section thickness
Tissue folds
Decalcification

Table 2 Imaging system factors which may impact the digital image

Light source (LED, halogen, environmental light interference)
Calibration of imaging system (white balance, illumination, color, focus, tissue detection)
Optical pathway (alignment, lens defects, lens aberration, lens contamination)
Magnification of scan, depth of field (Z-stack)
Hardware platform variability
File compression/file type (lossy or lossless)
Vibration during scan
Stitching/tiling artifact

specified in the FDA submission must match what the lab does in practice. If any of these elements are different, then it would be considered off-label use. In this context, a lab can still perform image analysis as a lab developed test (LDT); however, an internal validation must be performed. These requirements narrow the potential market size for a specific algorithm considerably. The vendors which produce antibodies, staining platforms, and whole slide scanners are in the best position to

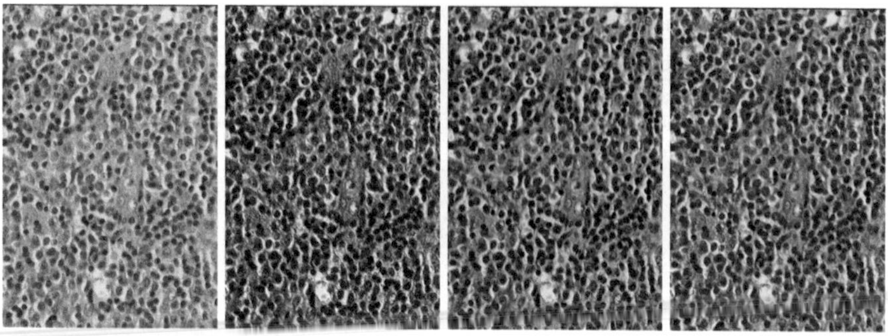

Fig. 1 The same glass slide scanned across various different commercially available scanners. There are differences in color, detail, and sharpness which will impact some image analysis techniques

market algorithms for clinical use. The implementation of these algorithms may be more streamlined if the lab already has the antibodies and specified hardware. To understand why, it is important to distinguish assay verification from assay validation. Verification applies to commercially available in vitro diagnostic tests (IVD). Verification means the laboratory has followed the package insert instructions and confirmed the assay performs according to vendor specifications. Validation applies to lab-developed tests. The validation documentation is more rigorous, requiring the laboratory to confirm that the assay performs according to the predetermined performance criteria and is safe and effective for its intended use.

WSI Scanner as a Medical Device

Slide scanners are medical devices which produce a digital image that is used by pathologists to render a diagnosis. The performance of the scanner is highly dependent on the mechanical and optical design. A single scanner needs to be able to produce high-quality scans consistently. The same slide should produce similar scans on different scanners of the same model and on the same scanner on repeated scans which is a measure of precision. In contrast, accuracy represents how well the device represents the color, clarity, and microscopic details present in the glass slide. Another way to think about precision and accuracy is that precision is a measure of repeatability while accuracy is a measure of how well the image represents ground truth. Currently there is no standard definition for ground truth in a whole slide image. For regulatory purposes accuracy has been measured by how well the diagnoses from digital images correlate with diagnoses performed on the same glass slide with a traditional microscope. A predefined standard that could be used commercially would be helpful to the industry. The standard would ultimately need to be able to quantify microscopic details which serve as proxy for resolving diagnostic features in tissue (nucleoli, nuclear grooves, mitotic figures). There is also a need to measure autofocus capabilities since tissue folds and undulations are part of

Table 3 Potential areas for WSI benchmarking

Accuracy	Metric	Utility
Color	Standardized metric of color reproduction	May also be used to perform white balance or tune color output across scanners and across runs
Fine detail resolution	Standardized metric of resolution performance	May be used to benchmark scanner performance or indicate need for maintenance
Autofocus	Standardized metric of focal plane optimization	May be used to benchmark scanner performance or indicate need for maintenance
Tissue detection	Standardized metric to detect faintly stained or small pieces of tissue	May be used to benchmark scanner performance or indicate need for maintenance

routine slide preparation. In addition, basic tissue detection may be an important performance metric. Standardized color slides have been used in a research setting to improve color reproduction between scanners [5]. Table 3 highlights some of the potential areas for slide scanner benchmarking. Development of these metrics may allow performance comparison among different vendors and may also make it easier to demonstrate devices are substantially equivalent from the perspective of regulatory agencies.

A few other major considerations in production use of digital pathology include scanner robustness and usability. Scanners need to be available for production use with minimal downtime and a low maintenance burden. In addition, a scanner that can automatically detect the area of interest and determine focus points would be more appealing for production use than a scanner that requires manual intervention to determine these parameters.

Economics

WSI scanners may vary widely in cost and features. Some desktop models may be available for under 25K while larger scanners integrated with slide storage servers, service contracts, and infrastructure can exceed 300K. Most institutions are going to need multiple scanners to accommodate the daily volume of slides and to build in redundancy for potential machine downtime. Image analysis packages also have a wide range of features and costs which may range from zero cost for open-source solutions such as ImageJ/Fiji and QuPath to several thousand dollars per year for some commercial solutions. One of the larger image analysis use cases is seen in quantitative immunohistochemistry. In 2020 the CPT code for a semi-quantitative/ quantitative immunohistochemistry manual read is 88360 and 88361 for a read using computational approaches [6]. The expected CMS reimbursement rates for 2020 are shown in Table 4. Considering the extra costs of hardware, software, storage, service contracts, personnel, and time to run computational image analysis,

Table 4 Reimbursement for semi-quantitative/quantitative IHC [6]

CPT code	Description	Technical	Professional	Total
88360	Quantitative IHC – manual	83.37	44.03	127.40
88361	Quantitative IHC – computational	82.65	46.56	129.21
IHC differential		−0.72	2.53	1.81

the economics require extremely high volume to even approach break-even numbers. For those using open-source or zero-cost software, the break-even calculation should also include the time spent to develop, modify, and validate/verify algorithms.

Digital Images Dissected

Every digital image is comprised of pixels. The term pixel is a hybrid of the terms picture (pix) and element (el) [7]. To gain a firm understanding of digital images and to really understand image analysis, further consideration of pixels is essential. The term pixel is often used interchangeably to describe characteristics of the image capture device, the digital file, and the physical display. In each of these situations, a pixel represents two parameters in the construction of an image: the coordinates and the color. The coordinate metric is the physical location of the pixel in a plane as determined by horizontal and vertical values. Color in digital images can be represented by several color spaces which include RGB, CMYK, CIE Lab, HSV, etc. [8, 9]. Work in different color spaces can be achieved by converting the image to the desired color space. For example, an RGB image can be converted to CIE Lab. Segregation of color components can also be achieved with color deconvolution. For the purposes of this chapter, examples will be described within the RGB space (red, green, blue) since it is the most common color space and conceptually easy to understand. Table 3 contains sample colors and component values for the RGB color space.

RGB Space

The RGB characteristics of a pixel describe the amount of red, green, and blue which are mixed together to represent one color. The scale for RGB space in computer terms is 0–255 for each channel: red, green, blue. In an electronic display, each pixel is composed of one red, one green, and one blue diode. Based on different intensities of each diode, different color combinations can be achieved. The value of 0 represents the minimum value or no color for that channel while 255 represents maximum color for that channel. Using these parameters basic colors can be defined as in Table 5 and Fig. 2.

Table 5 Example pixel values in RGB color space

Pixel color	Red value R	Green value G	Blue value B
White	255	255	255
Gray	122	122	122
Black	0	0	0
Red	255	0	0
Green	0	255	0
Blue	0	0	255
Yellow	255	255	0
Purple	255	0	255
Cyan	0	255	255

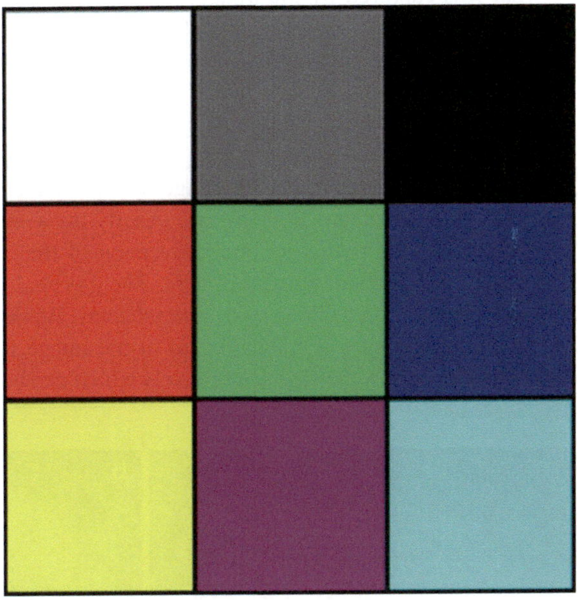

Fig. 2 Colors corresponding to Table 5

Pixels in Digital Detectors

Images are somewhat dependent on the properties of the camera which captured the image. For the purposes of discussion, an image sensor is either a charge-coupled device (CCD) or a complementary metal oxide semiconductor (CMOS) which converts light into a digital signal. The image sensor is composed of millions of photo diodes. The photo diodes convert light to a digital signal that can be processed and stored as a file for later display on a monitor. For instance, a 20 megapixel camera would have about 20 million photo diodes/pixels available to capture an image. A common microscopy camera has a CMOS sensor with 5760 × 3600 pixels/photo detectors on the chip. This totals about 20.7 million pixels with each pixel representing a 5.86 micron square in physical space [10]. While the concept is similar, this camera may differ in performance characteristics from a camera used in a whole slide scanner. In addition to the width and height properties present in the detector array, various detectors have different sensitivities to light conditions and speed of capture. One may gain additional understanding of the use of CCDs in microscopy by referencing the tutorial provided by Nikon at microscopyu.com [11].

Pixels in Digital Files

Digital pixels are the building blocks of digital images. Digital images are an archive of what was captured by the image detector. File formats will differ in how they store pixels, but they generally allocate space for storing pixel coordinates and color values. In the image file, the array of pixel values allows the reconstitution and display of the digital image. The files may also hold a color profile which helps with image display. The exact same image file can be used to show an image on two different display devices such as on a phone and a computer display. The operating system for each device reads the image file and renders it on the screen. The color elements and coordinate elements are exactly the same in each file (it is the same file). However, the rendering and conversion of the image to light are somewhat dependent on the display and software. The physical size of the image will obviously be different on a phone vs desktop display. While some of that size difference may be due to settings and scaling to fit the image to the display, there are also actual differences in the size of the pixels which can be seen in Fig. 3.

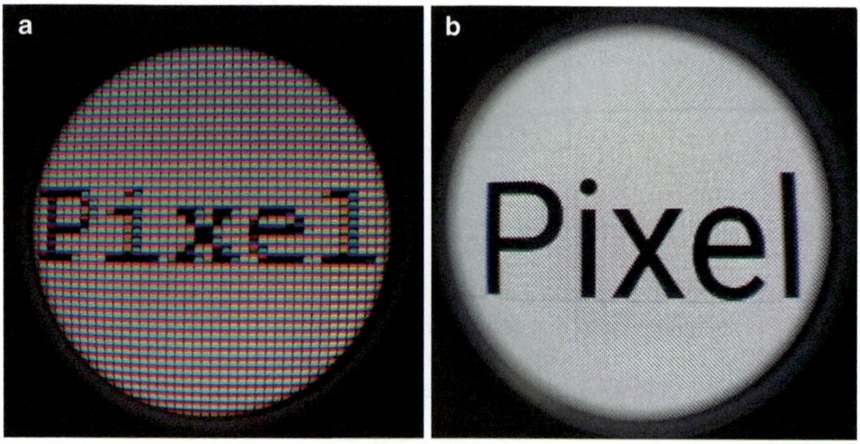

Fig. 3 (**a**) Magnified pixels from a desktop monitor 1920 × 1200 (24 inch diagonal, pixel pitch 0.27 mm, 94.07 pixels per inch). (**b**) Magnified pixels from a phone with screen resolution of 2560 × 1440 (5.7 inch diagonal, pixel pitch 0.049 mm, 518 pixels per inch)

There are also impacts on pixel values based on file type. A lossless file type such as BMP, PNG, or RAW preserves the original pixel values. If the file is alternatively saved in a lossy file type such as JPG, the original pixel values will be averaged based on the compression algorithm. While the images between a lossless and lossy file type may look the same, the process of file compression will change the pixel values and accordingly may impact image analysis algorithms. There are also some file types which may be either lossy or lossless depending on how the file was saved (JPEG2000, TIF).

Pixels in Digital Displays

Digital displays are an integral part of everyday life. They are present in phones, laptops, stand-alone computer monitors and television sets. Each of those displays has an electronic representation of color driven by pixels. Each pixel is actually composed of red, green, and blue diodes packed very closely together. A standard computer monitor is composed of a planar array of pixels. The array has a width and a height with coordinates x and y (x = width, y = height). At the time of this writing, a common monitor configuration known as 4K has a width of 3840 pixels with a height 2160 pixels. The native monitor resolution actually specifies the number of pixels physically present in the display expressed as width × height (3840 × 2160 in the current example). A monitor may display resolutions lower than the native resolution using the display settings on the computer. This may make the objects displayed on the monitor appear larger and blocky. Two monitors which are both 3840 by 2160 will have the same number of pixels, but they may differ with respect to pixel size. The spatial configuration of pixels is referred to as pixel pitch (pp) which is a measure of the distance between the centers of two adjacent pixels [12]. Smaller measures of pixel pitch indicate more densely packed pixels which is often found in higher quality displays that can display the same image in a smaller space. The monitor on a desktop computer and a smartphone may both have similar resolutions, but they have very different physical dimensions. Figure 3a shows the three colored diodes (red, green, blue) in each pixel in a standard desktop display with a pixel pitch of 0.27 mm. Figure 3b shows the more densely packed, smaller pixels from a phone display with pixel pitch of 0.049 mm. It is important to note that the representation of color in the display can be adjusted by hardware and software. However, for the purposes of image analysis, the digital file contains the color values and color profile where most calculations are performed.

WSI Images vs Other Images

In contrast to the digital images we commonly see from digital cameras and smartphones, the images captured from whole slide scanners can be huge. A slide scanned at 40× magnification could be 220,000 × 100,000 pixels and several gigabytes in size. Even CT and MRI images used in radiology are very small in comparison to digital pathology images. Radiology images are comprised of multiple image slices of a relative small proportion (1024 × 1024 pixels). The size of the radiology images can be calculated by multiplying the dimensions of one individual slice by the total number of slices. The total number of slices in CT and MRI images is recorded in the DICOM image header, and each image is the same size. In contrast, pathology WSI images are captured with many small fields of view that are stitched together in a larger single plane. In addition, pathology images may vary greatly in size based on the amount of tissue captured, whereas radiology images are consistently the same dimensions for the same type of study.

While the WSI scanner captures at one magnification and one plane, the pathologist needs to be able to see various magnifications. Most commercial scanners capture at 20× or 40× with some vendors offering options to capture at 100× (oil immersion). The magnification used at the time of scanning will impact the number of pixels and will impact many image analysis techniques. This has to be considered when running algorithms for research or clinical purposes. An algorithm developed and validated on 20× scans cannot be run on 40× scans without additional validation.

Pathologists often use many different magnifications to evaluate a sample and make a diagnosis. The common lenses on a traditional microscope include 2×, 4×, 10×, 20×, and 40×. Down sampling is performed to provide different levels of magnification in the WSI file. For example, if the original image is 75,000 × 75,000 pixels, then a down sampled image may be 50,000 × 50,000 images. This conceptually creates two levels; however, the WSI file may contain even more levels. Digital pathology vendors will often store these down sampled images in one file with the thumbnail and macro images. This eases file management and also speeds viewing by avoiding the overhead of down sampling on the fly while the image is being viewed [13].

Image Analysis Benefits

Many researchers and pathologists use image analysis techniques. While the options and approaches for image analysis are broad, they generally share one common theme: to quantify features in an image in a standardized, repeatable fashion. Manual methods are subject to intra- and inter-reader variability, fatigue, and variable application of scoring rules. Additional considerations for manual reads are listed in Table 6.

Table 6 Examples of factors which may impact results

Manual interpretation factors which may impact results
Intra-observer variability
Inter-observer variability
Inconsistent application of scoring rules
Fatigue
Experience
Variations in field of view/microscope configuration

In contrast, computational techniques can apply the same rules to each specimen which may improve result repeatability.

Pathologists may also find interest in algorithms performing some of the more tedious scoring procedures. The H-score is defined as the sum of the percentage of cells at staining intensities 0–3. This requires an estimate of percentage of tumor cells (PTC) at each intensity of staining (0+, 1+, 2+, 3+) with the application of a formula to achieve the end result. The formula for H-score is sum of PTC at 0, PTC at 1, PTC at 2, and PTC at 3. An image analysis algorithm could help pathologists save a lot of time in this determination. The complexity may increase in the research setting where H-scores may be calculated for the nuclear, cytoplasmic, and membranous compartments simultaneously.

If the algorithm gets too complex, image analysis techniques may struggle with validation. PD-L1 scoring is an area where strong clinical expertise is needed in conjunction with strong image analysis knowledge. The variety of antibody clones for PD-L1 tied to different pharmacologic agents is only a small component of the complexity. Each clone may have a variety of scoring techniques with different cutoffs in a different tumor types [14]. This complexity makes manual scoring of PD-L1 and comparison of results across clones difficult. Even validating one clone can be challenging. The PD-L1 combined positive score (CPS) for gastric, cervical, and urothelial cancers requires identification of which cell compartment is staining in which cell type and in some cases which grade of tumor (low-grade and high-grade papillary urothelial patterns are handled differently) [15]. This also requires assessment of proximity of inflammatory cells to tumor for proper handling of tumor-associated (TA) positive lymphocytes and macrophages. The CPS is calculated as follows: the sum of tumor cells with membrane staining, positive TA lymphocytes with membrane or cytoplasmic staining, and positive TA macrophages with membrane or cytoplasmic staining divided by the total number of viable tumor cells. Of note, positive staining plasma cells, eosinophils, neutrophils, stromal cells, and non-tumor-associated inflammatory cells are excluded. The exceptions to cell compartment staining, cell type, and inflammatory cell proximity to tumor are intriguing but make algorithmic approaches difficult for a comprehensive solution. Algorithmic approaches may help reduce workload by performing scoring in settings where the sample is clearly positive or negative. Algorithms may also be of benefit in cases where tumor can be easily distinguished from non-tumor. Furthermore, retrospective analysis using algorithmic approaches may be useful for finding additional relationships in the data.

Computational methods can be run on very large data sets in a relatively short period of time where manual methods may be impractical. In some instances algorithms can run in the background for quality assurance or overnight as a tool to help pathologists produce more consistent results. There are some pathologists who fear that algorithms may do such a good job that the practice of pathology will change leading to fewer jobs and more automation. This perspective should be balanced with a closer look at some of the pitfalls in image analysis.

Image Analysis Concerns

While computational approaches may improve precision, it should not be assumed that the results are automatically more accurate. Algorithms need to be carefully tuned and verified for appropriate results in a wide variety of contexts. Figure 4 shows how an algorithm can inaccurately represent a cell population and skew the results. Figure 4a shows invasive breast tumor with some glandular elements nestled deep in an inflammatory infiltrate. For estrogen and progesterone scoring, these glandular elements need to be included, but Fig. 4b shows only some of these nests are detected. In addition, the dense lymphocyte infiltrate is being counted as negative (blue) which should be excluded from the score. Overdetection of non-target objects and underdetection of target objects can each markedly skew quantitative results. This would be a challenging case to annotate which may be helpful in concept for excluding the inflammatory infiltrate. Other issues may arise with cell detection. For example, a single tumor nucleus may be detected as many nuclei, or the opposite problem may occur where many adjacent cells are detected as one. For these reasons, a pathologist experienced in image analysis should oversee the annotations and algorithm results to avoid some of these pitfalls. Algorithms do not work in all scenarios, and performing a manual score may be the only way to address some of the more challenging cases. Table 7 lists some of the common artifacts which may impact image analysis.

In addition to the target detection issues and artifacts, there are some other pitfalls to consider when implementing image analysis solutions. One of the biggest objections to image analysis raised by pathologists is that it takes time to annotate the image, wait for the algorithm run, and then come back to the case to report the result. These extra steps are an unwelcome disruption to workflow. It is much easier for a pathologist to render a manual score on a glass slide and be done with the result so that other tasks can be handled. The reimbursement schedule listed in

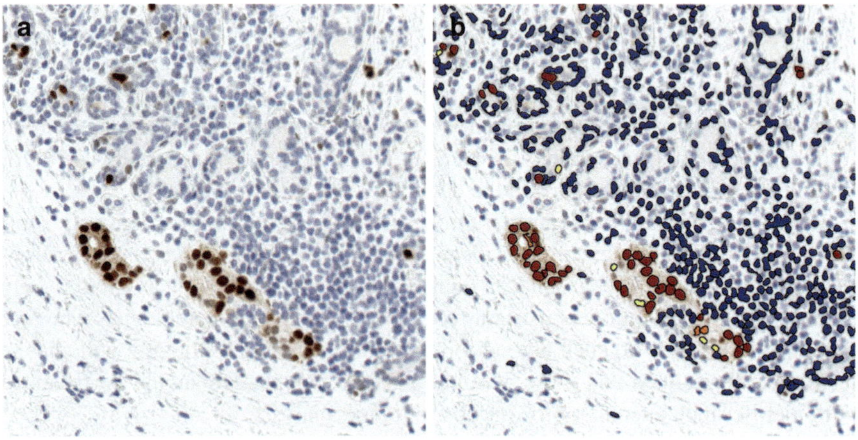

Fig. 4 (**a**, **b**) Inaccurate markup

Table 7 Common artifacts that may impact image analysis

Image	Potential impact
Tissue folds	May increase the color density or introduce artifactual lines into the tissue
Poor focus	Out-of-focus regions may impact edge detection and may homogenize pixel values over a broad area
Color variation	May be introduced by the scanner. May also be impacted by stainer variability
Dust/dirt/pigment	Pixel values in will usually register darker than tissue
Tissue ink/marking pen	Pixel values will usually register differently than tissue
Stitching artifact	May introduce artificial edges
Magnification	Algorithm designed to detect features at 40× may not work well with a 20× image
Coverslip issues	Air bubbles, dirt, debris, scratches, and glue may obscure the image

Table 4 certainly supports the argument that the extra time to run image analysis may actually be negatively impacting revenue. Some of the logistics underlying time concerns may change in a fully digital workflow.

Parallel Processing

One of the challenges in performing image analysis is processing time. There are many factors that may influence run time including hardware, processor load, algorithm design, image size, number of processing steps, etc. More recently, algorithms have benefited from the parallelization offered by running the algorithm on graphics processing units (GPUs). Within that space, there are two primary contenders: CUDA which is an Nvidia technology and OpenCL which was originally developed by Apple but is now open source. Without delving too much in to the technical details of these technologies, an improvement in processing speed can be realized by running portions of the algorithm in parallel. Using these technologies does require that the software is specifically designed to run on these architectures. A discussion of the benefits and differences between the technologies and the algorithm design for building on such technologies is beyond the scope of this chapter.

Tiling

The size of whole slide images makes them difficult to analyze as a single image. Most WSI systems capture small images during scanning and stitch them together to make one larger image. The approach to analyzing the image is often the reverse of the stitching procedure. A few image analysis packages will handle these procedures behind the scenes. There is an open-source plug-in for ImageJ/Fiji called SlideJ which was developed by a team at the University of Udine, Italy [16]. This plug-in handles native formats of some of the major WSI vendors. SlideJ allows an ImageJ/Fiji macros to be applied across the entire slide (https://github.com/MITEL-UNIUD/SlideJ). The SlideJ GitHub site hosts some demonstration macros in addition to the SlideJ plug-in. By default it works at the highest resolution of the target image. The setting can be modified using the "Series" variable. There is also a feature to account for overlap between tiles. Overlap becomes very useful when analyzing objects which span the interface between two tiles. If an object is present on both tiles, it may be cut in half and detected as two separate objects. This may not be a major issue if the number of tiles is low or the number of objects spanning tiles is low. It may however affect calculations and results which are based on object size.

Annotations

Many image analysis solutions allow the use of annotations to help focus the algorithm results. Annotations provide an alternative to running the algorithm on the entire whole slide image. This can have a big impact on reducing the algorithm run time by eliminating areas which are not relevant to the result. Annotations may also increase the performance characteristics for specificity and sensitivity of the result. In general, annotations can be classified as including specific regions or excluding specific regions. For most pathology tissues, the target of interest would include tumor tissue. The areas to be excluded are generally non-tumor portions of the slide which may be stroma, vessels, benign epithelium, necrosis, non-tissue/white space, blood, debris, margin ink or marking pen ink, printed regions of the slide, etc. This may be more difficult to address in practice as areas of tumor may be interrupted by areas which should be excluded. For practical purposes, annotations should be simple and easily repeated. If the annotations are high in number, time-consuming, or complex in nature, there is a negative impact on the precision/repeatability of the algorithm. If annotations cannot be easily reproduced by another user, then the algorithm results may in fact be invalid. In practice many pathologists find the manual process of drawing annotations time-consuming and tedious. Regulatory standards in the United States allow performance of annotations by non-pathologist staff members, but pathologist approval of the annotations is required [4].

Image Analysis Tools

The purpose of image analysis is to quantify, measure, or categorize some aspect of a digital image. There are several tools that may be used to assist in this regard. Open-source tools include QuPath and ImageJ/Fiji and Open Microscopy Environment (OME). Commercial tools include Aperio Algorithm Framework, HALO, Visiopharm, Definiens, ImagePro, and inForm. Each of these tools has its own learning curves and intended uses. Some of them come prepackaged with specific algorithms geared toward pathology use. They may offer algorithms for quantifying immunohistochemistry staining of nuclei or membrane staining, for example.

Some of them are geared for specific image formats. To avoid the vendor-specific file formats, storage techniques, and algorithm approaches, it is easiest to consider images from the properties they all share, pixels.

Pixel-Based Methods

Detecting pixels which meet certain criteria is the most basic approach to image analysis. Filters can be applied to separate the red, green, and blue channels to consider the values of one channel at a time. This reduces the complexity and essentially gives the equivalent of a grayscale image with pixel values ranging from 0 to 255. The complexity can be reduced even further by thresholding which sets a level at which pixels are included or excluded. The pixels above threshold are positive. The pixels below threshold are negative. After thresholding, the working image is now in binary format, and the image can be analyzed for particles/objects. Some useful ImageJ functions are presented in Table 8, and many more are available within ImageJ's documentation [17]. Similar functions are available in many image analysis packages.

Many vendors include a positive pixel count algorithm in the base package. In concept, the algorithm processes and categorizes pixels based on predefined parameters. While a pixel level analysis provides a lot information about the underlying data, establishing a clinically relevant cutoff based on individual pixels alone may be more difficult because the biologic and clinical areas of interest are usually represented by cells not pixels. Useful applications applying pixel-based approaches are still possible and may include representing the output as an intensity heatmap or averaging pixel values over an area of interest. Pixel intensity values are often used as building blocks for other algorithms.

Object-Based Methods

In contrast to pixel-based algorithms which use the intrinsic pixel values in the image, an object-based algorithm first attempts to categorize groups of pixels into an object. The object may be a nucleus, nucleolus, membrane, or an entire cell. Object-based algorithms are more difficult to code because there is biologic

Table 8 Image analysis functions

Procedure	Utility
Split channels	Separate red, green, and blue channels
Threshold	Set minimum value for pixels of interest
Remove outliers	Remove objects which are less than a specific pixel size
Watershed	Split adjacent objects into separate objects
Dilate	Grow regions of binary image (fill holes)
Erode	Shrink regions of binary image
Analyze particles	Quantify features and number of particles

heterogeneity in cells and structures which becomes even more pronounced when looking at tumors which by definition have lost some of their regulatory mechanisms. Object-based algorithms are more analogous to how a pathologist would perform IHC scoring in a clinical scenario. As an example, imagine a scenario requiring quantification of nuclear staining intensity in a digital slide. The pixel intensity averaged over the entire nucleus could be used to determine a per cell score. The scoring paradigm should be chosen to match the purpose of the algorithm. There are a few approaches to scoring which can be broadly categorized into binary, categorical, or continuous scales. A binary scale classifies all objects into positive or negative based on a cutoff or threshold value. A categorical scale sets predefined limits which pertain to certain categories that may be based on intensity such as negative, low, medium, and high. A continuous scale scoring paradigm may be more linear in nature.

Scoring of predictive markers for breast tumors uses object-based methods to determine a percentage of positive cells which is often used in combination with an intensity score. The clinical decision points in predictive markers for breast cancer are based on the percentage of positive tumor cells so it is important that nuclear detection efforts differentiate tumor nuclei from non-tumor nuclei. Algorithms may require fine-tuning and tweaking to filter out non-tumor cells such as lymphocytes, stromal cells, and DCIS. If these cell types are not excluded, the denominator becomes artificially enlarged which drives the positivity percentage down. Therefore, tumor isolation and nuclear detection must be performed prior to performing stain intensity scoring. HER-2 scoring uses cell detection to identify tumor cells prior to making determinations on membrane stain intensity. Many clinical scoring paradigms using visual methods use a quantitative estimate of the percentage positive tumor cells. Table 9 shows some example scoring paradigms and the clinical scenarios.

Architecture-Based Methods

Architecture-based analysis abstracts information about the objects and begins to look at relationships of objects to one another. This is parallel to how many pathologists approach histologic patterns. Some architectures are easy to conceptualize like a vessel, stroma, adipose tissue, epithelial surface, or a germinal center. These architectures are based on arrangement of cells in addition to their cellular morphologic features. Architecture approaches may be used to detect fibrosis, invasive tumor, epithelial surfaces, major tissue types such as bone and adipose, and disruptions in architecture such as effacement of a node. These approaches may extract data from the pixel and object levels to help identify differences in tissue architecture. Alternatively pattern recognition software may be used to train algorithms to classify patterns based on a training set.

Table 9 Example scoring paradigms

Scoring factors	Clinical scenario
Positive cell count	CD34-positive blast index Ki-67 proliferative index Kappa to Lambda ratio determination CD138 plasma cell index
Cell count and stain intensity	ER scoring PR scoring HER-2 scoring H-scoring
Cell count and stain density	FISH/CISH scoring
Cell count and cell type	PD-L1 scoring Marrow cellularity Myeloid to erythroid ratio scoring Tumor percentage of section Inflammatory infiltrate index
Non-cellular staining	Fibrosis Congo red/amyloid Cirrhosis
Cell morphology	Eosinophil count *H. pylori* detection Hodgkin lymphoma detection Follicular lymphoma grading Breast tumor grading

Future Directions

The application of computer-assisted diagnosis is a rapidly expanding area of medical informatics. This is being driven by multiple factors, but the growing digitization of health data is a key essential element. Analysis of digital images is just one application. The application of artificial intelligence (AI) techniques to digital pathology may vastly change how we practice pathology. There are long-standing products already using AI within the laboratory. CellaVision's DM96 has been FDA cleared since 2004 for classification of peripheral blood white blood cell images using a neural network with confirmation by a medical technologist [18]. Cell classifiers could be developed for other body fluids such as bone marrow aspirates, cerebrospinal fluid, pleural fluid, peritoneal fluid, or synovial fluid. The applications extend to solid tumors and other areas of medical imaging as well. An AI system performing image analysis on diabetic retinopathy images was granted de novo classification approval by the FDA in 2018 which allows the device to be legally marketed [19]. Of note, the de novo pathway is the same pathway used to allow marketing of the first WSI scanner system for clinical use in the United States in 2017.

AI technology is well suited to address some of the difficulties of object classification prior to running quantitative algorithms. Neural networks (NN) are established by training on a large set of images that have been previously classified. During training the network determines features and weights that optimally stratify the training set into the predetermined categories. A validation set is then run to test the performance on images that have not been seen by the NN before. Generally the training, validation, and test images represent small subsamples of a whole slide image. Using these techniques, computational models for pathology can be established that can be used to classify future images. A potential application of AI tools may include categorizing whole slide images into various tumor classes for final approval by a pathologist. There may be applications which triage the cases to specific pathologists for the day based on AI technologies. For example, an excised lymph node may be triaged to a surgical pathologist if metastatic disease is detected or sent to a hematopathologist if a lymph node showing a lymphoma pattern is detected. Realizing maximal benefit from AI technology would require a fully digital workflow with AI algorithms running as soon as the slide is digitized.

In a very large reference center, the volume of cases may support triaging cases within a given specialty. For example, a bone marrow with myelodysplastic features may be triaged to a specific pathologist while a plasma cell myeloma or benign marrow may be triaged to separate pathologists. A GI biopsy may be scanned and sent to hematopathology if the findings support MALT lymphoma or a GI pathologist if the findings were suspicious of adenoma or cancer. Case triaging may help pathologists become more efficient by providing a consistent mix of cases where the pathologist carries domain expertise. The algorithms may improve over time by comparing the preliminary classification to the final classification. In addition, if the cases are classified by AI with preliminary diagnoses, the concept could be extended to placing orders for panels of tests for further work up. The systems may also be able to monitor workload so that cases which need a lot of work can be evenly distributed. Digital queues may even be monitored to prevent sending new cases to an overburdened pathologist.

It must also be considered that there is a time element to running any algorithm. Very strong computational capabilities will be needed if AI algorithms are running on every slide coming out of the lab. Each slide processed by an AI algorithm may take several minutes or more depending on the size of the slide and the features which are being detected. Very small features on a very large slide will increase the amount of time required to run the algorithm. The time factor can be shifted to non-working hours or run in parallel with other procedures so as not to increase the turnaround time before a final interpretation is rendered. There are also cloud resources which can be leveraged to spread computational tasks over more hardware. However, cloud-based systems relating to digital pathology will need a fast and reliable mechanism to upload slides securely and in compliance with all regulations. Building local AI resources is also possible to avoid the security issues and network delays inherent in loading slides to the cloud. However, local resources may come at a higher initial expense.

Conclusion

The next several years in digital pathology will certainly be exciting. As adoption of digital workflows continues, the opportunities to use image analysis will increase. The combination of AI techniques with traditional image analysis techniques may yield results which are superior to either of the techniques applied independently. The use of these techniques may complement the expertise of pathologists to provide improvements in diagnostic accuracy, efficiency, and patient care.

References

1. https://www.selectscience.net/product-news/aperio-scanscope-systems-ce-marked-as-a-primary-in-vitro-diagnostic-aid/?artID=25313. Accessed 09/07/2021.
2. https://www.fda.gov/news-events/press-announcements/fda-allows-marketing-first-whole-slide-imaging-system-digital-pathology. Accessed 09/07/2021.
3. https://www.cap.org/covid-19/remote-sign-out-faqs. Accessed 09/07/2021.
4. CAP Anatomic Pathology checklist 2018.
5. Bautista PA, Hashimoto N, Yagi Y. Color standardization in whole slide imaging using a color calibration slide. J Pathol Inform. 2014;5:4.
6. https://www.cms.gov/apps/physician-fee-schedule/search/search-criteria.aspx. Accessed 09/07/2021.
7. https://en.wikipedia.org/wiki/Pixel. Accessed 09/07/2021.
8. https://en.wikipedia.org/wiki/List_of_color_spaces_and_their_uses. Accessed 09/07/2021.
9. Hunt RWG. The reproduction of colour. 6th edn, © 2004 John Wiley & Sons, Ltd. ISBN: 0-470-02425-9.
10. https://www.olympus-lifescience.com/en/camera/color/dp74/#!cms[tab]=%2Fcamera%2Fcolor%2Fdp74%2Fspecifications. Accessed 09/07/2021.
11. https://www.microscopyu.com/tutorials/ccd-resolution-for-optical-microscopy. Accessed 09/07/2021.
12. http://www.planar.com/blog/2018/2/23/what-is-pixel-pitch-and-why-does-it-matter/. Accessed 09/07/2021.
13. Zarella MD, Bowman D, Aeffner F, et al. A Practical Guide to Whole Slide Imaging: A White Paper From the Digital Pathology Association. Arch Pathol Lab Med. 2019;143(2):222–34. https://doi.org/10.5858/arpa.2018-0343-RA.
14. Ionescu DN, Downes MR, Christofides A, Tsao MS. Harmonization of PD-L1 testing in oncology: a Canadian pathology perspective. Curr Oncol. 2018;25(3):e209–16. https://doi.org/10.3747/co.25.4031.
15. https://www.agilent.com/cs/library/usermanuals/public/29276_22C3_pharmdx_uc_interpretation_manual_us.pdf. Accessed 09/07/2021.
16. Della Mea V, Baroni GL, Pilutti D, Di Loreto C. SlideJ: an ImageJ plugin for automated processing of whole slide images. PLoS One. 2017;12(7):e0180540. https://doi.org/10.1371/journal.pone.0180540.
17. https://imagej.nih.gov/ij/docs/index.html. Accessed 09/07/2021.
18. Lee LH, Mansoor A, Wood B, Nelson H, Higa D, Naugler C. Performance of CellaVision DM96 in leukocyte classification. J Pathol Inform. 2013;4:14. Published 2013 Jun 29. https://doi.org/10.4103/2153-3539.114205.
19. Abràmoff MD, Lavin PT, Birch M, Shah N, Folk JC. Pivotal trial of an autonomous AI-based diagnostic system for detection of diabetic retinopathy in primary care offices. NPJ Digit Med. 2018;1:39. Published 2018 Aug 28. https://doi.org/10.1038/s41746-018-0040-6.

Whole Slide Imaging: Deep Learning and Artificial Intelligence

Asmaa Aljuhani, Arunima Srivastava, James P. Cronin, Jany Chan, Raghu Machiraju, and Anil V. Parwani

Abbreviations

AI	Artificial intelligence
CNN	Convolutional neural networks
DL	Deep learning
DNN	Deep convolutional neural networks
HSV	Hue, saturation, value
ML	Machine learning
RGB	Red, green, blue

A. Aljuhani (✉) · A. Srivastava · J. Chan
Department of Computer Science and Engineering, College of Engineering, The Ohio State University, Columbus, OH, USA
e-mail: aljuhani.2@osu.edu; srivastava.92@osu.edu; chan.206@osu.edu

J. P. Cronin
Department of Veterinary Biosciences, College of Veterinary Medicine, The Ohio State University, Columbus, OH, USA

Department of Internal Medicine, College of Medicine, The Ohio State University, Columbus, OH, USA
e-mail: james.cronin@osumc.edu

R. Machiraju
Department of Computer Science and Engineering, College of Engineering, The Ohio State University, Columbus, OH, USA

Department of Biomedical Informatics, College of Medicine, The Ohio State University, Columbus, OH, USA

Department of Pathology, College of Medicine, The Ohio State University Wexner Medical School, Columbus, OH, USA
e-mail: machiraju.1@osu.edu

A. V. Parwani
Department of Pathology, College of Medicine, The Ohio State University Wexner Medical School, Columbus, OH, USA
e-mail: anil.parwani@osumc.edu

A. V. Parwani (ed.), *Whole Slide Imaging*,
https://doi.org/10.1007/978-3-030-83332-9_13

ROC	Receiver operating characteristic
ROI	Regions of interest
TIFF	Tagged Image File Format
WSI	Whole slide image

Introduction

Converging waves of increasingly sophisticated machine learning (ML), whole slide images (WSIs), and computing power have artificial intelligence (AI) (Fig. 1) poised to transform the practice of pathology. The ongoing collaboration of researchers from computer vision, AI, and pathology domains is driving this revolution. A recent explosion of ML models for the analysis of WSIs has produced state-of-the-art biomarker discoveries and impressive disease recognition capabilities [1]. ML has the potential to address the worsening global undersupply of pathologists [2] and the thorny issue of interpathologist variability [3]. Additionally, ML can be used to optimize the diagnostic pathologist's workflow via (1) attention direction to regions of interest (ROI) and (2) automated quantification of time-intensive tasks (e.g., mitotic indices). From the discovery perspective, ML can identify novel features of WSIs with prognostic and therapeutic significance in a variety of neoplastic and metabolic conditions [4, 5].

ML can be unsupervised or supervised. *Unsupervised* models do not introduce labeling bias when learning patterns in data. Rather, the model identifies distinct patterns in the data and forms clusters with unique patterns. Unsupervised learning is useful in an exploratory analysis in which ground truth is unknown. In comparison, *supervised* learning utilizes manually assigned labels from ground truth that identify relevant features of the dataset. Supervised models are conducive to iterative improvement, as the presence of labels helps optimize the model. The performance of the

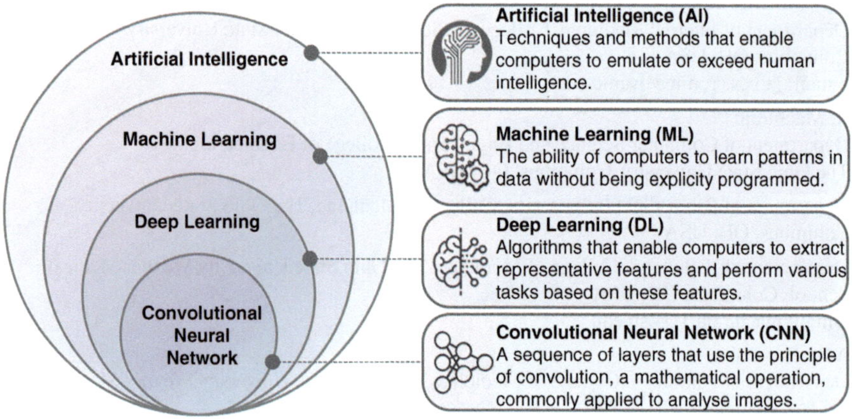

Fig. 1 The hierarchical relationship of different artificial intelligence concepts

supervised model depends on the (1) features, (2) labels, and (3) core algorithm used in training.

Deep learning (DL) is a subcategory of ML (Fig. 1) known for its ability to achieve high performance from complex visual inputs, such as WSIs [6]. DL algorithms utilize networks several layers in depth, progressively extracting higher level features from the raw input with each additional layer. DL algorithms iteratively improve by maximizing the separation between classes. With each iteration, data are propagated through the network to determine the corresponding output. The machine-predicted output is then compared to the actual output, and a penalty score is assigned so that the algorithm can learn to map the sample output to the correct class. Once the algorithm determines the discriminant features for each class, it is often able to generalize to unseen data without the need to handcraft additional features.

The convolutional neural network (CNN) is typically a *supervised* method under the DL umbrella (Fig. 1) that has recently been applied to digital pathology. CNNs are generally used to analyze images, where they assign weights to different regions and structures to model and classify groups. CNNs use the principle of convolution, in which a mathematical operation on two functions is used to produce a third that highlights essential structures (i.e., changes in signal or an underlying smoothness). CNNs are composed of three main types of layers: convolution layers, pooling layers, and fully connected layers. Stacking these layers forms a CNN architecture. The more layers added, the "deeper" the network becomes, hence the name deep convolutional neural networks (DNNs).

In this chapter, we highlight challenges in implementing CNNs in digital pathology (section "Challenges in Implementing Convolutional Neural Networks in Digital Pathology"), discuss data quality and transformation (section "Data Quality and Transformation"), inform annotation and labeling (section "Annotation and Labeling"), demystify CNNs (section "Convolutional Neural Networks"), explore fine-tuning CNNs (section "Further Steps for Fine-Tuning the CNN"), and list modern applications for AI in digital pathology (section "Applications of AI in WSI").

Challenges in Implementing Convolutional Neural Networks in Digital Pathology

Computational modeling of WSIs poses many unique challenges. CNNs are data-driven and require large datasets for training, validating, and testing. The development of large, high-quality datasets is impeded by several barriers to entry in digital pathology, including cost, expertise, and resistance to change. There are multiple steps in data pre-processing with the goal of maintaining data quality and optimizing data transformation. A compatible image format is imperative for downstream analysis, and investigators should consider the entire pipeline before selecting the image format. Different scanners can use propriety data formats for both image generation and annotation, which can add unique challenges for pre-processing and analysis. Investigators can choose from a variety of color spaces, transformations, and contrasts to suit their purpose. The images must then be tiled and filtered with care to maintain the representation of all structures of interest. Normalization is required to counteract batch effects, which can increase image variability due to disparate sample handling. The challenge of isolating distinct morphologic features can be overcome via stain deconvolution, a powerful computational technique for isolating the relative contributions of hematoxylin and eosin staining.

After image pre-processing, pathologist expertise is required to annotate key features for training. Pathology is a highly specialized field, and different organs and diseases require pathologists with a variety of specializations in order to generate accurate annotations. Furthermore, image annotation is time-consuming and requires multiple pathologists to reach a consensus [7]. For any computational modeling endeavor to be executed successfully in the histology domain, the modeling approach must be designed with the input of an expert pathologist at every stage. Hence, each modeling effort should begin with the well-understood integration of pathologists. Pathologist expertise to annotate data, construct models, and verify results is of utmost importance to ensure usability and adoption of AI in pathology.

Ultimately, careful consideration of the parameters for the modeling algorithms, the feature sets, and the neural network architecture are all essential pieces in the overall success of a digital pathology modeling experiment. From the size of the tiles (must contain enough of the relevant tissue substructures but not so much as to add unnecessary variation and noise) to the complexity of the ML model (less training data with more complex models leads to overfitting), all decisions impact the results and should be made after careful consideration and comprehensive validation [8].

Data Quality and Transformation

Sample Size

In computer-aided pathology, the size of the dataset is a crucial factor underlying model performance. The more data fed into the algorithm, the more accurately it will be able to model the full range of the disease of interest. Variation in the form of disease presentation and processing techniques must be captured in training to ensure robust results.

Image Format

Digital pathology relies on scanning hardware to convert glass slides into specific image formats with high resolutions. Automated image processors use existing standard formats or unique proprietary formats with associated tools and viewers [9]. Generally, the difference between formats stems from different metadata tags used, as well as the file compression type. Investigators should be aware that downstream analysis depends on how well computational tools handle the chosen image format. For example, fast rendering in the viewer, ease of annotations, and data management are dependent on the file format. Converting from a scanner-specific format to a standard format may be possible. However, lossy compression methods that degrade the data may be required to achieve a smaller size that is capable of easy viewing.

A standard image format for WSIs is the TIFF (Tagged Image File Format) with lossless compression to maintain image details via storage as multi-resolution (or "pyramidal") representations [10]. Scanner-specific formats include SVS (based on TIFF) from Aperio scanners [11] and MRXS from the Zeiss MIRAX series [12] and 3DHISTECH Pannoramic series [13]. These files typically contain multiple images that range from full-resolution to a low-resolution thumbnail [14]. Any or all these images can be extracted, and the investigator's choice will depend on the resolution needed for analysis.

Color Space, Transformation, and Contrast

Many downstream analyses, such as segmentation and object counting, are based on native *color space*. Thus, *transformation* of an image to a different color space affects the results of these endeavors. Different color spaces focus on distinct image quality characteristics. To illustrate, RGB (red, blue, green) and HSV (hue, saturation, value) are shown in Fig. 2. The number of possible color spaces is too vast to list here, and an investigator's selection will be informed by their objective. A straightforward and commonly used transformation is color to grayscale. This transformation has one feature per pixel: color intensity. Standard ML enables edge detection and segmentation using color intensity and can facilitate precise homogeneous region identification [15]. Similarly, a change in the *contrast* of an image can enable the detection of larger, more apparent objects. A change in contrast essentially changes the difference in luminance between objects in the image. In a grayscale image, darker objects become darker and lighter objects become lighter, in some cases rendering subtle details more apparent [16].

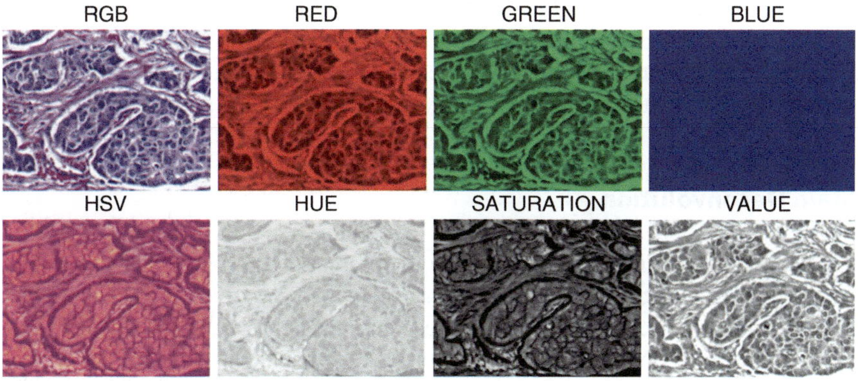

Fig. 2 RGB vs. HSV color spaces and their individual channels for a digital image of breast cancer

Tiling and Filtering the Image

In most cases, the whole image should be *tiled* for faster processing, meaning the whole image is segmented into smaller, rectangular regions or *tiles*, and irrelevant parts of the image should be *filtered*. The size of the tiles needs to be appropriate for the analysis being performed. Since the tile analyses are done in lieu of analyzing the entire WSI, the tiles need to be representative of the structures present in the whole tissue. Thus, the location, size, and magnification should facilitate each tile containing relevant structures [17].

Images can be *filtered* in multiple ways. We can filter artifacts (e.g., white space) or biological entities that do not pertain to the question (e.g., non-tumor region). The easiest way to perform filtration is to compute a measure per tile, which denotes whether the tile is useful or not. For example, if we aimed to analyze any areas which were not predominantly white space, we could average the RGB values of all pixels in each tile and use a threshold to demarcate the tiles to be included in the analysis. An alternative method is to extract specific ROIs from each tile and discard the rest of the image.

Normalization

A standard step in any data modeling protocol is data *normalization*, and computational modeling of WSIs is no different. Normalization is required whenever a set of images is to be analyzed together. This step is imperative as WSIs exhibit considerable variation and are highly prone to batch effects. Sources of variability include histology lab personnel, staining procedures, lab instruments, scanners, and digitization protocols [18]. Most normalization techniques transform all slides in the dataset to mimic a preselected reference slide [19]. The reference slide needs to be an accurate representation of the staining and structures across all slides. Hence, choosing a reference slide poses a challenge. Normalization techniques include pixel-wise standardization of image colors, brightness, and contrast. There are multiple proposed computational methods to perform normalization, and newer, more sophisticated methods are being developed using neural networks [20]. Approaches include color space transformation in the RGB space and color deconvolution that isolates the contribution of the two stain vectors, hematoxylin and eosin.

Stain Deconvolution

Since hematoxylin and eosin dyes adhere to different tissue components, an important step of many analysis protocols is to separate these two dyes in the image. This results in two grayscale images, one of each stain (Fig. 3). For some downstream analyses, such as counting nuclei, distinguishing epithelium and stroma, and assessing the nuclear to cytoplasmic ratio, single-channel grayscale is a powerful technique.

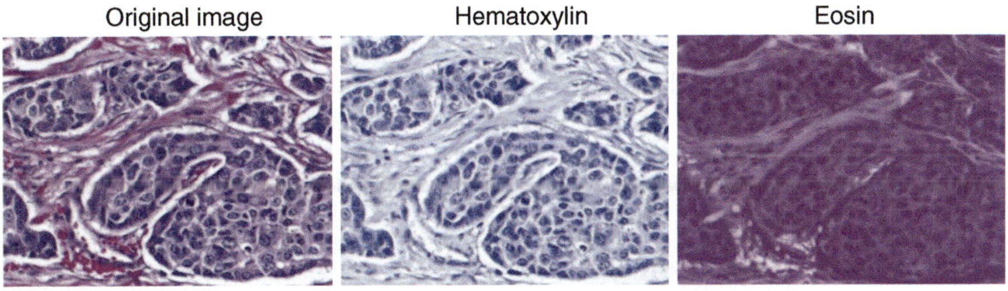

Fig. 3 An example of applying color deconvolution on a digital image of breast cancer

There are a variety of methods for stain deconvolution [21]. Most use a *stain matrix*, which, when multiplied with the color space channels, will produce a stain channel. These channels are specific to each image (or a set of images if they are normalized) and can be transformed into a grayscale image that represents stain intensity.

Annotation and Labeling

Annotation

Pathologists evaluate various structural, textural, and morphological markers to find evidence of disease. This expertise is achieved through years of training. Similarly, CNNs must be trained to identify diagnostic features and to ignore irrelevant noise and artifacts. This is accomplished via *annotation* of key morphological features. The specific features that are labeled depend on the problem to be addressed. For example, annotation of mitotic cells can inform a model predicting tumor grade in breast cancer [22].

Ideally, annotation protocols are determined at the inception of the computational modeling project with consideration of the clinical question/problem. Depending on the task, various implementations may be suitable, such as point annotations (that identify the centroid of the pathology marker), shape annotations (that define a bounding pre-defined shape around the pathology marker), or granular outline annotations (that precisely segment out the pathology marker). A categorical label needs to be assigned to each annotation. An annotation tool that allows for viewing the WSI, efficient annotation, and exportation is required. Annotation tools and software are commercially available with some provided by the image scanner manufacturers [23]. There are several open-source tools that support WSIs in a variety of formats, including QuPath, HistomicsTK, and ASAP. The annotations are exported in easily interpretable text formats such as JSON and XML [24]. Some annotation tools provide options for automated analysis, image normalization, and segmentation to aid in more efficient annotation of many images.

Recent crowdsourcing initiatives for histology annotation have been successful in aggregating labels for large datasets [25]. This has helped to address limitations in dataset sample size. Such initiatives facilitate computational modeling solutions that could be benchmarked and repurposed by computational pathologists to better understand and model in-house data [22].

Clinical and Histopathologic Labels

In contrast to annotation, which assigns labels to specific morphologic features, each WSI may be assigned a diagnostic label for training. Labels are shared by all the tiles emanating from the WSI. Examples of diagnostic labels include disease subtype, grade, sequencing data, drugs administered, and survival. These labels are extracted from patient records or derived by a subject matter expert who reviews the data before processing. Using labeling for sequencing data, we can identify recurring patterns that characterize genetic subtypes of the disease [26].

Convolutional Neural Networks

Prior to DL, traditional classification approaches required researchers to manually harvest domain-specific features. This process of extracting handcrafted features required extensive tuning to accommodate the variability of the data, and applicability to other problems (i.e., analyzing different diseases) was limited. Addressing this challenge, DL follows a *domain agnostic* approach, combining the process of automated feature extraction with the identification of discriminating markers. Thus, the process of harvesting discriminatory features becomes automated.

Deep convolutional neural networks (DNNs) (Fig. 4) have a dominant learning ability due to multiple feature extraction stages that allow them to learn representative features of the data. This powerful capability has earned DNNs steady popularity in analyzing large, high-resolution WSIs across a variety of cancer subtypes [27], as well as many other conditions, such as Alzheimer's disease [28].

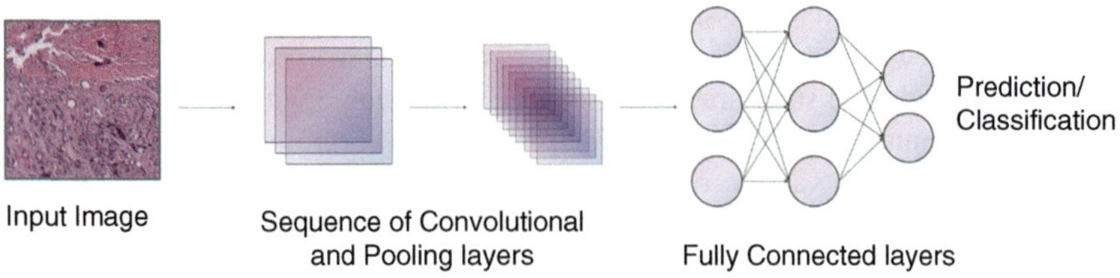

Fig. 4 The common structure of DNN models. An image is passed through a series of convolutional and pooling layers. These layers extract representative features that are used in the fully connected layers to classify the input image

Anatomy of a CNN

Neurons, the basic building block of the neural network, are assigned to one of three possible layers: *input*, *hidden*, or *output*. If every input neuron is connected to every output neuron and vice versa, the layers are considered **fully connected**. The input layer receives a pre-processed image as a matrix and passes it to the first hidden layer. The hidden layers perform mathematical computations to extract relevant image features. Lastly, the output layer returns the predicted value for the input image based on the features identified in the hidden layers.

Each connection between neurons is associated with a **weight** that prescribes the importance of the value from a neuron in the preceding layer. These are called the model's **parameters**. At the beginning of the training process, these weights are assigned randomly. Throughout the learning process, the model adjusts these weights based on how accurately it predicts the actual outputs. A loss function is used to evaluate the learning ability of the model. Ideally, the generated loss function is close to zero, which means the labels generated by the model are highly correlated with the actual labels.

Hidden Layers

The convolutional layer is the first layer to extract features from an input image. It preserves the dimensions of the input. It is based on a mathematical operation that takes two inputs, such as an image and a filter, and produces a convolved feature output. Applying different types of filters can generate the following transformations: edge detection, smoothing, and sharpening the input image.

The pooling layer is used to reduce the dimensionality of the input image to shorten training time and combat overfitting. There are different types of special pooling: max pooling, average pooling, and sum pooling.

The activation layer operates to minimize a loss function. This layer is to classify the output into different classes. The choice of activation function is dependent on the desired output. For example, sigmoid is preferred for binary classification while softmax is typically used for multiple classes [29].

Further Steps for Fine-Tuning the CNN

Feature Identification

A feature is defined as any measurable property of the WSI that is characteristic of the phenomenon being observed. For example, features can define a cell nucleus, inflammatory cells, extracellular matrix, etc. Choosing discriminative, informative, and independent features is a crucial component of developing a powerful CNN. The inherent statistics of the feature set, such as variation and distance between data points in the feature space (e.g., Euclidean space), will be used by the CNN to predict the most appropriate label (*supervised* models) or grouping (*unsupervised* models) for individual data points.

Validation and Performance

For model *validation*, common measurements like accuracy, precision, recall, F-score, and mean squared error evaluate correctness in different contexts. To assess the *performance* of a model, one can utilize K-fold validation, randomization of the input data, or titration with noise to compare the penultimate results. Techniques such as the *receiver operating characteristic* (ROC) curves make these measures and the changes easy to interpret and contextualize.

Applications of AI in WSI

Detection and Segmentation

CNNs facilitate the *detection* of disease-relevant structures and the subsequent *segmentation* of ROIs with high probability. This capability allows CNNs to be used as pre-screening and augmentation tools during histopathologic diagnosis of digitized slides. The CNN-guided discovery focuses the pathologist's attention on ROIs, thereby optimizing the pathologist's workflow. Moreover, identification and quantification of disease markers become standardized, thus reducing interpathologist variability.

The nucleus has been the target of many early studies in CNN segmentation. Investigators have successfully used several unique approaches and architectures to identify nuclear ROIs. For example, a PMap approach using CNNs gauges the probability of each pixel's proximity, according to its intensity, to cell nuclei to determine nuclei locations [30]. Alternatively, Mask R-CNN utilizes a region proposal network, first zeroing in on the areas that may contain nuclei and iteratively finding their exact boundaries for nuclei detection [31].

In addition to cellular features, detection of unique cellular phenomena, such as mitoses, is enabled by CNN segmentation. A standard method for quantifying mitotic figures is the mitotic count. Counting mitoses requires the pathologist to (1) identify the tumor region with highest mitotic activity, (2) differentiate mitoses from nuclear pyknosis, and (3) count mitotic events in at least ten representative, non-overlapping high-power fields. Each of these challenges is both time-consuming and highly prone to interobserver variability. DL networks that use spatial context to identify mitosis using a max pooling CNN have achieved significant success in mitosis identification [32]. A CNN feature set combined with domain-specific hand-crafted features gave rise to a computationally economical model which successfully identified mitosis [27].

CNNs have also been used to identify broad areas that contain multiple ROIs. For instance, to recognize tissue alternations of nonalcoholic fatty liver disease, a CNN model attained almost 95% accuracy, paving the way for more feasible and rapid diagnosis [33]. A CNN trained on patch annotations to identify ROIs and post-process the segmentation with a fully connected conditional random field can be used to build a generalizable method for identifying regions of diagnostic relevance in histology images [34].

Artifact Discovery

There are a variety of *artifacts* in histology slides that can impede accurate computational diagnosis and hamper experts when using digitized WSIs. To address this challenge, CNNs can be used as quality control and correction tools. For example, a tool trained on different amounts of blurry histology and immunohistochemistry images can reliably identify artifactual ROIs. Tools such as these may soon be integrated with scanners to automatically re-scan artifactual ROIs and optimize the preparation process prior to pathologist interpretation [35].

Classification (Diagnosis and Grading)

Diagnosis and grading are *classification* tasks conducted by the pathologist in daily practice. There are many examples of CNNs achieving success in this domain, showcasing the potential to reduce interpathologist discordance and hasten accurate diagnosis. For example, a CNN-based method presented an accuracy of 98% when using confidence-based scoring from a deep network to classify histology tissue of skin cancer into four main classes [36]. Another model, performing predictions on patches of WSIs using CNNs and subsequently aggregating these, was able to deliver whole slide classification close to pathologist decisions for subtypes of cancers [37]. Extending the classification paradigm, tumor grades can be identified using CNNs, as is evidenced by studies in the kidney [38], brain [39], and prostate [40]. A CNN training framework with the relevant labeled images can go a step further and directly prognosticate using WSIs from cancer [41].

Summary

This is an exciting time in pathology diagnostics. CNNs are powerful tools for complex image analysis, making them ideal for digital pathology applications. The workflow of CNN development on WSIs has several challenges, and the perspective of the pathologist is welcome at every stage of model development. As it is widely deployed and adopted in clinical settings, WSI technology will allow pathologists to rapidly access and share images easily. Once well integrated with clinical workflows, WSI will be increasingly used in CNNs and AI applications for feature selection, tumor diagnosis, tumor grading, and developing image-based prognostic assays. Progress in CNN- and AI-based tool development will be further accelerated as overall WSI adoption for primary diagnosis and other clinical applications moves forward.

References

1. Srinidhi CL, Ciga O, Martel AL. Deep neural network models for computational histopathology: a survey. arXiv:191212378 [cs, eess] [Internet]. 2019 Dec 27 [cited 2020 Jul 27]. Available from: http://arxiv.org/abs/1912.12378.
2. Robboy SJ, Weintraub S, Horvath AE, Jensen BW, Alexander CB, Fody EP, et al. Pathologist workforce in the United States: I. development of a predictive model to examine factors influencing supply. Arch Pathol Lab Med. 2013;137(12):1723–32.
3. Dasari S, Chakraborty A, Truong L, Mohan C. A systematic review of interpathologist agreement in histologic classification of lupus nephritis. Kidney Int Rep. 2019;4(10):1420–5.
4. Bychkov D, Linder N, Turkki R, Nordling S, Kovanen PE, Verrill C, et al. Deep learning based tissue analysis predicts outcome in colorectal cancer. Sci Rep. 2018;8(1):3395.
5. Signaevsky M, Prastawa M, Farrell K, Tabish N, Baldwin E, Han N, et al. Artificial intelligence in neuropathology: deep learning-based assessment of tauopathy. Lab Invest. 2019;99(7):1019–29.
6. Lakhani P, Gray DL, Pett CR, Nagy P, Shih G. Hello world deep learning in medical imaging. J Digit Imaging. 2018;31(3):283–9.
7. Gurcan MN, Boucheron LE, Can A, Madabhushi A, Rajpoot NM, Yener B. Histopathological image analysis: a review. IEEE Rev Biomed Eng. 2009;2:147–71.
8. Komura D, Ishikawa S. Machine learning methods for histopathological image analysis. Comput Struct Biotechnol J. 2018;16:34–42.
9. Zarella MD, Bowman D, Aeffner F, Farahani N, Xthona A, Absar SF, et al. A practical guide to whole slide imaging: a white paper from the digital pathology association. Arch Pathol Lab Med. 2019;143(2):222–34.
10. Besson S, Leigh R, Linkert M, Allan C, Burel J-M, Carroll M, et al. Bringing open data to whole slide imaging. In: Reyes-Aldasoro CC, Janowczyk A, Veta M, Bankhead P, Sirinukunwattana K, editors. Digital pathology [Internet]. Cham: Springer International Publishing; 2019 [cited 2020 Jul 27]. p. 3–10. (Lecture Notes in Computer Science; vol. 11435). Available from: http://link.springer.com/10.1007/978-3-030-23937-4_1.
11. Grove LBD of LMI 1700 LLB, Fax: +1 847-236-3009 I 60089 USOP +1 844 534 2262. Scan – Aperio digital pathology slide scanners [Internet]. Leica Biosystems. [cited 2020 Jul 27]. Available from: https://www.leicabiosystems.com/digital-pathology/scan/.
12. Carl Zeiss: MIRAX LIVE [Internet]. Microscopy news. 2017 [cited 2020 Jul 27]. Available from: https://microscopy-news.com/products/systems/carl-zeiss-mirax-live/.
13. Digital pathology | Epredia [Internet]. [cited 2020 Jul 27]. Available from: https://epredia.com/digital-pathology-solutions/.
14. Aperio format [Internet]. [cited 2020 Jul 27]. Available from: https://openslide.org/formats/aperio/.
15. Canny J. A computational approach to edge detection. IEEE Trans Pattern Anal Mach Intell. 1986;PAMI-8(6):679–98.
16. Ibrahim H, Pik Kong NS. Brightness preserving dynamic histogram equalization for image contrast enhancement. IEEE Trans Consum Electron. 2007;53(4):1752–8.
17. Gertych A, Swiderska-Chadaj Z, Ma Z, Ing N, Markiewicz T, Cierniak S, et al. Convolutional neural networks can accurately distinguish four histologic growth patterns of lung adenocarcinoma in digital slides. Sci Rep [Internet]. 2019 Feb 6 [cited 2020 Jul 27];9. Available from: https://www.ncbi.nlm.nih.gov/pmc/articles/PMC6365499/.
18. Khan AM, Rajpoot N, Treanor D, Magee D. A nonlinear mapping approach to stain normalization in digital histopathology images using image-specific color deconvolution. IEEE Trans Biomed Eng. 2014;61(6):1729–38.
19. Zanjani FG, Zinger S, Bejnordi BE, van der Laak JAWM, de With PHN. Stain normalization of histopathology images using generative adversarial networks. In: 2018 IEEE 15th International Symposium on Biomedical Imaging (ISBI 2018); 2018. p. 573–7.

20. Pontalba JT, Gwynne-Timothy T, David E, Jakate K, Androutsos D, Khademi A. Assessing the impact of color normalization in convolutional neural network-based nuclei segmentation frameworks. Front Bioeng Biotechnol. 2019;7:300.
21. Alsubaie N, Trahearn N, Raza SEA, Snead D, Rajpoot NM. Stain deconvolution using statistical analysis of multi-resolution stain colour representation. PLoS One. 2017;12(1):e0169875.
22. Chang JM, McCullough AE, Dueck AC, Kosiorek HE, Ocal IT, Lidner TK, et al. Back to basics: traditional Nottingham grade mitotic counts alone are significant in predicting survival in invasive breast carcinoma. Ann Surg Oncol. 2015;22 Suppl 3:S509–15.
23. Grove LBD of LMI 1700 LLB, Fax: +1 847–236-3009 I 60089 USOP +1 844 534 2262. Aperio ImageScope - pathology slide viewing software [Internet]. Leica Biosystems. [cited 2020 Jul 27]. Available from: https://www.leicabiosystems.com/digital-pathology/manage/aperio-imagescope/.
24. ASAP - Automated slide analysis platform [Internet]. [cited 2020 Jul 27]. Available from: https://computationalpathologygroup.github.io/ASAP/.
25. Grote A, Schaadt NS, Forestier G, Wemmert C, Feuerhake F. Crowdsourcing of histological image labeling and object delineation by medical students. IEEE Trans Med Imaging. 2019;38(5):1284–94.
26. Coudray N, Ocampo PS, Sakellaropoulos T, Narula N, Snuderl M, Fenyö D, et al. Classification and mutation prediction from non-small cell lung cancer histopathology images using deep learning. Nat Med. 2018;24(10):1559–67.
27. Wang H, Cruz-Roa A, Basavanhally A, Gilmore H, Shih N, Feldman M, et al. Mitosis detection in breast cancer pathology images by combining handcrafted and convolutional neural network features. J Med Imaging (Bellingham). 2014;1(3):034003.
28. Tang Z, Chuang KV, DeCarli C, Jin L-W, Beckett L, Keiser MJ, et al. Interpretable classification of Alzheimer's disease pathologies with a convolutional neural network pipeline. Nat Commun. 2019;10(1):2173.
29. Krizhevsky A, Sutskever I, Hinton GE. ImageNet classification with deep convolutional neural networks. In: Pereira F, Burges CJC, Bottou L, Weinberger KQ, editors. Advances in neural information processing systems 25 [Internet]. Curran Associates, Inc.; 2012 [cited 2020 Jul 27]. p. 1097–1105. Available from: http://papers.nips.cc/paper/4824-imagenet-classification-with-deep-convolutional-neural-networks.pdf.
30. Höfener H, Homeyer A, Weiss N, Molin J, Lundström CF, Hahn HK. Deep learning nuclei detection: a simple approach can deliver state-of-the-art results. Comput Med Imaging Graph. 2018;70:43–52.
31. Jung H, Lodhi B, Kang J. An automatic nuclei segmentation method based on deep convolutional neural networks for histopathology images. BMC Biomed Eng. 2019;1(1):24.
32. Cireşan DC, Giusti A, Gambardella LM, Schmidhuber J. Mitosis detection in breast cancer histology images with deep neural networks. Med Image Comput Comput Assist Interv. 2013;16(Pt 2):411–8.
33. Arjmand A, Angelis CT, Christou V, Tzallas AT, Tsipouras MG, Glavas E, et al. Training of deep convolutional neural networks to identify critical liver alterations in histopathology image samples. Appl Sci. 2020;10(1):42.
34. Chan L, Hosseini M, Rowsell C, Plataniotis K, Damaskinos S. HistoSegNet: semantic segmentation of histological tissue type in whole slide images. In: 2019 IEEE/CVF International Conference on Computer Vision (ICCV); 2019. p. 10661–70.
35. Senaras C, Niazi MKK, Lozanski G, Gurcan MN. DeepFocus: detection of out-of-focus regions in whole slide digital images using deep learning. PLoS One. 2018;13(10):e0205387.
36. Ianni JD, Soans RE, Sankarapandian S, Chamarthi RV, Ayyagari D, Olsen TG, et al. Tailored for real-world: a whole slide image classification system validated on uncurated multi-site data emulating the prospective pathology workload. Sci Rep. 2020;10(1):3217.
37. Hou L, Samaras D, Kurc TM, Gao Y, Davis JE, Saltz JH. Patch-based convolutional neural network for whole slide tissue image classification. In: 2016 IEEE Conference on Computer Vision and Pattern Recognition (CVPR); 2016. p. 2424–33.

38. Khoshdeli M, Borowsky A, Parvin B. Deep learning models differentiate tumor grades from H E stained histology sections. In: 2018 40th Annual International Conference of the IEEE Engineering in Medicine and Biology Society (EMBC); 2018. p. 620–3.
39. Ertosun MG, Rubin DL. Automated grading of gliomas using deep learning in digital pathology images: a modular approach with ensemble of convolutional neural networks. AMIA Annu Symp Proc. 2015;2015:1899–908.
40. Li W, Li J, Sarma KV, Ho KC, Shen S, Knudsen BS, et al. Path R-CNN for prostate cancer diagnosis and gleason grading of histological images. IEEE Trans Med Imaging. 2019;38(4):945–54.
41. Kather JN, Krisam J, Charoentong P, Luedde T, Herpel E, Weis C-A, et al. Predicting survival from colorectal cancer histology slides using deep learning: a retrospective multicenter study. PLoS Med. 2019;16(1):e1002730.

Index

A. V. Parwani (ed.), *Whole Slide Imaging*,
https://doi.org/10.1007/978-3-030-83332-9

GPSR Compliance

The European Union's (EU) General Product Safety Regulation (GPSR) is a set of rules that requires consumer products to be safe and our obligations to ensure this.

If you have any concerns about our products, you can contact us on ProductSafety@springernature.com

In case Publisher is established outside the EU, the EU authorized representative is:

Springer Nature Customer Service Center GmbH
Europaplatz 3
69115 Heidelberg, Germany

Batch number: 10732090

Printed by Printforce, the Netherlands